1992
YEAR BOOK OF
CARDIOLOGY®

The 1992 Year Book® Series

Year Book of Anesthesia and Pain Management: Drs. Miller, Abram, Kirby, Ostheimer, Roizen, and Stoelting

Year Book of Cardiology®: Drs. Schlant, Collins, Engle, Frye, Kaplan, and O'Rourke

Year Book of Critical Care Medicine®: Drs. Rogers and Parrillo

Year Book of Dentistry®: Drs. Meskin, Currier, Kennedy, Leinfelder, Matukas, and Rovin

Year Book of Dermatologic Surgery: Drs. Swanson, Salasche, and Glogau

Year Book of Dermatology®: Drs. Sober and Fitzpatrick

Year Book of Diagnostic Radiology®: Drs. Federle, Clark, Gross, Madewell, Maynard, Sackett, and Young

Year Book of Digestive Diseases®: Drs. Greenberger and Moody

Year Book of Drug Therapy®: Drs. Lasagna and Weintraub

Year Book of Emergency Medicine®: Drs. Wagner, Burdick, Davidson, Roberts, and Spivey

Year Book of Endocrinology®: Drs. Bagdade, Braverman, Horton, Kannan, Landsberg, Molitch, Morley, Odell, Rogol, Ryan, and Sherwin

Year Book of Family Practice®: Drs. Berg, Bowman, Davidson, Dietrich, and Scherger

Year Book of Geriatrics and Gerontology®: Drs. Beck, Abrass, Burton, Cummings, Makinodan, and Small

Year Book of Hand Surgery®: Drs. Amadio and Hentz

Year Book of Health Care Management: Drs. Heyssel, Brock, King, and Steinberg, Ms. Avakian, and Messrs. Berman, Kues, and Rosenberg

Year Book of Hematology®: Drs. Spivak, Bell, Ness, Quesenberry, and Wiernik

Year Book of Infectious Diseases®: Drs. Wolff, Barza, Keusch, Klempner, and Snydman

Year Book of Infertility: Drs. Mishell, Paulsen, and Lobo

Year Book of Medicine®: Drs. Rogers, Bone, Cline, Braunwald, Greenberger, Utiger, Epstein, and Malawista

Year Book of Neonatal and Perinatal Medicine®: Drs. Klaus and Fanaroff

Year Book of Nephrology: Drs. Coe, Favus, Henderson, Kashgarian, Luke, Myers, and Strom

Year Book of Neurology and Neurosurgery®: Drs. Currier and Crowell

Year Book of Neuroradiology: Drs. Osborn, Harnsberger, Halbach, and Grossman

Year Book of Nuclear Medicine®: Drs. Hoffer, Gore, Gottschalk, Sostman, Zaret, and Zubal

Year Book of Obstetrics and Gynecology®: Drs. Mishell, Kirschbaum, and Morrow

Year Book of Occupational and Environmental Medicine: Drs. Emmett, Brooks, Harris, and Schenker

Year Book of Oncology®: Drs. Young, Longo, Ozols, Simone, Steele, and Weichselbaum

Year Book of Ophthalmology®: Drs. Laibson, Adams, Augsburger, Benson, Cohen, Eagle, Flanagan, Nelson, Reinecke, Sergott, and Wilson

Year Book of Orthopedics®: Drs. Sledge, Poss, Cofield, Frymoyer, Griffin, Hansen, Johnson, Simmons, and Springfield

Year Book of Otolaryngology–Head and Neck Surgery®: Drs. Bailey and Paparella

Year Book of Pathology and Clinical Pathology®: Drs. Gardner, Bennett, Cousar, Garvin, and Worsham

Year Book of Pediatrics®: Dr. Stockman

Year Book of Plastic, Reconstructive, and Aesthetic Surgery: Drs. Miller, Cohen, McKinney, Robson, Ruberg, and Whitaker

Year Book of Podiatric Medicine and Surgery®: Dr. Kominsky

Year Book of Psychiatry and Applied Mental Health®: Drs. Talbott, Frances, Freedman, Meltzer, Perry, Schowalter, and Yudofsky

Year Book of Pulmonary Disease®: Drs. Bone and Petty

Year Book of Sports Medicine®: Drs. Shephard, Eichner, Sutton, and Torg, Col. Anderson, and Mr. George

Year Book of Surgery®: Drs. Schwartz, Jonasson, Robson, Shires, Spencer, and Thompson

Year Book of Transplantation: Drs. Ascher, Hansen, and Strom

Year Book of Ultrasound: Drs. Merritt, Mittelstaedt, Carroll, and Nyberg

Year Book of Urology®: Drs. Gillenwater and Howards

Year Book of Vascular Surgery®: Dr. Bergan

Roundsmanship '92–'93: A Student's Survival Guide to Clinical Medicine Using Current Literature: Drs. Dan, Feigin, Quilligan, Schrock, Stein, and Talbott

Editor-in-Chief

Robert C. Schlant, M.D.

Professor of Medicine (Cardiology), Department of Medicine, Division of Cardiology, Emory University School of Medicine; Chief of Cardiology, Grady Memorial Hospital, Atlanta, Georgia

Editors

John J. Collins, Jr., M.D.

Professor of Surgery, Harvard Medical School; Vice Chairman, Department of Surgery; Director, Sub-Department of Thoracic and Cardiac Surgery, Brigham and Women's Hospital, Boston, Massachusetts

Mary Allen Engle, M.D.

Stavros S. Niarchos Professor of Pediatric Cardiology, Professor of Pediatrics, Director of Pediatric Cardiology, The New York Hospital–Cornell Medical Center, New York, New York

Robert L. Frye, M.D.

Chairman, Department of Medicine, Rose M. and Maurice Eisenberg Professor, Mayo Clinic and Foundation, Rochester, Minnesota

Norman M. Kaplan, M.D.

Professor of Internal Medicine, Head of the Hypertension Division, University of Texas Southwestern Medical Center, Dallas, Texas

Robert A. O'Rourke, M.D.

Charles Conrad Brown Distinguished Professor in Cardiovascular Disease; Director of Cardiology, The University of Texas Health Science Center, San Antonio, Texas

1992

The Year Book of CARDIOLOGY®

Editor-in-Chief
Robert C. Schlant, M.D.

Editors
John J. Collins, Jr., M.D.
Mary Allen Engle, M.D.
Robert L. Frye, M.D.
Norman M. Kaplan, M.D.
Robert A. O'Rourke, M.D.

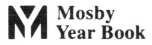
Mosby
Year Book

St. Louis   Baltimore   Boston   Chicago   London   Philadelphia   Sydney   Toronto

Editor-in-Chief, Year Book Publishing: Kenneth H. Killion
Sponsoring Editor: Nancy Puckett
Manager, Literature Services: Edith M. Podrazik
Senior Information Specialist: Terri Santo
Senior Medical Writer: David A. Cramer, M.D.
Assistant Director, Manuscript Services: Frances M. Perveiler
Associate Managing Editor, Year Book Editing Services: Connie Murray
Senior Production/Desktop Publishing Manager: Max F. Perez
Proofroom Manager: Barbara M. Kelly

Editorial Office:
Mosby–Year Book, Inc.
200 North LaSalle St.
Chicago, IL 60601

International Standard Serial Number: 0899-8019
International Standard Book Number: 0-8151-7778-X

Table of Contents

Journals Represented

Mosby–Year Book subscribes to and surveys nearly 900 U.S. and foreign medical and allied health journals. From these journals, the Editors select the articles to be abstracted. Journals represented in this YEAR BOOK are listed below.

American Heart Journal
American Journal of Cardiology
American Journal of Diseases of Children
American Journal of Epidemiology
American Journal of Hypertension
American Journal of Medicine
American Journal of Physiology
American Journal of the Medical Sciences
Angiology
Annals of Internal Medicine
Annals of Surgery
Annals of Thoracic Surgery
Archives of Disease in Childhood
Archives of Internal Medicine
Archives of Neurology
Atherosclerosis
Blood
British Heart Journal
British Journal of Surgery
British Medical Journal
Canadian Journal of Cardiology
Cardiovascular Research
Catheterization and Cardiovascular Diagnosis
Chest
Circulation
Circulation Research
Clinical Genetics
European Heart Journal
European Journal of Clinical Pharmacology
European Journal of Pediatrics
Health Affairs
Hypertension
International Journal of Cardiology
Journal of Cardiac Surgery
Journal of Cardiovascular Electrophysiology
Journal of Clinical Investigation
Journal of Clinical Pharmacology
Journal of Geriatric Psychiatry
Journal of Heart Transplantation
Journal of Heart and Lung Transplantation
Journal of Hypertension
Journal of Internal Medicine
Journal of Pediatrics
Journal of Psychosomatic Research
Journal of Thoracic and Cardiovascular Surgery
Journal of the American College of Cardiology
Journal of the American Medical Association
Journal of the American Society of Echocardiography

Lancet
Mayo Clinic Proceedings
New England Journal of Medicine
New York State Journal of Medicine
Obstetrics and Gynecology
Pediatric Cardiology
Pediatric Dermatology
Pediatric Pathology
Pediatric Research
Pediatrics
Proceedings of the National Academy of Sciences
Psychosomatic Medicine
Radiology
Stroke
Therapeutic Drug Monitoring

STANDARD ABBREVIATIONS

In many articles in this edition, at least one of the following terms is used: acquired immunodeficiency syndrome (AIDS), acute myocardial infarction (AMI), atrioventricular (AV), coronary artery bypass graft (CABG), central nervous system (CNS), cardiopulmonary resuscitation (CPR), cerebrospinal fluid (CSF), computed tomography (CT), electrocardiogram (ECG), human immunodeficiency virus (HIV), left anterior descending (LAD), left ventricular (LV), left ventricular ejection fraction (LVEF), magnetic resonance (MR) imaging (MRI), myocardial infarction (MI), New York Heart Association (NYHA), right ventricular (RV), and ventricular tachycardia (VT). Rather than spell out these terms in full each time they appear, their abbreviations will be used.

Publisher's Preface

As publishers, we feel challenged to seek ways of presenting complex information in a clear and readable manner. To this end, the 1992 YEAR BOOK OF CARDIOLOGY now provides structured abstracts in which the various components of a study can easily be identified through headings. These headings are not the same in all abstracts but, rather, are those that most accurately designate the content of each particular journal article. We are confident that our readers will find the information contained in our abstracts to be more accessible than ever before. We welcome your comments.

Introduction

This 1992 YEAR BOOK OF CARDIOLOGY, is the 32nd in the series. The 6 editors have selected and provided comments on 318 clinically relevant articles in cardiology. In many instances, additional references are provided with the comments.

All of the editors again thank the staff at Mosby–Year Book for assistance, patience, and understanding. We are especially indebted to Ms. Nancy Gorham and Ms. Nancy Puckett.

Robert C. Schlant, M.D.

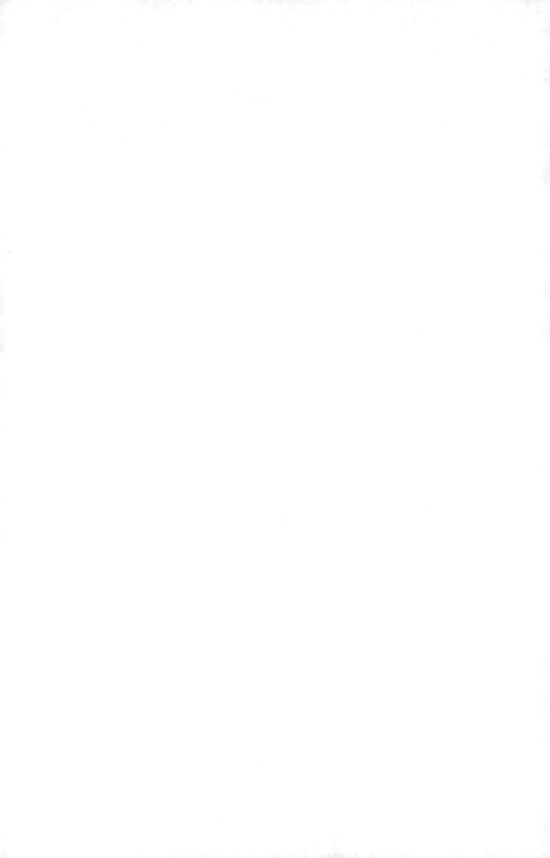

1 Coronary Artery and Other Heart Diseases, Heart Failure

Introduction

This year's YEAR BOOK on coronary disease contains fascinating work that continues to provide a perspective of clinical studies related to coronary artery disease. The breadth and quality of clinical investigation continues to be most remarkable and is a credit to the cardiovascular community. I have included a number of papers dealing with health policy issues, which were quite fascinating. In addition, in my judgment, the epidemiology of coronary artery disease is of real importance to the clinician managing patients with this disease. The advances with interventional therapies continues to be most impressive. Fortunately, important properly controlled studies are under way, and we have included a number of important observational studies in the chapter.

Robert L. Frye, M.D.

Thrombolytic Therapy

Impact of Field-Transmitted Electrocardiography on Time to In-Hospital Thrombolytic Therapy in Acute Myocardial Infarction

Karagounis L, Ipsen SK, Jessop MR, Gilmore KM, Valenti DA, Clawson JJ, Teichman S, Anderson JL (LDS Hosp, Salt Lake City)
Am J Cardiol 66:786–791, 1990
1–1

Background.—Thrombolytic reperfusion is now an established treatment for acute myocardial infarction (AMI). Delays in giving this treatment can occur during transport and after arrival at the hospital. Paramedic transmission of an in-field, 12-lead ECG to physicians at the hospital may reduce delays in diagnosis and treatment. The feasibility and impact of field-transmitted ECG on the prehospital and early hospital care of patients with suspected AMI was investigated.

Methods.—Randomized and open trials were done with a portable ECG system coupled with a cellular phone programmed to transmit ECGs automatically to the base hospital. Patients consecutively served by the 6 units of the Salt Lake City Emergency Rescue System were included. Thirty-four patients were randomly assigned to in-field ECG and 37 to no ECG.

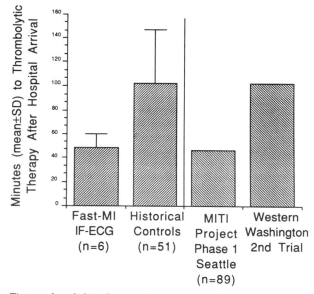

Fig 1–1.—Times to thrombolytic therapy after hospital arrival. **Left,** patients with acute myocardial infarction who received an in-field ECG (IF-ECG) compared with recent historical control patients (**right**) not getting IF-ECG; **right,** a literature comparison also showing treatment times for patients receiving IF-ECG (**left hand bar**) and historical control subjects without IF-ECG (**right hand bar**). (Courtesy of Karagounis L, Ipsen SK, Jessop MR, et al: *Am J Cardiol* 66:786–791, 1990.)

Results.—Mean time on scene was 16.4 minutes for the ECG group and 16.1 for the control group, a nonsignificant difference. Average times of transport were 18.2 and 17.6 minutes, also a nonsignificant difference. Six patients in the ECG group showed AMI and qualified for and received thrombolytic treatment a mean of 48 minutes after hospital arrival. Mean times to treatment for 51 historical control patients and 6 patients in the control group were 103 minutes and 68 minutes (Fig 1–1).

Conclusions.—In-field ECG produces negligible delays in paramedic time and results in significant reduction in time to in-hospital thrombolysis. It may also make in-field treatment possible. In-field ECG may therefore be an important addition to the treatment of patients with AMI.

▶ This is a very important study documenting the advantage of paramedic transmission of 12-lead electrocardiograms at the earliest possible time in patients with acute myocardial infarction. All struggle with the problem of reducing the time to availability of thrombolytic therapy or other approaches to opening the infarct-related artery in patients with myocardial infarction, and these data are strongly supportive of such efforts.—R.L. Frye, M.D.

Effect of Age on Use of Thrombolytic Therapy and Mortality in Acute Myocardial Infarction

Weaver WD, Litwin PE, Martin JS, Kudenchuk PJ, Maynard C, Eisenberg MS, Ho MT, Cobb LA, Kennedy JW, Wirkus MS, MITI Project Group (Univ of Washington)
J Am Coll Cardiol 18:657–662, 1991   1–2

Background.—Relatively few elderly patients have received thrombolytic therapy for suspected acute myocardial infarction. There is concern over a higher risk of bleeding in this population—especially intracerebral hemorrhage.

Objective.—The outcome of thrombolytic therapy was related to age in a series of 3,256 consecutive patients hospitalized for acute infarction. Twenty-eight percent of patients were aged 65–74 years, and the same proportion were aged 75 years and older.

Findings.—Mortality rose markedly with advancing age, to 17.8% in patients aged 75 years and older. Both complicating illness and a nondiagnostic ECG were more frequent in older patients. No patient younger than age 47 years died while hospitalized (Fig 1–2). In patients aged 65 years and older, adverse events were related to both a history of heart failure and older age. Thrombolytic therapy did not improve the outcome; however, only 12% of patients older than age 65 years received this treatment, making it difficult to detect this effect.

Discussion.—Elderly persons often have acute myocardial infarction after having complications from ischemic heart disease. Treatment decisions are difficult because of the frequency of nonspecific ECG abnormalities, the occasional absence of chest pain, and the high rate of complicating illness.

▶ This is a nice report of the experience in the MITI Project and provides a perspective for the clinician faced with the problem of treating the elderly patient-

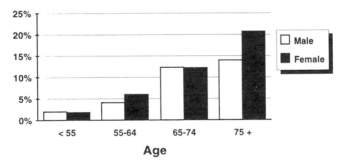

Age

Fig 1–2.—Mortality rates by age for the 3,256 patients with acute myocardial infarction. No patient younger than age 47 years died during hospitalization, whereas the overall mortality rate in patients, aged 75 years and older, was 18%. Gender-specific mortality rates were similar in all but the last stratum. The median age of men and women in the group, aged 75 years and older, was 80 and 82 years, respectively. Age-adjusted mortality rates for men and women were not significantly different (9.1% and 11.3%, respectively). (Courtesy of Weaver WD, Litwin PE, Martin JS, et al: *J Am Coll Cardiol* 18:657–662, 1991.)

with acute myocardial infarction, specifically in relation to use of thrombolytic therapy.—R.L. Frye, M.D.

Racial Differences in Responses to Thrombolytic Therapy With Recombinant Tissue-Type Plasminogen Activator: Increased Fibrin(ogen)olysis in Blacks
Sane DC, Stump DC, Topol EJ, Sigmon KN, Clair WK, Kereiakes DJ, George BS, Stoddard MF, Bates ER, Stack RS, Califf RM, and the Thrombolysis and Angioplasty in Myocardial Infarction Study Group (Duke Univ; Univ of Vermont; Univ of Michigan; Christ Hosp, Cincinnati; Riverside Methodist Hosp, Columbus, Ohio, et al)
Circulation 83:170–175, 1991   1–3

Introduction.—Black Americans have a poorer prognosis after acute myocardial infarction (AMI) than do white Americans. This difference has been attributed in part to a higher prevalence of baseline risk factors in blacks. Studies investigating race-dependent differences in treatment responses after AMI have shown that blacks and whites have similar reductions in mortality with propranolol therapy and similar survival rates after coronary artery bypass grafting (CABG). However, race-related differences in the response to thrombolytic therapy have never been studied.

Patients.—Twenty-four black patients and 352 white patients with AMI were treated with intravenous infusion of recombinant tissue-type plasminogen activator (rt-PA) at a mean of 3 hours after the onset of chest pain. At 90 minutes after initiation of rt-PA therapy, patients underwent coronary arteriography and left ventriculography. The rt-PA antigen, fibrinogen, fibrin(ogen) degradation products, and fragment D-dimer were assayed at baseline and at 3, 5, 8, and 12 hours after rt-PA therapy was begun.

Results.—At 90 minutes after initiation of thrombolytic therapy, patency rates of infarct-related arteries were 91% for blacks and 72% for whites. The difference was significant. However, blacks and whites had similar survival to discharge and were equally likely to undergo CABG. Peak rt-PA antigen levels did not differ significantly between blacks and whites, but there was a trend toward higher rt-PA levels in blacks during and at the end of the rt-PA infusion. Baseline fibrinogen levels in both groups were similar, but blacks had significantly lower nadir fibrinogen levels and higher peak fibrin(ogen) degradation product levels than did whites, reflecting greater fibrinogen depletion.

Conclusion.—The greater patency rates in black patients with AMI after thrombolytic therapy and a greater fibrinogen depletion at equivalent rt-PA levels suggest either race-related altered pharmacologic action of rt-PA or an increased sensitivity to fibrinolysis.

▶ These observations from TAMI are of great interest and point to the need for further detailed basic studies to explain these differences in responsiveness to thrombolytic therapy between whites and blacks. See also Abstract 1–23.— R.L. Frye, M.D.

A Prospective, Randomized Trial Comparing Combination Half-Dose Tissue-Type Plasminogen Activator and Streptokinase With Full-Dose Tissue-Type Plasminogen Activator

Grines CL, Nissen SE, Booth DC, Gurley JC, Chelliah N, Wolf R, Blankenship J, Branco MC, Bennett K, DeMaria AN, and the Kentucky Acute Myocardial Infarction Trial Group (Univ of Kentucky, Lexington; VA Med Ctrs, Lexington; United Hosp, Grand Forks, ND; Geisinger Med Ctr, Danville, Pa)
Circulation 84:540–549, 1991   1–4

Rationale.—A pilot study has suggested that combining half-dose tissue-type plasminogen activator (t-PA) with full-dose streptokinase yields a high patency rate for infarct vessels with a low rate of reocclusion. Nevertheless, the value of combining thrombolytic agents in treating myocardial infarction remains uncertain.

Study Design.—In a prospective trial, 216 patients were randomized within 6 hours of myocardial infarction to receive either combination therapy or a conventional full dose of 100 mg of t-PA over 3 hours. Combination treatment included 50 mg of t-PA and 1.5 MU of streptokinase infused concomitantly through separate intravenous lines. Heparin and aspirin therapy were continued until follow-up catheterization on day 7.

Results.—Early patency rates were higher after combined treatment than with t-PA alone (79% vs. 64%). Patency exceeded 95% in both groups after angioplasty for failed thrombolysis. Serum fibrinogen was markedly depleted after combined treatment. Reocclusion was less frequent in patients who were given combined thrombolytic treatment, as were reinfarction and the need for emergency bypass surgery. Estimates of infarct-zone function suggested greater myocardial salvage from combined treatment. Hospital mortality and the occurrence of serious bleeding were similarly frequent in the 2 treatment groups.

Conclusions.—Combining half-dose t-PA with streptokinase has yielded favorable results in patients seen within 6 hours of myocardial infarction. Bleeding is not more of a problem than with full-dose t-PA alone, and the costs are less.

▶ This innovative approach of combining t-PA with streptokinase looks most promising, and the investigators are to be congratulated on an important contribution. Further study in larger trials will be eagerly awaited.—R.L. Frye, M.D.

Thrombolysis in Myocardial Infarction (TIMI) Phase II Trial: Outcome Comparison of a "Conservative Strategy" in Community Versus Tertiary Hospitals

Feit F, Mueller HS, Braunwald E, Ross R, Hodges M, Herman MV, Knatterud GL, the TIMI Research Group (New York Univ School of Medicine; Albert Einstein College of Medicine, Bronx, NY; Harvard Med School, Boston; Maryland Research Inst, Baltimore; Hennepin County Med Ctr, Minneapolis, et al)
J Am Coll Cardiol 16:1529–1534, 1990   1–5

Background.—Early thrombolytic therapy after myocardial infarction can recanalize the affected artery, salvage the left ventricular myocardium, and reduce mortality. In the conservative strategy arm of the Thrombolysis in Myocardial Infarction Phase II (TIMI-II) trial, patients were treated with intravenous recombinant tissue-type plasminogen activator (rt-PA) followed by coronary angiography. Angioplasty, if feasible, was performed only for recurrent spontaneous or exercise-induced ischemia.

Methods.—Of 1,461 patients assigned to this conservative strategy, 1,155 were admitted to a tertiary hospital with on-site coronary angiography and angioplasty, and 306 were admitted to a community hospital that required transfer to the tertiary hospital for angiography and angioplasty. Coronary angiography was carried out if ischemic pain recurred spontaneously or on exercise. Angioplasty was done at the same time if there was severe residual stenosis and suitable anatomy. Patients were followed up to an end point of 42 days.

Results.—Angiography was done in 48% of the patients initially admitted to the tertiary hospital and 32% of those initially admitted to the community hospital, despite the similar baseline characteristics of the 2 groups. As a result, use of several procedures was greater at the tertiary than at the community hospital, including coronary angioplasty, 18% vs. 11% of patients; coronary artery bypass surgery, 12% vs. 8%; and blood transfusion, 12% vs. 5.5%. Despite these differences, there were no significant differences in mortality, recurrent myocardial infarction, or left ventricular function.

Conclusions.—A conservative strategy for patients with acute myocardial infarction treated with rt-PA appears to be applicable to the community hospital setting. Such hospitals need to make arrangements for expeditious transfer of patients with recurrent myocardial ischemia. Higher thresholds for community hospital patients to undergo coronary angiography appear to be appropriate.

Hemorrhagic Events During Therapy With Recombinant Tissue-Type Plasminogen Activator, Heparin, and Aspirin for Acute Myocardial Infarction: Results of the Thrombolysis in Myocardial Infarction (TIMI), Phase II Trial

Bovill EG, Terrin ML, Stump DC, Berke AD, Frederick M, Collen D, Feit F, Gore JM, Hillis LD, Lambrew CT, Leiboff R, Mann KG, Markis JE, Pratt CM, Sharkey SW, Sopko G, Tracy RP, Chesebro JH (Univ of Vermont; Maryland Med Research Inst, Baltimore; Genentech, Inc, San Francisco; St Francis Hosp, Roslyn, NY; Univ of Leuven, Belgium; et al)

Ann Intern Med 115:256–265, 1991   1–6

Introduction.—Thrombolytic therapy often is effective in early acute myocardial infarction, but hemorrhagic complications continue to occur, and rates as high as 30% are reported when invasive procedures are part of the protocol.

Study Design.—A multicenter trial included 3,339 patients with ischemic chest pain who received recombinant tissue plasminogen activator in a dose of 150 or 100 mg. Patients were assigned randomly to either an invasive approach (coronary angiography with percutaneous angioplasty, if feasible, 18–48 hours after the start of thrombolysis) or conservative management. Those patients assigned to conservative management had angiography if ischemia recurred. Patients also were randomized to immediate intravenous β-blocker therapy or deferred treatment.

Results.—Among patients given 100 mg of recombinant tissue-type plasminogen activator (rt-PA), hemorrhage was more frequent in those assigned to invasive management than in those managed conservatively (18.5% vs. 12.8%). Hemorrhage correlated with the degree of fibrinogen breakdown, the peak rt-PA level, thrombocytopenia, an activated partial thromboplastin time exceeding 90 seconds, and signs of cardiac decompensation. Patients weighing 70 kg or less and women had hemorrhagic events more frequently. Intracranial bleeding was more common in patients given the higher dose of rt-PA, and a greater hemostatic defect developed in these patients.

Conclusions.—Many factors contribute to the occurrence of hemorrhage in patients given thrombolytic treatment for myocardial infarction. Invasive management was associated with more frequent hemorrhage in this study.

▶ These additional studies from the TIMI II Trial (Abstracts 1–5 and 1–6) provide important data to guide the management of patients with acute myocardial infarction receiving thrombolytic therapy. The use of percutaneous transluminal coronary angioplasty after thrombolytic therapy should be based on evidence of recurring ischemia.—R.L. Frye, M.D.

Myocardial Infarction With Minimal Coronary Atherosclerosis in the Era of Thrombolytic Reperfusion

Kereiakes DJ, Topol EJ, George BS, Stack RS, Abbottsmith CW, Ellis S, Candela RJ, Harrelson L, Martin LH, Califf RM, and the Thrombolysis and Angioplasty in Myocardial Infarction (TAMI) Study Group (Christ Hosp Cardiovascular Research Ctr, Cincinnati; Univ of Michigan, Ann Arbor; Riverside Methodist Hosp, Columbus, Ohio; Duke Univ, Durham, NC)

J Am Coll Cardiol 17:304–312, 1991   1–7

Introduction.—Most patients who have an acute myocardial infarction (AMI) have significant underlying coronary atherosclerosis and will show a persistent high grade of residual coronary stenosis of the infarct-related artery after successful intravenous thrombolytic therapy. However, a small percentage of AMI patients with insignificant underlying coronary atherosclerosis show a minimal coronary lesion after successful recanalization. The incidence of minimal residual atherosclerotic coronary obstruction among patients with AMI successfully treated with intravenous thrombolysis was evaluated.

Patients.—During a 3-year period, 810 patients with AMI were successfully treated with intravenous recombinant tissue-type plasminogen activator (rt-PA), combined intravenous rt-PA and urokinase, or high-dose intravenous urokinase. All patients underwent coronary angiography of the infarct-related artery and left ventriculography 90 minutes after initiation of thrombolytic therapy. Residual coronary stenosis was quantitated with an automated edge detection computer algorithm. The findings in 783 patients were assessable.

Findings.—Initial 90-minute angiography showed high-grade residual coronary stenosis greater than 50% in 740 patients (94.5%) and no significant residual stenosis in 43 patients (5.5%). However, 42 patients had further resolution of obstruction to less than 50% at follow-up angiography 7–10 days later. In all, 85 patients (10.9%) had insigificant atherosclerotic coronary obstruction after successful intravenous thrombolysis for AMI. Patients with minimal residual coronary obstruction were significantly younger, had less multivessel coronary disease, had better initial left ventricular ejection fraction, and had lower in-hospital mortality than did patients with significant residual coronary obstruction after intravenous thrombolysis. However, despite improved hospital survival and a more benign hospital course, patients with minimal residual stenosis experienced a similar incidence of death and recurrent nonfatal AMI in the long-term follow-up period compared with patients with high-grade residual coronary obstruction.

Conclusion.—New strategies to prevent coronary rethrombosis in patients with minimal atherosclerosis after thrombolytic therapy for AMI should be evaluated in a long-term follow-up study.

▶ This is a fascinating study. One wonders about methods to assess stability of plaques in the coronary arteries that may not be hemodynamically significant. It would be of interest to know whether the late terminal events occurred in the original infarct-related artery.—R.L. Frye, M.D.

Precordial ST Segment Depression Predicts a Worse Prognosis in Inferior Infarction Despite Reperfusion Therapy
Bates ER, Clemmensen PM, Califf RM, Gorman LE, Aronson LG, George BS, Kereiakes DJ, Topol EJ, the Thrombolysis and Angioplasty in Myocardial Infarction Study Group (Univ of Michigan; Duke Univ; Riverside Methodist Hosp, Columbus, Ohio; Christ Hosp, Cincinnati)
J Am Coll Cardiol 16:1538–1544, 1990   1–8

Background.—Precordial ST segment depression and rates of complication similar to those seen with anterior myocardial infarction are associated with inferior infarction and a larger infarct size. The effect of precordial ST segment depression on angiographic and clinical outcomes after reperfusion therapy and selective coronary angioplasty was studied in patients with inferior myocardial infarction.

Methods.—Patients were separated into 3 groups for analysis. Group I comprised 289 patients with anterior infarction, group II included 135 patients with inferior infarction and precordial ST segment depression, and group III consisted of 159 patients with inferior infarction and no precordial ST segment depression. The study involved infusions of intravenous recombinant tissue-type plasminogen activator, coronary angiography with rescue coronary angioplasty if appropriate, and post-thrombolytic therapy with heparin, lidocaine, aspirin, dipyridamole, and diltiazem.

Results.—Precordial ST segment depression was seen in 71% of infarct-related circumflex arteries and in 40% of right coronary arteries. Acute patency rates were not statistically different; however, a trend toward different patency rates at day 7 was noted, partly resulting from insignificantly higher rates of reocclusion in group III. In patients with inferior infarction, infarct zone regional wall motion was lower in those with precordial ST segment depression, both acutely and at day 7. Patients in group II also tended to have a lower ejection fraction at these times than those in group III. Their complication rates also tended to be higher. Mortalities were 8% for group I, 6% for group II, and 5% for group III.

Conclusions.—In patients who have inferior myocardial infarction with precordial ST segment depression, ventriculographic and clinical outcomes appear to be worse, despite reperfusion therapy. These patients also appear to have a higher complication rate and worse left ventricular function, despite having a lower rate of reocclusion than similar patients without precordial changes.

▶ I was surprised that there was not a more obvious benefit with thrombolytic therapy in those patients with ST segment depression in the precordium. This is an important issue, and we need more controlled studies in an attempt to identify those with inferior myocardial infarction who benefit from thrombolytic therapy.—R.L. Frye, M.D.

Timing and Mechanism of In-Hospital and Late Death After Primary Coronary Angioplasty During Acute Myocardial Infarction

Kahn JK, O'Keefe JH Jr, Rutherford BD, McConahay DR, Johnson WL, Giorgi LV, Shimshak TM, Ligon RW, Hartzler GO (Cardiovascular Consultants, Inc., Kansas City, Mo)
Am J Cardiol 66:1045–1048, 1990   1–9

Background.—Early myocardial reperfusion after acute myocardial infarction (AMI) reduces hospital mortality and confers a sustained survival advantage, but its effect on patterns of death is unknown. To determine the mechanism and timing of in-hospital and late deaths, 614 patients who underwent coronary angioplasty were studied.

Methods.—The procedures were performed in 445 men and 169 women (mean age, 59) over an 8-year period. None of the patients had thrombolytic therapy before coronary angioplasty. Follow-up data were obtained by reviewing records for patients who died in the hospital and by mail or telephone for discharged patients.

Results.—Forty-nine patients died in the hospital, a rate of 8%, 4 dying in the catheterization laboratory. Twenty-two patients died of cardiogenic shock and 5 of acute vessel reclosure. Death was sudden in 8 patients and was preceded by elective coronary artery bypass surgery in 8 patients. Only 2 patients had cardiac rupture after failed angioplasty; this did not occur in any of the 574 patients who had successful reperfusion. Failed infarct angioplasty, cardiogenic shock, 3-vessel coronary artery disease, and age of 70 years or older were multivariate predictors of in-hospital death. Fifty five patients died over a mean follow-up period of 32 months. Of these, 36 died of cardiac causes, including 23 who died of arrhythmic death and 13 who died of circulatory failure. Actuarial survival after hospital discharge was 95% at 1 year and 87% at 4 years. Ninety-six percent of patients were free of cardiac death at 1 year and 92% at 4 years. Three-vessel disease, baseline ejection fraction of 40% or less, age greater than 70 years, and female gender were multivariate predictors of late death.

Conclusions.—The status of the left ventricle and the extent of coronary artery disease appear to be determinants of death after coronary angioplasty for AMI. This procedure may reduce the incidence of cardiac rupture.

▶ Another excellent observational study from Hartzler and colleagues. Fortunately, at least 2 randomized trials are comparing primary percutaneous transluminal coronary angioplasty versus thrombolytic therapy in patients with AMI. The results of these trials will be eagerly awaited.—R.L. Frye, M.D.

A Comparison Between Heparin and Low-Dose Aspirin as Adjunctive Therapy With Tissue Plasminogen Activator For Acute Myocardial Infarction

Hsia J, Hamilton WP, Kleiman N, Roberts R, Chaitman BR, Ross AM, Heparin–Aspirin Reperfusion Trial (HART) Investigators (George Washington Univ, Washington, DC; Baylor College of Medicine; St Louis Univ)
N Engl J Med 323:1433–1437, 1990   1–10

Methods.—The Heparin–Aspirin Reperfusion Trial is a collaborative trial that compares early intravenous heparin with oral aspirin as adjunct treatment when recombinant tissue plasminogen activator (rt-PA) is used for coronary thrombolytic treatment during acute myocardial infarction. Within 6 hours of onset of symptoms (average, 3.1 hours) suggestive of myocardial ischemia, 205 patients began receiving rt-PA, 100 mg, intravenously, administered over a 6-hour period in combination with either immediate and continuous intravenous heparin, starting with a 5,000 U bolus, or immediate and daily oral aspirin, 80 mg.

Results.—At 7–24 hours after the start of rt-PA infusion, angiography revealed patent infarct-related arteries in 82% of heparin recipients, compared with only 52% of those assigned to aspirin; the difference was highly significant. By day 7, repeat angiography revealed no significant difference in the patency rates of patients receiving the 2 types of treatments (88% vs. 95% for heparin vs. aspirin). Hemorrhagic events occurred in 18 patients receiving heparin and 15 patients receiving aspirin, and recurrent ischemic events occurred in 8 and 2 patients, respectively. The difference was not significant.

Conclusions.—These findings indicate that treatment with rt-PA and early concomittant intravenous heparin is associated with higher coronary patency rates than with rt-PA and concomittant low-dose aspirin. It appears that the advantage of early heparin is in its ability to prevent reocclusion in the first 24 hours. These findings should be considered in the design and interpretation of clinical trials involving coronary thrombolytic treatment.

▶ This excellent study by the HART investigators is most important in the continuing debate regarding the appropriate use of aspirin and heparin. Fortunately, the GUSTO Trial that is in progress should provide additional important data on the issue of the importance of early intravenous heparin treatment in thrombolytic therapy.—R.L. Frye, M.D.

Sudden Death

Survivors of Acute Myocardial Infarction: Who Is at Risk for Sudden Cardiac Death?

Shen W-K, Hammill SC (Mayo Clinic and Found, Rochester, Minn)
Mayo Clin Proc 66:950–962, 1991   1–11

Introduction.—Coronary artery disease (CAD) accounts for 40% of all deaths in the United States annually, approximately half of which are sudden cardiac deaths. Of the approximately 400,000 sudden cardiac deaths per year, 300,000 occur in patients with CAD. Reducing the high risk of sudden cardiac death requires accurate identification of high-risk patients and effective preventive therapy.

Risk Factors.—Extensive studies in patients with CAD who have had a myocardial infarction (MI) have shown that left ventricular dysfunction, frequent ventricular ectopic activity, and nonsustained ventricular tachycardia (VT) are markers for sudden cardiac death. However, the sensitivity and specificity of those markers vary, and their positive predictive power is less than satisfactory. The role of premature ventricular complexes as an independent risk factor is also uncertain.

Diagnostic Methods.—The value of programmed ventricular stimulation as a predictor for future malignant VT or sudden cardiac death in patients with MI who have experienced spontaneous sustained VT or who have been resuscitated from cardiac arrest is well established, but its value in the general population of patients who have had infarction is unclear. Current noninvasive diagnostic techniques lack the predictive power to identify patients at high risk for sudden cardiac death.

Preventive Therapy.—A recent review of 10 clinical trials that investigated the efficacy of anti-arrhythmic drugs in preventing sudden cardiac death showed that the currently available agents have limited efficacy, and that some anti-arrhythmic drugs may have potential lethal effects. In view of those findings, empirical anti-arrhythmic therapy is inadvisable. Implanted automatic defibrillators can significantly decrease the frequency of sudden death, as well as abort sudden death in patients with prior sustained VT. However, their more general use in asymptomatic postinfarction patients who are at high risk for sudden cardiac death has not been evaluated.

Conclusion.—The optimal diagnostic and therapeutic strategies to drastically lower the mortality from sudden cardiac death in patients with CAD and in patients who have had infarction remain to be determined.

▶ This is a nice summary of the approach to prevention of sudden death. As the authors indicate, much remains to be learned, but I think this approach will be of interest to clinicians treating such patients.—R.L. Frye, M.D.

Late Outcome of Survivors of Out-of-Hospital Cardiac Arrest With Left Ventricular Ejection Fraction ≥50% and Without Significant Coronary Arterial Narrowing

Kudenchuk PJ, Cobb LA, Greene HL, Fahrenbruch CE, Sheehan FH (Univ of Washington, Seattle)
Am J Cardiol 67:704–708, 1991   1–12

Introduction.—Out-of-hospital cardiac arrest in patients without evidence of major structural heart disease is uncommon. The cause of ventricular fibrillation (VF) in these patients remains obscure, but drug abuse, primary conduction system disease, coronary artery spasm, and subclinical myocarditis are potential etiologic factors. However, predictors of recurrent out-of-hospital cardiac arrest in these VF survivors are not well defined. The records of VF survivors in whom no major structural cardiac abnormalities were found after resuscitation were reviewed to identify predictors of mortality and recurrent out-of-hospital cardiac arrest.

Patients.—Of 1,195 survivors of out-of-hospital VF, 43 met the following study inclusion criteria: VF was the initial rhythm as documented by paramedics, coronary angiography and contrast left ventriculography were performed within 6 months of VF, the contrast left ventricular ejection fraction was .50 or greater, and there was no evidence of coronary artery stenosis of ≥50% luminal diameter.

Results.—There were 33 men and 10 women aged 20–73 years, with a mean age of 47 years. Thirteen patients (30%) had abnormal wall motion on left ventriculography and 20 patients (47%) had persistent ECG abnormalities. During an average follow-up of 86 months, 7 (16%) of the 43 patients had a recurrent out-of-hospital cardiac arrest. The presence of wall motion or ECG abnormalities identified those who were at increased risk of recurrent cardiac arrest. The risk for recurrent cardiac arrest within 5 years was 30% for patients with abnormal ECGs and 5% for those with normal ECGs. The difference was significant. Age was a negative independent predictor of recurrent cardiac arrest in that recurrence was more common among younger patients.

Conclusion.—Resuscitated survivors of cardiac arrest in whom no major structural heart disease is identified can be stratified for risk of recurrence by age and by abnormal ECG or left ventriculography findings. Younger patients and patients with persistent ECG or left ventricular wall motion abnormalities after cardiac arrest are at increased risk for recurrence.

▶ An interesting group of patients. The predictive value of resting ECG abnormalities and left ventricular ejection fraction is again demonstrated.— R.L. Frye, M.D.

Prevention and Epidemiology

The Case Against Childhood Cholesterol Screening
Newman TB, Browner WS, Hulley SB (Univ of California, San Francisco)
JAMA 264:3039–3043, 1990   1–13

Introduction.—Some government authorities and agencies have suggested that all children should be screened for cholesterol to prevent coronary heart disease (CHD). The published literature was reviewed to determine whether indications for childhood cholesterol screening should be broadened or narrowed.

Findings.—No available evidence clearly demonstrates that measurements of blood cholesterol levels in children actually predict who will have CHD in the future. A raised blood cholesterol level in childhood can predict an elevated cholesterol level 1–2 decades after the initial measurement. However, the estimated risks for CHD deaths before age 65 based on the quintile ratings of blood cholesterol levels are relatively small. As boys age, the risks for the 5 quintiles becomes more similar. The difference in risk for CHD deaths between boys in the fifth and fourth quintiles (.4% to 1.1%, depending on tracking assumptions) indicates that the potential results of a screening and intervention program are extremely limited. In nonresearch settings such as physicians' offices or shopping malls, blood cholesterol measurements can be grossly inaccurate. Although measurements of childhood cholesterol levels do not accurately predict adult risks for CHD, assessing a child's cholesterol level could be preventative if intervention programs instituted in childhood were more effective than those begun later. However, the few trials conducted suggest that dietary interventions have only reduced cholesterol levels by about 5%, compared with the 10% reductions in cholesterol usually seen in adults undergoing dietary treatment for high levels. On the other hand, children and young adults appear to have a higher mortality rate from accidents, violence, and suicide, which have been linked with cholesterol-lowering interventions in randomized trials. In addition, a low-fat and low-cholesterol diet in growing children may not be safe.

Conclusions.—The benefits from cholesterol screening may not outweigh the risks. Rather than supporting the recommendation for general cholesterol screening for all children, it is recommended that children not be screened for high cholesterol levels.

▶ This is a provocative analysis of cholesterol screening in childhood. There remains much that we do not know in this arena, and in my own practice, I have screened children only in families with premature vascular disease and lipid abnormalities.—R.L. Frye, M.D.

Postmenopausal Estrogen Therapy and Cardiovascular Disease: Ten-Year Follow-Up From the Nurses' Health Study
Stampfer MJ, Colditz GA, Willett WC, Manson JE, Rosner B, Speizer FE, Hennekens CH (Harvard Med School; Brigham and Women's Hosp, Boston; Harvard School of Public Health)
N Engl J Med 325:756–762, 1991   1–14

Background.—The influence of exogenous hormones on the risk of cardiovascular disease has long been debated. Two recent studies came to opposite conclusions about the benefit of estrogen use in the risk of coronary disease. The results for coronary disease and stroke from a 10-year follow-up of a large cohort were analyzed.

Methods.—A cohort of 48,470 postmenopausal women, aged 30 to 63, was followed. These women were participants in the Nurses' Health Study and did not have a history of cancer or cardiovascular disease when they were enrolled. During 337,854 person-years of follow-up, there were 224 strokes, 405 cases of major coronary disease, and 1,263 deaths from all causes.

Results.—After age and other risk factors were adjusted for, the overall relative risk of major coronary disease in women currently taking estrogen was .56. Women with natural or surgical menopause had a significantly reduced risk. The duration of estrogen use appeared to have no effect independent of age. The adjusted relative risks to current and former estrogen users compared with women who had never used estrogen were .89 for total mortality and .72 for cardiovascular mortality. When current users were compared with those who had never used estrogen, the risk of stroke was .97, with no marked differences according to type of stroke.

Conclusions.—Current estrogen use is associated with a reduced incidence of coronary heart disease and mortality from cardiovascular disease in postmenopausal women. It is not, however, associated with any change in the risk of stroke.

▶ This is a critically important study, which has provoked much discussion on the need for a properly controlled study of postmenopausal estrogen therapy on cardiovascular disease. I have no doubt that such trials will be underway shortly under the vigorous leadership of Dr. Bernadine Healy in her role as the Director of the National Institutes of Health.—R.L. Frye, M.D.

A Prospective Study of Aspirin Use and Primary Prevention of Cardiovascular Disease in Women
Manson JE, Stampfer MJ, Colditz GA, Willett WC, Rosner B, Speizer FE, Hennekens CH (Harvard Med School; Harvard School of Public Health)
JAMA 266:521–527, 1991   1–15

Background.—Both men and women with prior vascular occlusive disease can benefit from aspirin therapy, although it has not been possible to determine sex differences in efficacy. Two trials of primary prevention have included men only. A prospective cohort study was done in women to investigate the association between regular aspirin use and risk of a first cardiovascular event.

Methods.—The sample consisted of participants in the Nurses' Health Study who responded to a 1980 questionnaire. There were 87,678 patients in 11 states, ranging in age from 34 to 65. It was estimated that 98% of the women were white. Follow-up included 475,265 person-years, which represented 96.7% of the total potential follow-up. Main outcome measures were myocardial infarction, stroke, cardiovascular death, and important vascular events.

Results.—Forty percent of the women reported taking aspirin regularly. There were 240 nonfatal myocardial infarctions, 146 nonfatal

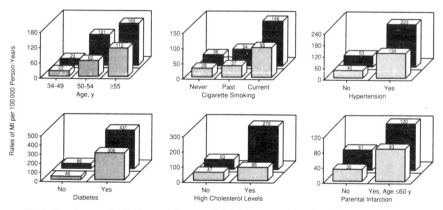

Fig 1–3.—Age-standardized rates of myocardial infarction (combined nonfatal MI and fatal coronary heart disease) among women who took 1 to 6 aspirin per week *(shaded bars)* compared with those who took no aspirin *(solid bars)* according to levels of coronary risk factors. All rates (except age-specific rates) are standardized to the age distribution of those women who took no aspirin. (Courtesy of Manson JE, Stampfer MJ, Colditz GA, et al: *JAMA* 266:521–527, 1991.)

strokes, and 130 deaths resulting from cardiovascular disease. Age-adjusted relative risk (RR) of a first myocardial infarction was .68 among women who took 1 to 6 aspirin per week compared with those who took no aspirin. A RR of .75 was obtained after simultaneous adjustment for coronary disease risk factors (Fig 1–3). Age-adjusted RR was .61 and multivariate RR was .68 among women aged 50 and older. Risk of stroke appeared to be unaffected. For cardiovascular death and important vascular events, multivariate RRs were .89 and .85, respectively. Very similar results were seen when subgroups of women taking 1 to 3 and 4 to 6 aspirin per week were examined separately, and no reductions in risk were seen in those who took 7 or more aspirin per week. The main reasons for taking aspirin were headache, arthritis, and musculoskeletal pain.

Conclusions.—Risk of a first myocardial infarction appears to be decreased in women who take 1 to 6 aspirin per week. Conclusive data must await a randomized trial. Aspirin may be considered for female patients only on the basis of clinical judgment, including the patient's cardiovascular risk status, the side effects, and the possible benefits.

▶ An important observation and one that will undoubtedly lead to a major randomized trial.— R.L. Frye, M.D.

A Prospective Study of Cholesterol, Apolipoproteins, and the Risk of Myocardial Infarction
Stampfer MJ, Sacks FM, Salvini S, Willett WC, Hennekens CH (Brigham and Women's Hosp, Boston; Harvard School of Public Health, Boston)
N Engl J Med 325:373–381, 1991   1–16

Background.—The relation between low high-density lipoprotein cholesterol (HDL-C) levels and an increased risk of coronary heart disease and myocardial infarction (MI) has been well established. However, the independent contributions to that risk by HDL_2 and HDL_3, the 2 principal subfractions of HDL, and by the apolipoproteins have not been clarified. Whether the HDL subfractions and the apolipoproteins are independent predictors of the risk of MI was investigated in participants in the ongoing Physicians' Health Study.

Methods.—Blood samples were prospectively collected at baseline from 14,916 men aged 40–84 years. Men with a history of coronary heart disease, MI, or stroke were excluded. Every man who suffered a confirmed MI was paired with a control study participant of the same age and with the same smoking status. Aliquots of stored plasma samples from the case subject and the control were then sent paired for laboratory analysis. The pooled plasma samples were analyzed for total cholesterol, HDL, HDL_2, HDL_3, and apolipoproteins.

Results.—After 5 years of follow-up, 246 men had a new MI. Case patients had significantly higher levels of total cholesterol, higher ratios of

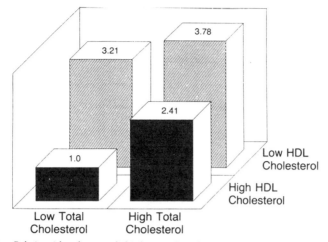

Fig 1–4.—Relative risks of myocardial infarction for subjects with values above and below the median for total and HDL cholesterol levels. The median for total cholesterol was 5.49 mmol/L, and that for HDL-C 1.22 mmol/L. The interaction of total cholesterol and HDL-C was statistically significant in a model that also included total cholesterol and HDL-C as separate terms ($P = .01$). (Courtesy of Stampfer MJ, Sacks FM, Salvini S, et al: *N Engl J Med* 325:373–381, 1991.)

total to HDL-C, and significantly lower levels of HDL, HDL_2, and HDL_3 cholesterol, apolipoprotein A-I, and HDL particles without apolipoprotein A-II. Case patients also had lower mean levels of apolipoprotein A-II and apolipoprotein A-II–containing HDL particles and higher levels of apolipoprotein B-100, but the differences were not statistically significant.

Higher HDL-C levels were associated with a substantial decrease in risk of infarction. The benefit of higher HDL levels was most pronounced in patients with lower total cholesterol levels (Fig 1–4). After multivariate analysis, the HDL-C level remained a powerful predictor of risk of MI. That inverse association was not limited to the contribution by HDL_2 cholesterol, as previously thought; HDL_3 cholesterol was even more strongly associated with a decreased risk of MI. Apolipoprotein A-I and A-II levels were also associated with decreased risk. However, in a model that included the total:HDL-C ratio, neither the 2 HDL subfractions nor the apolipoproteins added significantly to the value of the total:HDL-C ratio in predicting MI. In contrast, the total:HDL-C ratio remained a significant independent predictor of risk of MI.

Conclusion.— The HDL cholesterol level is an important predictor of risk of MI. The subfractions, HDL_2 and HDL_3, and apolipoproteins have protective effects, but none are independent predictors of risk of MI.

▶ This is a powerful study from the Harvard group and emphasizes the importance of HDL cholesterol in predicting risk of myocardial infarction. This certainly fits with my own clinical practice where we regularly see patients with myocardial infarction and near normal total cholesterol levels but very low HDL cholesterol.— R.L. Frye, M.D.

Prospective Study of Alcohol Consumption and Risk of Coronary Disease in Men

Rimm EB, Giovannucci EL, Willett WC, Colditz GA, Ascherio A, Rosner B, Stampfer MJ (Harvard Univ, Boston; Brigham and Women's Hosp, Boston)
Lancet 338:464–468, 1991   1–17

Introduction.—Several different types of studies have reported an inverse association between alcohol consumption and the risk of coronary artery disease (CAD). However, some suggest that the inverse association is an artifact attributable to preexisting disease or the inclusion of heavy drinkers in reference groups of nondrinkers who are lying about their alcohol intake. Few studies of alcohol intake and CAD have taken dietary intake into consideration.

Methods.—A 131-item semiquantitative food frequency questionnaire that included questions about alcoholic beverage consumption was mailed to a cohort of 51,529 men aged 40–75 who are enrolled in an ongoing study of dietary causes of heart disease and cancer. All men are health professionals. Questions on medical history, heart disease risk factors, and dietary changes over the past 10 years were also included in the survey. The data from 44,059 men were available.

Results.—Analysis of the replies revealed that 23.4% of the men consumed alcoholic beverages either never or less than once per month, 26.4% drank more than 15 g of alcohol or 1 drink per day, and 3.5% drank more than 50 g of alcohol or 3–4 drinks per day. There were 350 confirmed new cases of CAD. After adjustment for coronary risk factors, including dietary intake of cholesterol, fat, and dietary fiber, increasing alcohol consumption was inversely related to CAD incidence. The exclusion of current nondrinkers or of those with disorders potentially related to CAD, which might have led them to reduce their alcohol intake, did not substantially affect the relative risks.

Conclusion.—The findings provide additional support for the hypothesis that moderate alcohol intake reduces the risk of CAD. The inverse association between moderate alcohol consumption and risk of CAD is not an artifact attributable to preexisting disease or differences in dietary habits, but is causal.

▶ These additional studies from Harvard support the moderate use of alcohol in terms of reducing the risk of coronary heart disease. This finding remains of great interest but of limited value in terms of therapy because one is reluctant to push alcohol intake in this particular group of patients, particularly if there is any tendency to hypertension or rhythm disturbances.—R.L. Frye, M.D.

Long-Term Mortality After 5-Year Multifactorial Primary Prevention of Cardiovascular Diseases in Middle-Aged Men

Strandberg TE, Salomaa VV, Naukkarinen VA, Vanhanen HT, Sarna SJ, Mietti-

nen TA (Univ of Helsinki, Finland; Natl Public Health Inst, Helsinki, Finland; Jorvi Hosp, Espoo, Finland)
JAMA 266:1225–1229, 1991   1–18

Background.—A randomized primary prevention trial was begun in 1974–1980 to assess the value of intensive dietetic and hygienic measures, hypolipidemic therapy with clofibrate and/or probucol, and antihypertensive therapy mainly with β-blockers and diuretics. Ten-year follow-up data now are available on the 612 initially healthy men who were assigned to primary prevention and 610 control subjects.

Findings.—Half the subjects in the intervention group received antihypertensive medication and 45% were given hypolipidemic medication. Overall mortality was 10.9% in the intervention group and 7.5% in the control group (Fig 1–5). The rates of mortality from coronary heart disease were 5.6% in the intervention group and 2.3% in the control group (Fig 1–6). Multiple logistic regression analysis failed to explain the excess cardiac mortality.

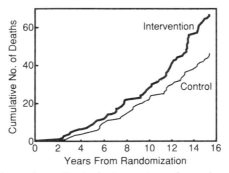

Fig 1–5.—Cumulative total mortality in the intervention and control groups during the 15-year follow-up. $P = .048$ for the difference between the groups. (Courtesy of Strandberg TE, Salomaa VV, Naukkarinen VA, et al: *JAMA* 266:1225–1229, 1991.)

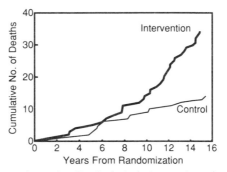

Fig 1–6.—Cumulative incidence of cardiac deaths in the intervention and control groups during the 15-year follow-up. $P = .0035$ for the difference between the groups. (Courtesy of Strandberg TE, Salomaa VV, Naukkarinen VA, et al: *JAMA* 266:1225–1229, 1991.)

Implications.—Coronary mortality increased in this study despite effective reduction of cardiovascular risk factors. The findings may relate only to this particular population, and they do not invalidate the concept of multifactorial primary prevention. They do, however, mean that ongoing research is needed on selecting methods for primary prevention of cardiovascular disease.

▶ This provocative study emphasizes the need for continued attention to the consequences of lipid-lowering drugs as part of a primary prevention effort. The increase in total and coronary heart disease mortality rates are of real concern, and this issue must be resolved before imposing screening and drug interventions in the presumably healthy population.—R.L. Frye, M.D.

Screening for Total Cholesterol: Do the National Cholesterol Education Program's Recommendations Detect Individuals at High Risk of Coronary Heart Disease?
Bush TL, Riedel D (The Johns Hopkins Univ)
Circulation 83:1287–1293, 1991   1–19

Background.—The National Cholesterol Education Program recommends total cholesterol screening of all adults older than age 20 years to identify persons at high risk of coronary heart disease because of lipid abnormalities. However, total cholesterol screening may fail to identify persons with acceptable cholesterol values who are at high risk for coronary heart disease because of high low-density lipoprotein (LDL) cholesterol levels or low high-density lipoprotein (HDL) cholesterol levels. The sensitivity of total cholesterol level as a screening tool was assessed.

Methods.—Data from the Lipid Research Clinics Program were used to simulate a population-based cholesterol screening program, following the recommendations of the National Cholesterol Education Program. The simulated study population consisted of 5,827 persons, aged 20–39 years, for whom complete information on cholesterol and lipoprotein levels was available. Persons were considered to be at high risk of coronary heart disease if they had LDL levels greater than 160 mg/dL or HDL levels less than 35 mg/dL.

Results.—Of 5,827 screened individuals, 1,163 (20%) had LDL levels equal to or greater than 160 mg/dL, and 718 (12%) had HDL levels less than 35 mg/dL. Men were more likely than women to have elevated LDL and low HDL levels. When the National Cholesterol Education Program guidelines were applied, 21% of those with high LDL levels and 66% of those with low HDL levels would not be referred for immediate treatment. Overall, 41% of those at high risk for coronary heart disease because of lipid abnormalities would not be promptly evaluated. The sensitivity of the National Cholesterol Education Program guidelines for promptly identifying individuals with lipoprotein abnormalities in this simulated population sample was 59%.

Conclusion.—The National Cholesterol Education Program guidelines for screening for lipid abnormalities need to be studied. Estimating the cost-benefit ratio of routine screening for lipoproteins, particularly for HDL cholesterol, should be a first step in the reviewing process.

▶ Another paper documenting the importance of cost-benefit analysis. Before embarking on these huge programs, the cost-effectiveness should be considered, and this includes implementation of the National Cholesterol Education Program.—R.L. Frye, M.D.

Practice Guidelines and Cholesterol Policy
Garber AM, Wagner JL (Stanford Univ; U.S. Office of Technology Assessment, Washington, DC)
Health Affairs 10:52–66, 1991   1–20

Background.—The National Cholesterol Education Program was organized in 1985 by the National Institutes of Health and charged with creating national guidelines for the identification and treatment of persons at high risk of coronary heart disease because of increased serum cholesterol levels. The National Cholesterol Education Program appointed an Adult Treatment Panel comprised of scientific and medical experts that was directed not to consider costs in drafting its recommendations.

Guidelines.—The Adult Treatment Panel guidelines recommend that all adults, aged 20 years and older, be screened for blood cholesterol levels at least once every 5 years. Serum low-density lipoprotein (LDL) cholesterol levels are to be measured in persons with a serum cholesterol level of 200 mg/dL or greater. A cholesterol-lowering diet is recommended for persons with a history of coronary heart disease, those with 2 cardiac risk factors and an LDL cholesterol level of 130 mg/dL or greater, or for those with fewer than 2 risk factors but an LDL level of 160 mg/dL or greater. Drug therapy should be considered after 6 months if diet therapy has failed to lower either the LDL or the total serum cholesterol level.

Effectiveness.—A review of published studies on the effectiveness of cholesterol reduction in preventing CHD has shown that lowering serum cholesterol level can prevent CHD in asymptomatic men but does not increase survival. In men who already have CHD or who have survived a heart attack, cholesterol-lowering diets and drug therapy can slow or reverse the accumulation of atherosclerotic deposits in the coronary arteries. However, the effects of cholesterol-lowering treatment in women of any age, in men with borderline cholesterol elevations, in younger men, and in men who are aged 65 years and older, are still unknown.

Costs.—In 1991 United States dollars, annual nationwide screening alone would cost about $424 million if all young adults were to comply, $299 million for screening the middle-aged individuals, and $146 million for screening all elderly persons. Drug treatment and follow-up would run into the billions of dollars, even though the overall effectiveness of such treatment is still largely unproven.

Conclusion.—The implementation of health care guidelines designed without any consideration of costs represents poor use of available health care dollars. The new Agency for Health Care Policy and Research, charged with the development of condition-specific national treatment guidelines, hopefully will identify and eliminate ineffective practices to prevent further waste of the nation's health dollars.

▶ I have included this health policy paper because of the increasing concern regarding allocation of health care resources. The need for careful consideration of costs with these vast primary prevention programs must be included in the data when considering the appropriateness of this sort of an approach.— R.L. Frye, M.D.

Cost Effectiveness of Incremental Programmes for Lowering Serum Cholesterol Concentration: Is Individual Intervention Worth While?
Kristiansen IS, Eggen AE, Thelle DS (Univ of Tromsø, Norway)
BMJ 302:1119–1122, 1991   1–21

Introduction.—There is strong evidence to suggest that lowering serum cholesterol levels will reduce the incidence of coronary heart disease. Three strategies that can lower serum cholesterol levels are population-based promotion of better eating habits, individual dietary treatment, and individual diet therapy combined with drug therapy. The relative cost-effectiveness of the various cholesterol-lowering programs used in Norway was evaluated.

Methods.—In Norway, 200,000 men aged 40–49 years are currently targeted by the Norwegian cholesterol-lowering program. This program advocates dietary treatment for persons with serum cholesterol levels ranging from 6 mmol/L to 7.9 mmol/L, and combined dietary and drug treatment for persons with serum cholesterol levels of 8 mmol/L or greater. The marginal cost-effectiveness was calculated for each approach, using the ratio of net treatment costs to life-years gained, as well as the ratio of net treatment costs to quality of life-years saved. The net treatment cost was calculated as the cost of treatment for a high cholesterol level minus the savings in treatment costs for coronary heart disease.

Outcome.—The calculated discounted total net cost for a population-based strategy that promotes better eating habits was estimated at £36,700 with a gain of 3,100 discounted life-years, resulting in a marginal cost-effectiveness ratio of £12 per life-year gained for men who were 40–49 years of age at the time of entry into the program. For an individual strategy based on dietary treatment, the cost would escalate to about £12,400 per life-year gained, and to £111,549 per life-year gained if drug therapy were to be added for half of those with serum cholesterol levels of 8 mmol/L or greater. Although the cost per life-year saved by the population-based strategy would be negligible, the marginal net cost of dietary treatment would be substantial compared with the extra life-years saved and even higher with the addition of drug therapy. Analysis of the respective calculated costs revealed that individual cholesterol-lowering treatment would be less cost-effective than the treatment of coronary heart disease.

Conclusions.—Mass educational programs to lower serum cholesterol are cost-effective and responsible. However, the guidelines for individual diet therapy should be implemented more selectively than currently recommended. Drug therapy should be limited to persons with genetic hypercholesterolemia and those who are otherwise at very high risk of arteriosclerotic disease.

An Economic Evaluation of Lovastatin for Cholesterol Lowering and Coronary Artery Disease Reduction
Hay JW, Wittels EH, Gotto AM Jr (Stanford Univ, Stanford, Calif; Baylor College of Medicine, Houston)
Am J Cardiol 67:789–796, 1991   1–22

Background.—Reduction of total serum cholesterol level and its low-density lipoprotein components are important in preventing coronary artery disease (CAD). The cost-effectiveness of cholesterol reduction using drug intervention will affect decisions regarding allocation of resources toward cholesterol screening, monitoring, and preventive intervention. Lifetime lovastatin therapy was used as an intervention model for cholesterol lowering in adults between ages 35 and 55 years. This analysis examines costs and benefits of CAD risk reduction using lovastatin.

Methods.—The measure of the costs and benefits of cholesterol lowering, from the perspective of an individual patient, is the present expected value of the cost per life-year saved. The net costs consist of the intervention plus side effect costs, minus the reductions in expected medical costs. The Framingham Study data and United States vital statistics were used in calculations.

Findings.—The effect of cholesterol lowering on CAD risk is impacted by the level of other disease risk factors besides age, sex, and initial cholesterol level. The cost per life-year saved ranged from $9,000 to $106,000 for average-risk men and $35,000 to $297,000 for average-risk women. The cost per life-year saved ranged from $6,000 to $53,000 in high-risk men and from $19,000 to $160,000 in high-risk women (Fig 1–7).

Conclusions.—Results were more favorable than previous studies of alternate medication therapies for hypercholesterolemia. Current cholesterol medication could be economically justified, particularly for persons with high levels of primary CAD risk factors. In the age range 35–55 years, the incidence of CAD is lower for women, so the benefits of intervention are not as great. Studies on the outcome efficacy of lovastatin and other cholesterol reduction interventions will aid in establishing

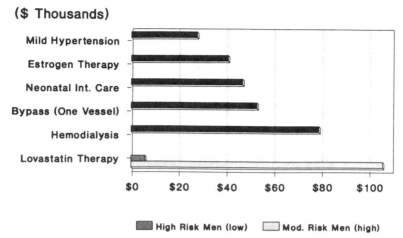

($ Thousands)

Fig 1–7.—Cost per life-year saved for various medical interventions. Lovastatin values were derived in the present study; other values are conversions to 1989 U.S. dollars from 1983 U.S.-dollar or pound-sterling costs reported by Drummond MF: *Health Policy* 7:309–324, 1987. *Abbreviations: int*, intensive; *mod*, moderate. (Courtesy of Hay JW, Wittels EH, Gotto AM Jr: *Am J Cardiol* 67:789–796, 1991.)

guidelines for efficient allocation of health care resources in reducing CAD risk.

▶ These two papers (Abstracts 1–21 and 1–22) explore an increasingly important issue in preventive cardiology. Whereas the investigators of lovastatin therapy (Abstract 1–22) present an optimistic view of the cost-effectiveness of drug therapy, others have failed to document such a favorable economic conclusion (1). The data from Abstract 1–21 support mass education programs but demonstrate significantly increasing costs for screening and then individual programs of treatment. Both studies document that the most cost-effective use of drugs is in high-risk patients (i.e., those with highest levels of cholesterol and other risk factors).—R.L. Frye, M.D.

Reference

1. Kinosion BP, Eisenberg JM: *JAMA* 259:2249, 1988.

Ethnic Immunity to Coronary Heart Disease?
Vermaak WJH, Ubbink JB, Delport R, Becker PJ, Bissbort SH, Ungerer JPJ (Univ of Pretoria; Inst for Biostatics, Pretoria, South Africa)
Atherosclerosis 89:155–162, 1991   1–23

Background.—Dietary fat intake frequently is regarded as a major determinant of coronary heart disease. Coronary heart disease remains rare in westernized black Africans, despite high rates of risk factors (e.g., hypertension, obesity, and smoking).
Study Group.—A group of young black and white men exposed to the

same physical and social environment for 2 years or longer and ingesting the same Western diet were assessed. Twenty-seven black and 26 white men aged 18–25 years participated in the study when working in nature conservation in a remote area of Namibia. Sixty-one black and 66 white healthy term neonates also were studied.

Findings.—Levels of total cholesterol in cord blood were 12% lower in black than in white neonates. Levels of low-density lipoprotein (LDL) cholesterol were 18% lower in the black group, and apolipoprotein B levels were 22% lower. Comparing the male adults, total cholesterol levels were 11% lower in black men, LDL cholesterol levels were 19% lower, and apolipoprotein B levels were 40% lower than in white men. Black men had high-density lipoprotein cholesterol levels that were 20% higher than in white men.

Conclusions.—Ethnic (genetic) factors appear to be important in determining the response of urban African men to their diet. Such factors may help to explain why these men are relatively resistant to coronary heart disease.

▶ These data on a comparison of coronary heart disease in South African whites and blacks are quite interesting. Such studies may provide further insights to be considered in explaining ethnic differences in rates of coronary disease as well as different responses to treatment. Note also Abstract 1–3, which demonstrates a difference in responsiveness of blacks and whites in the United States to thrombolytic therapy.—R.L. Frye, M.D.

Are Regional Variations in Ischaemic Heart Disease Related to Differences in Coronary Risk Factors? The Project 'Myocardial Infarction in Mid-Sweden'

Nerbrand C, Olsson L, Svärdsudd K, Kullman S, Tibblin G (Uppsala Univ, Sweden; Centre for Public Health Research, Karlstad, Sweden)
Eur Heart J 12:309–314, 1991   1–24

Purpose.—In a previous report, there was a pronounced geographic variation in total mortality and mortality rate from ischemic heart disease (IHD) in the east-west gradient of mid-Sweden. To explain the differences in the high mortality in the western part of the region and the low mortality in the east, a random mail questionnaire was distributed.

Methods.—Questionnaires were sent to a random sample of men, aged 45–64 years, in each of 40 communities. The questionnaire requested information on angina pectoris, myocardial infarction, medication for hypertension, smoking habits, physical activity during leisure time, stress, and food intake. Response rate was 88% (14,675 men). Ischemic heart disease cases were defined as those with a history of myocardial infarction and/or angina pectoris.

Findings.—High IHD prevalence in the west and low IHD prevalence in the east showed the same geographic variation as IHD mortality (Fig 1–8). In the 40 communities, there was a moderate variation in risk fac-

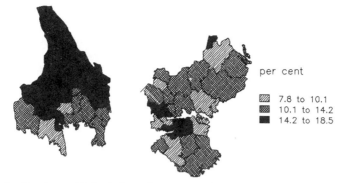

Fig 1–8.—Prevalence of ischemic heart disease expressed as cases per 100,000 population among men, aged 45–64 years, in 40 communities in mid-Sweden. *Filled areas* indicate the quartile of the communities with the highest prevalence, the *hatched area* indicates the quartile with the lowest prevalence, and the *checkered area* indicates the 2 mid-quartile communities. (Courtesy of Nerbrand C, Olsson L, Svärdsudd K, et al: *Eur Heart J* 12:309–314, 1991.)

tor levels of smoking habits, antihypertensive treatment, body mass index, food habits, stress, and physical activity during leisure time. Even with this variable accounted for, the geographic IHD variation was still substantial. Factors may include socioeconomics, drinking water qualities, mineral soil content, or other environmental factors.

Conclusion.—The large geographic variation in mid-Sweden of IHD mortality rate was also found for IHD prevalence. This variation was not caused by regional variations in diagnostic criteria, case fatality rate, or risk factors. Other factors of socioeconomics, drinking water qualities, mineral soil content, and other environmental factors will be systematically examined in this project.

Myocardial Infarction in Mexican-Americans and Non-Hispanic Whites: The San Antonio Heart Study

Mitchell BD, Hazuda HP, Haffner SM, Patterson JK, Stern MP (Univ of Texas Health Science Ctr at San Antonio)
Circulation 83:45–51, 1991   1–25

Introduction.—Although Mexican-American men have significantly higher frequencies of risk factors for coronary heart disease (CHD) than non-Hispanic white men, they experience lower cardiovascular (CV) mortality rates. This difference in CV mortality does not occur among Mexican-American women. The difference in CV mortality for men could be the result of a lower incidence of CV disease or a lower case fatality rate among Mexican Americans. The prevalence of CHD in Mexican Americans was compared with that in non-Hispanic whites in the San Antonio Heart Study.

Methods.—The population-based survey of cardiovascular disease was conducted between 1979 and 1988, and comprised 5,148 persons, aged 25–64 years, including 3,281 Mexican Americans and 1,867 non-Hispanic whites. All study participants were assessed for myocardial infarction (MI) by standard 12-lead electrocardiograms analyzed according to Minnesota Code criteria, and by a self-reported history of a physician-diagnosed heart attack. Diabetes, obesity, cigarette smoking, and lipid status were also assessed.

Results.—An analysis of risk factors for CHD revealed that Mexican Americans had a significantly higher prevalence of obesity and diabetes but lower total cholesterol levels and a lower prevalence of cigarette smoking than non-Hispanic whites. However, the difference in high-density lipoprotein cholesterol levels was only significant for women. After adjustment for age and diabetes status, the prevalence of MI was 21%–42% lower in Mexican-American men than in non-Hispanic white men, and mortality attributable to CV disease was 15%–36% lower in Mexican-American men than in non-Hispanic white men. The prevalence of MI was slightly higher in Mexican-American women than in non-Hispanic white women, but the difference was not statistically significant.

Conclusion.—The reduced rate of CV mortality in Mexican-American men reflects a lower incidence of MI rather than a reduced case fatality rate. It is hypothesized that genetic factors may confer relative protection against CHD in Mexican-American men.

Decline in Ischaemic Heart Disease in Iceland and Change in Risk Factor Levels
Sigfusson N, Sigvaldason H, Steingrimsdottir L, Gudmundsdottir II, Stefansdottir I, Thorsteinsson T, Sigurdsson G (Icelandic Heart Assoc, Reykjavik, Iceland; Icelandic Nutritional Council, Reykjavik; Reykjavik City Hosp)
BMJ 302:1371–1375, 1991   1–26

Purpose.—Mortality and morbidity trends from ischemic heart disease (IHD) in Iceland were analyzed in relation to changes in the 3 major risk factors for IHD and the consumption of saturated fats as documented in ongoing population surveys.

Methods.—Iceland has a total population of 250,000. More than half of the population lives in Reykjavik. Trends in morbidity attributable to IHD were assessed in 12,814 randomly selected residents aged 45–64 years living in the Reykjavik area. Data on smoking, serum cholesterol concentration, and systolic blood pressure, considered the 3 major risk factors for IHD, were obtained at survey visits. Secular trends in food consumption were compared with trends in serum cholesterol levels. Data on IHD mortality were obtained from death certificates issued from 1951 to 1988.

Results.—Total mortality from IHD decreased 17% to 18% after 1970 and decreased significantly after 1985. During 1981–1986, the myocardial infarction rate in men younger than 75 years fell by 23%. In women, mortality from IHD fell by 18% between 1970 and 1986–1988. There was an overall decrease in smoking, which decreased the risk of death from IHD by 13% for men and by 8% for women. The mean serum cholesterol level decreased by .42 mmol/L in men and by .75 mmol/L in women, which decreased the risk of death from IHD by 14% in men and by 17% in women. The mean systolic blood pressure decreased by 15.5 mm Hg in men and by 19.3 mm Hg in women, which decreased the risk of death from IHD by 17% in men and by 24% in women. Patterns of food consumption changed considerably during the observation period, resulting in a significant reduction in saturated fat consumption. The overall reduction in risk of IHD for persons aged 45–64 years was approximately 35%, which was similar to the observed decrease in mortality attributable to IHD for that age group.

Conclusion.—The observed reduction in the 3 major risk factors for IHD in Iceland during recent years has resulted in a concomitant similar reduction in mortality from IHD.

▶ The regional differences in coronary heart disease mortality remain unexplained and of great interest. There seems to be a lower mortality in the east of Sweden as compared with the west. This is in contrast to the United States, where the earliest declines in coronary heart disease mortality were experienced in the west, and in general, the declines in a more global sense have followed a west to east gradient. The excellent San Antonio Heart Disease Study (Abstract 1–25) continues to provide extremely interesting and important data. These ethnic differences must also be explained by those presuming to understand completely the basis for the decline in coronary heart disease mortality. Abstract 1–26 documents the existing dogma regarding declines in risk factors and coronary heart disease mortality. I believe we must also recognize the potential importance of "unrecognized" risk factors. An excellent reference for those interested in the general topic of declining coronary heart disease mortality is Higgins and Thom.—R.L. Frye, M.D.

Lipoprotein (a) and Coronary Heart Disease: A Prospective Case-Control Study in a General Population Sample of Middle Aged Men
Rosengren A, Wilhelmsen L, Eriksson E, Risberg B, Wedel H (Univ of Gothenburg, Sweden; Nordic School of Public Health, Gothenburg)
BMG 301:1248–1251, 1990   1–27

Background.—Concentrations of serum lipoprotein (a) are increased in patients with coronary heart disease and cerebrovascular disease, but the function of this lipoprotein remains largely unknown. It appears to be associated with coronary atherosclerosis and myocardial infarction. A prospective, case-control study was done to examine the association between serum lipoprotein (a) concentration and subsequent coronary heart disease.

Method.—The subjects were from a general population sample of 776 men aged 50 at baseline. Serum samples from these men were kept at −70°C for 6 years. Over this time, 31 men had a myocardial infarction or died of coronary heart disease. Of these, 26 had no history of previous infarction and had complete data. Their serum samples, along with those of 109 randomly selected controls from the same sample, were analyzed for lipoprotein (a). The controls also had no history of myocardial infarction at baseline.

Results.—Mean serum lipoprotein (a) concentrations were 277.7 mg/L in patients with heart disease and 172.7 mg/L in controls. The mean difference of 105 mg/L was significant. Men whose serum lipoprotein levels were in the highest fifth (over 365 mg/L) had more than twice the rate of coronary heart disease than men in the lower four fifths of concentrations had. According to logistic regression analysis, serum lipoprotein (a) concentration was significantly associated with coronary heart disease, independent of other risk factors. Twenty-three of 26 patients were smokers, had high serum lipoprotein (a) concentrations, or both.

Conclusions.—In middle-aged men, serum lipoprotein (a) concentration is an independent risk factor for myocardial infarction or death from coronary heart disease. The population attributable fraction may be calculated as 27%.

▶ This is the first prospective, case-control study documenting an independent predictive value of lipoprotein (a) for myocardial infarction or death from coronary heart disease. These data emphasize the importance of looking beyond levels of total cholesterol in assessing risk factors in individual patients. I continue to be impressed in my own practice with patients who have serious coronary heart disease but normal total cholesterol and low high density lipoprotein cholesterol. Studies of lipoprotein (a) in these patients and their families will be of great interest. Investigations into the molecular genetics of coronary disease are ongoing, and this will be a most exciting development in future years.—R.L. Frye, M.D.

Miscellaneous

Regression of Coronary Artery Disease as a Result of Intensive, Lipid-Lowering Therapy in Men With High Levels of Apolipoprotein B
Brown G, Albers JJ, Fisher LD, Schaefer SM, Lin J-T, Kaplan C, Zhao X-Q, Bisson BD, Fitzpatrick VF, Dodge HT (Univ of Washington, Seattle)
N Engl J Med 323:1289–1298, 1990   1–28

Background.—With the advent of more effective treatments for hyperlipidemia, new arteriographic methods for assessing atherosclerosis, and new insights into atherogenesis, the question of whether progression of atherosclerosis can be retarded or reversed with treatment of hyperlipidemia can be addressed. In a randomized, double-blind, placebo-controlled trial, the effect of intensive, lipid-lowering regimens on coronary atherosclerosis in men at high risk for cardiovascular events was assessed by quantitative arteriography.

Methods.—A group of 146 men, 62 years of age or younger, with elevated ($\geq$125 mg/dL) apolipoprotein B levels, documented coronary artery disease, and a family history of vascular disease participated in the 2.5-year trial. Patients were given dietary counseling and assigned to 1 of

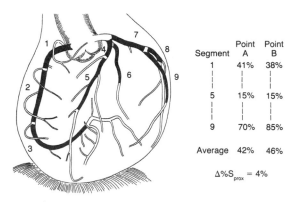

Segment	Point A	Point B
1	41%	38%
5	15%	15%
9	70%	85%
Average	42%	46%

$$\Delta\%S_{prox} = 4\%$$

Fig 1–9.—Location of 9 standard proximal segments of the coronary artery. The lesion causing the worst stenosis in each of these segments was measured, the average percent stenosis among these segments was computed, and the mean change in this value between the 2 studies (time points A and B) was determined. This estimate of the mean change in the severity of proximal stenosis $(\Delta\%S_{prox})$, here 4%, was made for each patient. (Courtesy of Brown G, Albers JJ, Fisher LD, et al: *N Engl J Med* 323:1289–1298, 1990.)

3 treatment groups: lovastatin, 20 mg twice a day, with colestipol, 10 g 3 times a day; niacin, 1 g 4 times a day, with colestipol, 10 g 3 times a day; or conventional treatment with placebo or with colestipol if the low-density lipoprotein (LDL) cholesterol level was elevated. The primary endpoint was the average change between the initial and follow-up coronary arteriography in the percent stenosis of the worst lesion in each of 9 proximal segments (Fig 1–9).

Results.—Among the 120 men who completed the trial, the levels of LDL and high-density lipoprotein (HDL) cholesterol changed only slightly in the conventional group but more substantially in the 2 intensively treated groups. Definite lesion progression as the only change occurred more frequently in conventionally treated patients (46%) than in those who received lovastatin and colestipol (21%) or niacin and colestipol (25%). Lesion regression as the only change was 3 times more common in the 2 groups of intensively treated patients (32% and 39%, respectively) than in conventionally treated patients (11%). Furthermore, intensive lipid-lowering treatment decreased the frequency of cardiovascular events, such as death, myocardial infarction, or revascularization for worsening symptoms. Clinical events occurred in 3 of 46 men treated with lovastatin and colestipol and 2 of 48 men receiving niacin and colestipol, compared with 10 of 52 men assigned to conventional treatment. Reductions in apolipoprotein B levels (or LDL cholesterol) and systolic blood pressure and increases in HDL cholesterol correlated independently with regression of coronary lesions.

Conclusions.—These data indicate that intensive lipid-lowering treatment of men with coronary artery disease who are at high risk for cardiovascular events reduces the frequency of progression of coronary lesions, increases the frequency of regression, and reduces the incidence of cardiovascular events.

▶ These quantitative studies on regression of atherosclerosis are of great interest and reflect increasing data to support aggressive lipid-lowering efforts in patients with documented coronary disease.—R.L. Frye, M.D.

Primary Angioplasty in Myocardial Infarction: Assessment of Improved Myocardial Perfusion With Technetium-99m Isonitrile
Behrenbeck T, Pellikka PA, Huber KC, Bresnahan JF, Gersh BJ, Gibbons RJ
(Mayo Clinic and Found, Rochester, Minn)
J Am Coll Cardiol 17:365–372, 1991   1–29

Background.—The kinetics of the new radiopharmaceutical compound technetium-99m-hexakis-2-methoxy-2-isobutylisonitrile (technetium-99m isonitrile) allow assessment of changes in myocardial perfusion

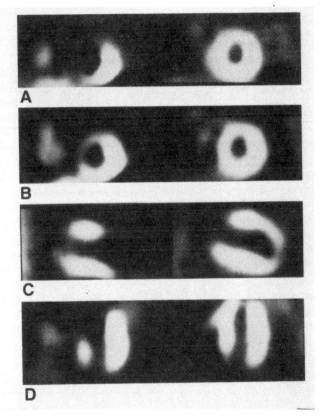

Fig 1–10.—Representative technetium-99m isonitrile tomographic images. **Left column,** acute phase images; **right column,** late images. **A,** short-axis slices at the midventricular level. The anterior wall is at **top** and the septum is at **left. B,** short-axis slices at the basal level, same orientation. **C,** vertical long-axis slices. Anterior wall is at **top** and apex is at **right. D,** horizontal long-axis slices. Septum is at **left** and apex is at **top.** In each panel there is improved perfusion in the septum and anterior wall with a residual defect at the apex. (Courtesy of Behrenbeck T, Pellikka PA, Huber KC, et al: *J Am Coll Cardiol* 17:365–372, 1991.)

without delays in therapy. This unique tool was used to evaluate the effectiveness of successful primary angioplasty in 17 consecutive acute myocardial infarction patients.

Methods.—The patients were 15 men and 2 women (median age, 61). There were 13 anterior, 1 lateral, and 3 inferior defects. The median time from onset of chest pain to start of therapy was 298 minutes. Eight patients with their first myocardial infarction and angiographically documented persistent coronary occlusion were studied as controls. Patients underwent tomographic imaging with technetium-99m isonitrile at rest immediately and 6 to 10 days later, before discharge.

Results.—On the initial images, the mean size of the defect before angioplasty was 47% of the left ventricle (Fig 1–10). On the late scans, the defects decreased in size significantly to 29%. Time to therapy and reduction in defect size were unrelated. A definite reduction in the size of the initial defect was seen in 12 patients, including 7 of the 11 who were treated after 4 hours. In controls, there was no significant difference in the size of the defect between initial (24%) and late (26%) scans.

Conclusions.—Technetium-99m isonitrile imaging can document myocardial salvage after primary angioplasty. The procedure was very effective in restoring vessel patency. Controlled clinical trials are needed to compare primary angioplasty and thrombolytic drug therapy.

Noninvasive Identification of Myocardium at Risk in Patients With Acute Myocardial Infarction and Nondiagnostic Electrocardiograms With Technetium-99m-Sestamibi

Christian TF, Clements IP, Gibbons RJ (Mayo Clin and Found, Rochester, Minn)
Circulation 83:1615–1620, 1991   1–30

Introduction.—A significant minority of patients with myocardial infarction have chest pain without ST segment elevation on the ECG. It is important to identify these patients at an early stage so that reperfusion therapy will succeed. This study determined whether imaging with 99mTc-Sestamibi is helpful in this group of patients.

Study Design.—Imaging was carried out in 14 patients who had chest pain but no ST elevation, and who developed enzymatic evidence of myocardial infarction within 24 hours. Imaging was done 1–6 hours after injection of 20–30 mCi of 99mTc-Sestamibi, using a rotating gamma camera.

Observations.—Eleven patients had coronary occlusion documented by angiography. The mean perfusion defect was 20% of the left ventricle, or 17% if 4 patients with past infarction were excluded. One patient lacked a perfusion defect, but in all other patients the images were consistent with the area supplied by the infarct vessel.

Conclusion.—Imaging with 99mTc-Sestamibi can help identify infarction patients who lack ECG evidence of myocardial damage at an early stage so that acute reperfusion can be carried out.

► These 2 papers (Abstracts 1–29 and 1–30) reflect important studies using a new imaging technique to determine myocardium at risk. Fortunately, as suggested in Abstract 1–29, Gibbons et al. will shortly be presenting results from a randomized trial comparing primary angioplasty and thrombolytic therapy in acute myocardial infarction using this imaging modality as the major endpoint. Abstract 1–30 illustrates the importance of such imaging in those patients without ECG changes of acute infarction.—R.L. Frye, M.D. ·

Prevention of Early Aortocoronary Bypass Occlusion by Low-Dose Aspirin and Dipyridamole
Sanz G, Pajarón A, Alegría E, Coello I, Cardona M, Fournier JA, Gómez-Recio M, Ruano J, Hidalgo R, Medina A, Oller G, Colman T, Malpartida F, Bosch X, Grupo Español para el Seguimiento del Injerto Coronario (GESIC)
Circulation 82:765–773, 1990   1–31

Background.—Although several studies have shown that platelet-inhibiting drugs can prevent aortocoronary vein graft occlusion, questions remain about this treatment and its timing. A multicenter, double-blind, placebo-controlled study was done to analyze the effectiveness of low-dose aspirin in preventing early aortocoronary vein graft occlusion.

Methods.—The study, conducted at 6 institutions, included 1,112 patients less than 71 years old who were undergoing elective aortocoronary bypass surgery with saphenous vein grafts. Patients were randomized into 3 groups and given 50 mg of aspirin, 50 mg of aspirin plus 75 mg dipyridamole, or placebo 3 times daily. For 48 hours before surgery, all patients received 100 mg dipyridamole 4 times daily. Assigned treatments were begun 7 hours after surgery. Eighty-three percent of patients were assessed with vein graft angiography within 28 days of surgery.

Results.—The occlusion rate of distal anastomoses was 18% in the

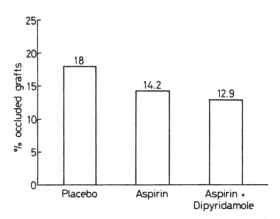

Fig 1–11.—Percentages of occluded grafts (distal anastomoses) in each treatment group. By cluster analysis, the *P* value for the comparison between aspirin and placebo was .058, and the value for that between aspirin plus dipyridamole and placebo was .017. (Courtesy of Sanz G, Pajarón A, Alegría E, et al: *Circulation* 82:765–773, 1990.)

placebo group. The 12.9% rate in patients who received aspirin plus dipyridamole was significantly lower, and the 14% rate in patients who received aspirin alone approached significance (Fig 1–11). The percentage of patients with occluded grafts was 33% in the placebo group, 27.1% in the aspirin group, and 24.3% in the aspirin plus dipyridamole group; only the latter difference was significant. The aspirin plus dipyridamole group had slightly more mediastinal drainage (713 mL vs. 670 mL in the placebo group). The 3 groups had similar hospital mortality and early reoperation rates, averaging 4.6% and 3.9%, respectively.

Conclusions.—The patency of early saphenous vein aortocoronary grafts apparently is safely improved by low-dose aspirin plus dipyridamole when given in addition to preoperative dipyridamole. These results provide the rationale for a trial comparing drug treatments directly.

▶ This is an excellent study documenting the effectiveness of low-dose aspirin combined with dipyridamole in reducing occlusion of saphenous vein grafts after coronary bypass surgery. Most would now seem to accept that aspirin alone is sufficient to accomplish the desired effect.—R.L. Frye, M.D.

Coronary Artery Bypass Grafting: The Relationship of Surgical Volume, Hospital Location, and Outcome
Zelen J, Bilfinger TV, Anagnostopoulos CE (State Univ of New York, Stony Brook)
NY State J Med 91:290–292, 1991   1–32

Background.—Some studies have suggested an inverse relationship between surgical volume and in-hospital mortality. Other studies have found that a patient's preoperative severity of illness affects postoperative morbidity and mortality. Mortality rates for coronary artery bypass grafting (CABG) in 3 high-volume and 5 low-volume institutions were compared.

Discussion.—In the Greater New York metropolitan area, low-volume centers and physicians achieved survival rates equal to those of high-volume centers and physicians. The urban or suburban location of a center did not affect the outcome. Although the development of preoperative criteria for the assessment of operative risk is desirable, criteria developed in one institution may not be applicable in another institution because of different treatments and populations.

Conclusion.—No differences were found in survival after CABG between hospitals with high and low volumes or urban and suburban locations.

▶ This provocative study from New York state is contrary to others that have reflected a higher mortality in low-volume institutions. The careful attention to risk stratification and monitoring coronary bypass surgery in New York is a model for other states to emulate. There is increasing pressure for public disclosure in the media of such differences. This requires a highly reliable risk stratification methodology, which seems to have been achieved in the New York studies.—R.L. Frye, M.D.

Prognostic Significance of a Predischarge Exercise Test in Risk Stratification After Unstable Angina Pectoris
Wilcox I, Freedman SB, Allman KC, Collins FL, Leitch JW, Kelly DT, Harris PJ
(Royal Prince Alfred Hosp, Camperdown, Australia)
J Am Coll Cardiol 18:677–683, 1991   1–33

Introduction.—Exercise stress testing in patients with unstable angina pectoris (UAP) was previously considered unsafe. Recent studies reported that exercise testing can be performed safely in patients with UAP who have responded to medical therapy. However, the prognostic significance of predischarge exercise testing in patients with UAP is not well documented. Whether predischarge exercise testing in medically treated UAP patients would add independent prognostic information to standard clinical and ECG information was studied prospectively.

Patients.—Exercise testing was performed before discharge from the coronary care unit in 107 patients with UAP whose condition had stabilized with medical therapy. Only patients who had been free of pain for at least 3 days and who had no other contraindication to exercise testing were included in the study. All patients were followed by personal or telephone interview 4 and 12 months after hospital discharge. The effects of 20 clinical, ECG, and exercise test variables on the risk of an adverse outcome were determined by univariate and multivariate analysis.

Results.—During a mean follow-up period of 12.8 months, 2 patients died, 8 had a nonfatal myocardial infarction, and 22 were readmitted with recurrent UAP. Multivariate analysis identified diabetes mellitus, rest pain after admission, evolutionary T wave changes, a low rate-pressure product during exercise testing, and a positive exercise ECG as significant independent predictors of death, nonfatal myocardial infarction, or readmission with UAP. Using these 3 clinical and 2 exercise test variables in a logistic regression model to define high and low risk groups predicted 93% of the adverse outcomes. Conversely, patients in the low risk group had only a 5% risk of an adverse outcome. Angina during exercise testing was the only variable associated with effort angina at the 4-month follow-up visit. This relation was no longer seen at 12 months.

Conclusion.—A symptom-limited exercise test performed before hospital discharge in patients with UAP whose condition has been medically stabilized and who do not need coronary revascularization provides additional independent prognostic information to known clinical and ECG risk factors.

▶ This careful study by the Royal Prince Alfred group in Australia deserves the careful attention of clinicians managing patients with unstable angina. Unstable angina appears to comprise an increasing proportion of patients with coronary artery disease evaluated in the hospital setting, and this attempt to risk stratify the group is most important.—R.L. Frye, M.D.

Effect of Iraqi Missile War on Incidence of Acute Myocardial Infarction and Sudden Death in Israeli Civilians

Meisel SR, Kutz I, Dayan KI, Pauzner H, Chetboun I, Arbel Y, David D (Tel Aviv Univ, Israel; Sapir Med Ctr, Kfar Saba, Israel)
Lancet 338:660–661, 1991   1–34

Introduction.—The Iraqi SCUD missile attacks on Israel provided a unique opportunity to study the effects of fear and the threat of annihilation on the incidence of acute myocardial infarction (AMI) and sudden cardiac death in a civilian population.

Study Design.—The number of patients admitted to the intensive coronary care unit (ICCU) of a 550-bed tertiary care hospital near Tel Aviv during the first week of the war, January 17–25, 1991, was compared with numbers admitted during 5 control periods. The incidence of sudden out-of-hospital cardiac death during January 1991 was compared with that during January 1990.

Results.—During the first week of missile attacks on Tel Aviv, 20 patients were admitted with AMI, compared with 7–9 patients with AMI admitted during any prewar control period. The peak incidence of AMI closely coincided with the onset of the Gulf war. The rate of admissions to the ICCU reverted to normal after the first week of war despite continuing missile attacks. The mean age, sex ratio, hospital mortality, or proportion of patients in whom AMI was the first symptom of coronary artery disease were similar for all periods. However, 50% of the patients admitted during the study period had an acute anterior MI, compared with a mean of 30% of the patients admitted during the control periods. In addition, 45% of patients admitted during the study period received thrombolytic therapy, compared with a mean of 33% of patients admitted during the control periods. Mortality rates were similar for all periods. During January 1991, there were 41 cases of sudden out-of-hospital death, compared with 22 during the same period in 1990.

Conclusion.—The effects of extreme emotional stress in patients with preexisting cardiac disease may be profound and potentially dangerous.

▶ This is a fascinating observation on cardiovascular events during the missile attacks on Israel. The mechanisms are nicely discussed and reemphasize the importance of stress in patients with coronary artery disease.—R.L. Frye, M.D.

Diltiazem Increases Late-Onset Congestive Heart Failure in Postinfarction Patients With Early Reduction in Ejection Fraction

Goldstein RE, Boccuzzi SJ, Cruess D, Nattel S, the Adverse Experience Committee, the Multicenter Diltiazem Postinfarction Research Group (Uniformed Services Univ of the Health Sciences, Bethesda, Md; Montreal Heart Inst)
Circulation 83:52–60, 1991   1–35

Introduction.—The Multicenter Diltiazem Postinfarction Trial (MD-PIT) found no overall increase in the frequency of late congestive heart failure (CHF) among postinfarction patients treated with diltiazem compared with placebo-treated patients. However, MDPIT data analysis did identify a diltiazem-related increase in the frequency of recurrent cardiac events compared with placebo-treated patients. Thus, the cardiac event data did not agree with the late CHF data. For this second data analysis, patients were divided by baseline ejection fraction (EF) and by treatment assignment, using the same criteria for EF dichotomization used in the primary data analysis (i.e., .40 or more and less than .40).

Methods.—The MDPIT was a randomized, double-blind, placebo-controlled trial of diltiazem including 2,466 postinfarction patients who were followed up for 12–52 months. The trial ended in 1987. To assess baseline left ventricular function, radionuclide ejection fraction was measured before hospital discharge in 2,159 patients.

Results.—Of 1,536 patients with a baseline EF of 40% or greater, 758 were treated with placebo and 778 with diltiazem. Of 623 patients with a baseline EF less than 40%, 326 were treated with placebo and 297 with diltiazem. Among the patients with a baseline EF of less than .40, late CHF appeared in 39 (12%) of the placebo-treated patients and in 61 (21%) of the diltiazem-treated patients. The occurrence of late CHF was 3.9% overall in patients with a baseline EF of .40 or greater. There was no difference in the frequency of late CHF between placebo-treated and diltiazem-treated patients. Thus, there was an unequivocal diltiazem-related increase in the frequency of late CHF in patients with an EF less than 40%. Furthermore, the more severe the reduction in baseline EF, the greater the increment in diltiazem-associated occurrence of late CHF relative to placebo. The diltiazem-related increase in late CHF occurred in patients who took concomitant β-blockers as well as in those who did not.

Conclusion.—Postinfarction patients with an EF lower than .40 are at increased risk for subsequent CHF when treated with diltiazem.

▶ These data are particularly important for those recommending or performing percutaneous transluminal coronary angioplasty (PTCA) in patients after myocardial infarction. In my own institution, with a very active angioplasty group, I have been interested to note the frequency with which diltiazem is used in post myocardial infarction patients who have had PTCA (rather than a β-blocker). The Multicenter Diltiazem Post Infarction Trial makes quite clear that post myocardial infarction patients with left ventricular ejection fraction less than 40% are at increased risk for cardiac events when treated with diltiazem. This is an important observation, and these investigators are to be commended for not only a superb trial but also the manner in which it has been analyzed.—R.L. Frye, M.D.

Thiamine Deficiency in Patients With Congestive Heart Failure Receiving Long-Term Furosemide Therapy: A Pilot Study
Seligmann H, Halkin H, Rauchfleisch S, Kaufmann N, Tal R, Motro M, Vered Z, Ezra D (Sheba Med Ctr, Tel Hashomer; Sackler School of Medicine, Tel Aviv; Bnai-Zion Med Ctr, Haifa; Hebrew Univ Hadassah Med School, Jerusalem, Israel)
Am J Med 91:151–155, 1991   1–36

Background.—Diuretic therapy is still a mainstay of management for chronic congestive heart failure. Thiamine deficiency has been demonstrated in furosemide-treated animals, and this deficiency might impair myocardial performance.

Study Design.—Thiamine status was determined in 23 patients with congestive failure who were on long-term furosemide therapy, and in 16 persons who did not have heart failure and were not given diuretics. Patients with congestive heart failure had been given furosemide for 3 to 14 months in daily doses of 80 to 240 mg. No patient had overt evidence of thiamine deficiency.

Observations.—Estimates of thiamine pyrophosphate effect on red cell transketolase activity indicated deficiency in all but 2 of the furosemide-treated patients but in only 2 of 16 control patients. Ten drug-treated patients had a deficiency greater than 24%. Only 1 patient had low urinary thiamine excretion. All 6 patients given parenteral thiamine supplementation responded. The left ventricular ejection fraction increased in several of these patients, but cardiac output did not change significantly.

Conclusions.—Long-term furosemide therapy can produce significant thiamine deficiency in patients with congestive heart failure, and cardiac performance may suffer as a result. The deficit can be corrected by thiamine supplementation.

▶ Quite frankly, I was unaware of this complication of furosemide therapy. It would appear that we should be alert to this possibility in our patients on chronic furosemide therapy who have congestive heart failure. Further careful clinical studies seem mandatory.—R.L. Frye, M.D.

Characteristics of Black Patients Admitted to Coronary Care Units in Metropolitan Seattle: Results from the Myocardial Infarction Triage and Intervention Registry (MITI)

Maynard C, Litwin PE, Martin JS, Cerqueira M, Kudenchuk PJ, Ho MT, Kennedy JW, Cobb LA, Schaeffer SM, Hallstrom AP, Weaver WD (Univ of Washington)
Am J Cardiol 67:18–23, 1991   1–37

Background.—There is increasing interest in the clinical course of acute myocardial infarction (AMI) in black patients. A prospective study was done to evaluate the clinical course of black patients with chest pain admitted to Seattle area coronary care units, particularly those with a discharge diagnosis of AMI.

Patients.—Over a 2-year period, 12,534 patients with chest pain of presumed cardiac origin were admitted to coronary care units in the metropolitan Seattle area. The analysis included 641 black and 11,893 white patients; those of other or unknown race were excluded. There were 2,870 patients with a discharge diagnosis of AMI, including 19% of the black patients and 23% of the white patients.

Results.—Black patients tended to be younger than white patients (58 vs. 66). Seventy-one percent of blacks and only 32% of whites were admitted to a central city hospital. Blacks were more likely to be discharged with a diagnosis of hypertension or, to a lesser extent, congestive heart failure. Among the AMI patients, blacks tended to be younger than whites (59 vs. 67). Two percent of the blacks and 10% of the whites had coronary artery bypass graft surgery, and 69% of blacks and 33% of whites had a prior hospitalization. Coronary angioplasty was done during hospitalization in 10% of blacks and in 18% of whites, and coronary artery bypass graft surgery was done in 4% of blacks and in 10% of whites. The races had equal use of thrombolytic therapy and cardiac catheterization. For blacks, hospital mortality was 7.4%, compared with 13.1% for whites. This difference was less apparent after logistic regression adjustment of key demographic and clinical variables.

Conclusions.—Black and white AMI patients in metropolitan Seattle appear to have similar outcomes, despite differences in age, hypertension, referral patterns, and the use of certain procedures. Coronary angioplasty and coronary bypass surgery were performed more often in blacks than in whites.

▶ These additional studies on characteristics of black patients with coronary disease is of great interest. Access to appropriate coronary angioplasty and bypass surgery in blacks is a major issue. We have much to learn regarding the basis for these differences.—R.L. Frye, M.D.

PTCA

Acute Complications of Percutaneous Transluminal Coronary Angioplasty for Total Occlusion
Plante S, Laarman G, de Feyter PJ, Samson M, Rensing BJ, Umans V, Suryapranata H, van den Brand M, Serruys PW (Erasmus Univ, Rotterdam, The Netherlands)
Am Heart J 121:417–426, 1991   1–38

Background.—Percutaneous transluminal coronary angioplasty (PTCA) patients with unstable angina who have a totally occluded artery at the time of the procedure may be at increased risk for acute complications from fragmentation and dislodgment of an occlusive thrombus. A retrospective study was done to evaluate the incidence of complications in patients with a totally occluded artery who underwent PTCA, with special focus on those with unstable angina pectoris.

Methods.—Over a 3-year period, 1,649 PTCA procedures were performed, 153 of them in patients with totally occluded coronary arteries. Procedures done for acute myocardial infarction or for re-stenosis were excluded, leaving 90 patients. Of these, 44 had stable angina and 46 had unstable angina. Patients were compared for age, gender, history of previous myocardial infarction in the area supplied by the occluded vessel, and estimated duration of maximal occlusion.

Results.—In patients with stable angina, the average estimated duration of occlusion was 87 days, compared with 10 days in the patients with unstable angina. None of the patients with stable angina had abrupt closure of the vessel during PTCA, but 17% of the patients with unstable angina did. The immediate angiographic success rates were 48% in patients with stable angina and 74% in patients with unstable angina. There was one myocardial infarction in the stable angina group, for a major complication rate of 2.5%. The rate in the unstable angina group was 20%. In patients who had unstable angina and nonocclusive stenosis during the same period, the complication rate was 8%.

Conclusions.—The risk of major complications is increased in patients with unstable angina who undergo PTCA of a totally occluded artery. This subset of patients may benefit from pretreatment with thrombolytic agents, but prospective trials are needed to evaluate the safety and usefulness of this approach.

▶ These are very important data from an experienced group of angioplasty operators and investigators addressing the problem of PTCA in the setting of total occlusion. The data on the patients with unstable angina are particularly noteworthy and emphasize the high complication rate that may be seen in such patients when PTCA is used in this setting for a totally occluded coronary artery. As noted in Abstract 1–33, it is increasingly important to identify subsets of patients under the broad and poorly defined category of "unstable angina." It does appear that there are patients with varying "natural histories" within this label, and these data emphasize some of the anatomical features that may be associated with high complication rates if angioplasty is used.— R.L. Frye, M.D.

Results of Percutaneous Transluminal Coronary Angioplasty in Patients ≥65 Years of Age (From the 1985 to 1986 National Heart, Lung, and Blood Institute's Coronary Angioplasty Registry)
Kelsey SF, Miller DP, Holubkov R, Lu AS, Cowley MJ, Faxon DP, Detre KM, Investigators from the NHLBI PTCA Registry (Univ of Pittsburgh)
Am J Cardiol 66:1033–1038, 1990   1–39

Background.—Initially, percutaneous transluminal coronary angioplasty (PTCA) was not done in patients age 60 years and older, but the use of this procedure in the elderly has expanded. To examine results of PTCA in the light of rapid technologic advances and expanding indications, the National Heart, Lung, and Blood Institute's voluntary PTCA registry was reopened in 1985. Risk profiles of elderly patients undergoing the procedure were compared with those of younger patients.

Methods.—Data came from 16 centers that participated in the initial registry. Patients were followed for 5 years. The cohort included 1,801 patients, 27% of whom were 65 or older (elderly) and 12% of whom were 75 and older (very elderly). In the 1979 cohort, 12% were elderly and 1% were very elderly.

Results.—Elderly patients were more likely than their younger counterparts to be women and to have unstable angina. They were also more likely to have histories of hypertension and congestive heart failure. Similar numbers of lesions and vessels were attempted with PTCA in the older and younger cohorts, despite the presence of more extensive vessel disease in the elderly patients. All groups had similar rates of angiographic success and complications in the catheterization laboratory. However, 5.4% of elderly patients required emergency coronary artery bypass graft (CABG) surgery and 3.9% required elective CABG, compared with 2.8% and 1.6%, respectively, of younger patients. In-hospital death rates were 3.1% in the elderly and .2% in younger patients. Elderly and younger patients had similar symptoms and cumulative rates of myocardial infarction, CABG, and repeat PTCA at 2-year follow-up. The 2-year death rates, however, were 8.8% for elderly patients and 2.9% for younger patients. After adjustment of relative risk of death for history of congestive heart failure, multivessel disease, unstable angina, history of hypertension, and female gender, relative risk remained significant but was reduced from 3.3 to 2.4.

Conclusions.—Success rates of PTCA in elderly patients are similar to those of younger patients, despite differences between the 2 groups. Mortality among elderly patients treated with PTCA appears to be no greater than in those treated with CABG. Thus, PTCA appears to be an attractive therapy for use in elderly patients.

▶ Important clinical information continues to be presented from the National, Heart, Lung, and Blood Institute Coronary Angioplasty Registry. As with coronary bypass surgery, more elderly patients are having PTCA in the management of coronary artery disease. Advances in both the experience of operators and the technology are reflected in success in more complicated patients. However, appropriate use of angioplasty is of increasing concern.— R.L. Frye, M.D.

Restenosis After Coronary Angioplasty: A Multivariate Statistical Model to Relate Lesion and Procedure Variables to Restenosis
Hirshfeld JW Jr, Schwartz JS, Jugo R, MacDonald RG, Goldberg S, Savage MP, Bass TA, Vetrovec G, Cowley M, Taussig AS, Whitworth HB, Margolis JR, Hill JA, Pepine CJ, and the M-Heart Investigators (Univ of Pennsylvania, Philadelphia; Cordis Corp, Miami; Dalhousie Univ, Halifax, Nova Scotia; Thomas Jefferson Univ, Philadelphia; Univ Hosp, Jacksonville, Fla, et al)
J Am Coll Cardiol 18:647–656, 1991   1–40

Introduction.—Re-stenosis after successful percutaneous transluminal coronary angioplasty (PTCA) remains a major problem. Re-stenosis rates ranging from 25% to 40% have been reported. The ability to predict the risk of re-stenosis for a particular patient or lesion remains poor. A multivariate statistical model was created to predict the probability of re-stenosis for a particular lesion. The data for this analysis were obtained from a placebo-controlled trial assessing the effect of methylprednisolone pretreatment on coronary re-stenosis after PTCA.

Methods.—Of 510 patients with 598 successfully dilated lesions after PTCA, 237 (39.6%) had re-stenosis as confirmed at angiographic re-study. Of the 4 preprocedure variables analyzed, the strongest association was found for re-stenosis and lesion location, with saphenous bypass grafts having the highest (68.2%) re-stenosis rate. Among native coronary artery segments, re-stenosis was most frequent in the left anterior descending artery (45.4%) and least common in the left circumflex (30.8%) and right (32.2%) coronary arteries. Lesion length and percent stenosis were also significantly related to re-stenosis. The relation between minimal lesion diameter and re-stenosis was weak. Analysis of procedure outcome variables found a complex relation between the balloon:artery diameter ratio and re-stenosis. Multivariate analysis confirmed that the probability of re-stenosis after PTCA was determined predominantly by the characteristics of the lesion.

Recommendation.—Future studies to evaluate anti–re-stenosis therapeutic measures should be rigorously controlled for the key variables of lesion location and lesion severity.

▶ This is a particularly important study, and emphasizes the reality of re-stenosis, a major limitation in PTCA. Noteworthy is the re-stenosis rate in graft PTCA and also in the left anterior descending artery, where many seem to feel that angioplasty is the treatment of choice. Whereas this may be true in patients who are highly symptomatic with angina and have anatomical lesions that are ideal, one would certainly need to pause with these data in urging angioplasty in patients with mild or no symptoms and left anterior descending disease.— R.L. Frye, M.D.

Safety and Cost Effectiveness of Combined Coronary Angiography and Angioplasty

O'Keefe JH Jr, Gernon C, McCallister BD, Ligon RW, Hartzler GO (Cardiovascular Consultants, Inc, Kansas City, Mo)
Am Heart J 122:50–54, 1991   1–41

Introduction.—Several studies have demonstrated the safety and efficacy of performing percutaneous transluminal coronary angioplasty (PTCA) at the time of initial diagnostic cardiac catheterization. Many centers presently perform urgent simultaneous PTCA and coronary arteriography in patients admitted with acute myocardial infarction. This retrospective study was undertaken to determine the safety, efficacy, and cost-effectiveness of elective simultaneous PTCA and coronary angiography.

Patients.—During a 4-year study period, 733 patients underwent nonurgent combined procedures. Indications were re-stenosis after previous angioplasty in 61%, unstable angina in 26%, and purely elective in 13%. A subset of 219 patients who had the combined procedures was analyzed and compared with 191 patients treated during the same year with PTCA as a traditional staged procedure. The mean duration of follow-up was 27 months.

Results.—Success and complication rates among patients who had the combined procedure were similar to those among patients who had PTCA as a staged procedure. Patients who underwent the combined procedure were hospitalized for a mean of 4.6 days. The average total in-hospital charge was $11,128. Patients who had the staged procedure were hospitalized for a mean of 8 days at an average cost of $13,160. Total time spent in the cardiac catheterization laboratory was shortened by 37%, and the total contrast agent load was 93 mL less for patients who underwent the combined procedure. All differences were statistically significant.

Conclusion.—Combining PTCA and angiography shortens hospital stay, reduces total charges for revascularization, and reduces radiation exposure without jeopardizing the safety or effectiveness of the procedure.

▶ This report from St. Luke's Hospital supports the combined approach to coronary arteriography and angioplasty. It certainly requires high quality images to be displayed in the procedure room to ensure appropriate planning of the PTCA intervention. A need for consultation and consent before the procedure is emphasized. This reflects the need to update and critically review existing ACC/AHA practice guidelines.—R. I. Frye, M.D.

Clinical and Angiographic Determinants of Primary Coronary Angioplasty Success

Savage MP, Goldberg S, Hirshfeld JW, Bass TA, Macdonald RG, Margolis JR, Taussig AS, Vetrovec G, Whitworth HB, Zalewski A, Hill JA, Cowley M, Jugo R, Pepine CJ, for the M-Heart Investigators (Thomas Jefferson Univ Hosp, Philadelphia)

J Am Coll Cardiol 17:22–28, 1991   1–42

Background.—Outcomes of percutaneous transluminal coronary angioplasty have improved to the point where the procedure is 90% successful in experienced centers. To assess clinical and anatomical factors determining initial success, a prospective study of 1,000 lesions in 826 patients was performed.

Methods.—The patients, 639 men and 187 women ranging in age from 31 to 85, were enrolled in the Multi-Hospital Eastern Atlantic Restenosis Trial (M-HEART). Patients received either intravenous methylprednisolone or placebo in double-blind fashion. All patients had at least one coronary artery stenosis with a reduction of 60% or more in diameter. A successful procedure was one in which residual stenosis was less than 50% and no major complications occurred.

Results.—Angioplasty was successful in 88.6% of lesions, and this rate was uniform in the 8 participating centers. Gender, age, race, and clinical features such as severity and duration of angina, history of myocardial infarction, pain at rest, transient ST segment elevation, and history of smoking or diabetes had no effect on outcome. There was a significant association between outcome and angiographic factors specific to the lesion. Success rates were 96% for stenoses of 60%–74%, 90% for stenoses of 75%–89%, 84% for stenoses of 90%–99%, and 69% for stenoses of 100%. The success rate was 82% in calcified lesions and 90% in noncalcified lesions. Outcomes were successful in 82% of thrombotic lesions and 90% of nonthrombotic lesions. Angioplasty was successful in 84% of right coronary artery lesions and 90% of lesions in other vessels. Other anatomical variables (proximal vs. distal lesion, vessel size, lesion eccentricity, lesion length, or translesional gradient) were not related to outcome. Significant independent predictors of success, according to multivariate logistic regression, were percentage of stenosis before angioplasty, location in right coronary artery, and calcification.

Conclusions.—Results of coronary angioplasty are not adversely affected by female sex, circumflex artery or distal locations, or eccentric morphology. The main determinants of outcome appear to be the severity of stenosis, calcification, thrombosis, and location of the lesion in the right coronary artery.

▶ The investigators of this multicenter trial are certainly to be complimented on a careful and detailed analysis of their database. All clinicians need to remain attentive to these angiographic factors that determine coronary angioplasty outcome.—R.L. Frye, M.D.

Relation of Stenosis Morphology and Clinical Presentation to the Procedural Results of Directional Coronary Atherectomy

Ellis SG, De Cesare NB, Pinkerton CA, Whitlow P, King SB III, Ghazzal ZMB, Kereiakes DJ, Popma JJ, Menke KK, Topol EJ, Holmes DR (Univ of Michigan, Ann Arbor; St Vincent's Hosp, Indianapolis; Cleveland Clinic Foundation; Emory Univ Hosp; Christ Hosp, Cincinnati; et al)
Circulation 84:644–653, 1991
1–43

Introduction.—Directional coronary atherectomy is now available for treating coronary stenoses. This study of 378 patients consecutively treated for 400 stenoses relates patient features and morphology of stenoses to the outcome of directional atherectomy.

Technique.—After placing a sheath percutaneously into the femoral artery, a special guiding catheter is advanced to the ascending aorta, and the coronary ostium is intubated. A coronary guidewire then is steered through the stenosis, and the atherectomy catheter is advanced across it and aligned toward the stenosis by gentle torquing. Predilatation by standard balloon methods occasionally is necessary.

Results.—The procedural success rate was 88%. Major ischemic complications occurred in 6% of patients. Less success was achieved with very angular stenoses and proximal tortuosity. Treatment of complex—probably thrombus-related—stenoses had a favorable outcome.

Discussion.—The overall outcome of directional atherectomy may be similar to that obtained with coronary angioplasty, but the results are closely associated with the morphology of coronary stenoses.

Effect of Lesion Characteristics on Outcome of Directional Coronary Atherectomy
Hinohara T, Rowe MH, Robertson GC, Selmon MR, Braden L, Leggett JH, Vetter JW, Simpson JB (Sequoia Hosp, Redwood City, Calif)
J Am Coll Cardiol 17:1112–1120, 1991   1–44

Background.—The benefits of balloon dilation in percutaneous transluminal coronary angioplasty can be limited by primary failure and acute occlusion, especially in complex lesions. Directional coronary atherectomy excises the pathologic tissue from the obstructive lesion rather than simply dilating the vessel. The safety and efficacy of directional coronary atherectomy for treatment of obstructive lesions in coronary arteries and the effect of lesion complexity on outcome were evaluated.

Methods.—Coronary atherectomy was performed on 447 lesions in 382 procedures. The patients had symptomatic disease and angiographic evidence of obstruction greater than 50%.

Results.—The combined atherectomy and angioplasty success rate was above 90%, and the risk of significant complications requiring coronary bypass surgery was 3.1%. Treatment of lesions with calcific deposits or lengthy lesions had a lower success rate and a higher complication rate. The most common complication was vessel occlusion during the procedure. The most serious potential complication unique to directional coronary atherectomy is perforation by excessive excision of tissue. One potential advantage is prevention of dissection by creating a smooth luminal surface.

Conclusion.—The technology of atherectomy is still evolving, but directional coronary atherectomy appears to be effective and safe for treatment of obstructive coronary artery disease. The success rate is high even in lesions that are eccentric, have ostial involvement, or have an abnormal contour. Lesions with calcific deposits or lengthy lesions have a lower success rate.

▶ These studies (Abstracts 1–43 and 1–44) are included because of the great interest in interventional techniques. Deserving emphasis is the need for properly controlled studies to evaluate the incremental value of those techniques over and above existing technology. Fortunately, such studies are in progress. An additional personal concern is the excisional momentum based on anatomy. We will need to be sure that the patient is best served with an intervention, particularly with the high re-stenosis rates currently observed.—R.L. Frye, M.D.

Differences in the Use of Procedures Between Women and Men Hospitalized for Coronary Heart Disease

Ayanian JZ, Epstein AM (Brigham and Women's Hosp, Boston; Harvard Med School)
N Engl J Med 325:221–225, 1991   1–45

Background.—Men and women with coronary heart disease have been found to have different usages of major diagnostic and therapeutic procedures. To determine the generalizability of these findings, a retrospective analysis was made of patients hospitalized for coronary heart disease.

Methods.—Abstracted discharge data for the states of Massachusetts and Maryland in 1987 were used. There were 49,623 discharges in Massachusetts and 33,159 in Maryland. Abstracts were analyzed for the use of coronary artery bypass surgery and percutaneous transluminal coronary angioplasty. Adjusted odds of use of a procedure were estimated by multiple logistic regression, controlling for main diagnosis, age, secondary diagnosis of congestive heart failure or diabetes mellitus, race, and insurance status.

Results.—Men had 28% higher adjusted odds than women of undergoing angiography in Massachusetts and 15% higher odds in Maryland. Odds of undergoing revascularization were 45% higher for men in Massachusetts and 27% higher for men in Maryland. These differences could be related to differing thresholds for hospital admission. Therefore, another analysis was done of 11,865 discharges in Massachusetts and 6,894 in Maryland with diagnosed acute myocardial infarction. In both states, differences in odds ratios of the sexes remained significant for both angiography and revascularization.

Conclusions.—Among patients hospitalized with the diagnosis of coronary heart disease, women apparently undergo fewer major procedures. The procedures may be overused in men or underused in women, or they may reflect suitable levels of care for both sexes. The causes of these differences and how they affect patients' outcomes should be determined.

Sex Differences in the Management of Coronary Artery Disease

Steingart RM, Packer M, Hamm P, Coglianese ME, Gersh B, Geltman EM, Sollano J, Katz S, Moyé L, Basta LL, Lewis SJ, Gottlieb SS, Bernstein V, McEwan P, Jacobson K, Brown EJ, Kukin ML, Kantrowitz NE, Pfeffer MA, the Survival and Ventricular Enlargement Investigators (Winthrop Univ Hosp, Mineola, NY; Univ of Texas Health Science Ctr, Houston; Mount Sinai School of Medicine, New York; Mayo Clin and Found, Rochester, Minn; Washington Univ, St. Louis, et al)
N Engl J Med 325:226–230, 1991   1–46

Background.—Coronary artery disease is the leading cause of death for women, surpassing all the neoplastic diseases combined. There appears to be a sex-related difference in the care of patients with this disease. Physicians are more likely to attribute anginal symptoms in women to noncardiac causes and to refer women for cardiac catheterization and coronary bypass surgery later in the course of their disease. The care received by women in a postinfarction intervention trial was compared to that received by men.

Methods.—The subjects were 1,842 men and 389 women who had been enrolled in the Survival and Ventricular Enlargement Study (SAVE). They had left ventricular ejection fractions of 40% or less after an acute myocardial infarction. The nature and severity of anginal symptoms and the use of antianginal and antiischemic interventions before enrollment were assessed.

Findings.—Before their index infarction, men and women had similar prevalences and frequencies of angina, but women reported greater functional disability. Despite reporting greater disability, women were less likely to be referred for cardiac catheterization. Men were twice as likely to undergo an invasive cardiac procedure, but for men and women who underwent catheterization, bypass surgery was performed with equal frequency.

Conclusion.—Women with coronary heart disease evidently undergo cardiac catheterization and coronary bypass surgery less often than men, although their functional disability may be greater. When clinical variables were controlled, men were twice as likely as women to undergo a cardiac procedure. Consequently, women were twice as likely to be excluded from therapeutic intervention trials because they did not have the cardiac catheterization required for enrollment.

▶ These two papers (Abstracts 1–45 and 1–46) have provoked a great deal of discussion regarding the influence of gender on use of cardiovascular procedures in management of patients with coronary artery disease. This is an important issue and deserves careful additional study. It is noteworthy that the debate regarding these procedures has shifted from inappropriate use to denial of clinically important services on the basis of gender bias. I suspect there are clinical differences that may account for some of this, as the investigators note, but other currently unrecognized factors may also have influenced decisions on use of these procedures.—R.L. Frye, M.D.

Safety and Efficacy of Percutaneous Transluminal Coronary Angioplasty in Patients With Left Ventricular Dysfunction
Stevens T, Kahn JK, McCallister BD, Ligon RW, Spaude S, Rutherford BD, McConahay DR, Johnson WL, Giorgi LV, Shimshak TM, Hartzler GO (St. Luke's Hosp, Kansas City, Mo)
Am J Cardiol 68:313–319, 1991   1–47

Background.—Patients with left ventricular (LV) dysfunction frequently have poor response to treatment and an increased risk of surgical revascularization. Although it was not originally considered for patients with LV dysfunction, percutaneous transluminal coronary angioplasty (PTCA) is now being investigated as a therapeutic option. The procedural risks and long-term outcomes after PTCA were examined in patients with LV dysfunction.

Methods.—Patients with an ejection fraction of 40% or less calculated from contrast ventriculography were considered to have LV dysfunction. Results of 845 elective PTCA procedures in patients with LV dysfunction were compared with those of 8,117 procedures in patients with an ejection fraction greater than 40%.

Results.—Risk and outcome in the patient group were confounded by worse LV function, older age, and more extensive coronary artery disease than in the control group. The angiographic success rate of 93% was lower than that in patients with relatively preserved LV function. Complete revascularization was achieved less frequently and procedural mortality was 4 times higher in patients with LV dysfunction. At mean follow-up of 33.5 months, 59% of patients were angina-free, and survivals at 1 and 4 years were 87% and 69%, respectively.

Conclusion.—Survival after PTCA appears to be similar to that after bypass surgery, making it a potentially effective treatment for coronary artery disease in patients with LV dysfunction.

▶ Those who may wish to expand their indications for PTCA to these patients with higher risk must bear in mind that the results presented are from a highly experienced group of expert angioplasty operators, and their results are not easily achieved by those with less experience.—R.L. Frye, M.D.

Effects of Nonionic Versus Ionic Contrast Media on Complications of Percutaneous Transluminal Coronary Angioplasty

Lembo NJ, King SB III, Roubin GS, Black AJ, Douglas JS Jr (Emory Univ, Atlanta)
Am J Cardiol 67:1046–1050, 1991   1–48

Background.—Although ionic contrast agents used during percutaneous transluminal coronary angioplasty (PTCA) are generally well tolerated, a small percentage of patients will have transient ischemic complications after injection of the contrast agent. Whether the use of nonionic contrast media would reduce the incidence of those complications compared with standard ionic contrast agents was investigated in 913 patients undergoing 1,058 separate PTCA procedures.

Methods.—The patients were randomly allocated to receive either ionic or nonionic contrast medium. Nonionic iopamidol was used in 507 PTCA procedures and meglumine sodium diatrizoate was used in 551 procedures. Hypotension was defined as a mean arterial pressure of less than 65 mm Hg. Bradycardia was defined as a heart rate of less than 40 beats per minute.

Results.—Contrast medium-associated hypotension occurred during 8.5% of the PTCA procedures in which iopamidol was used and during 9.5% of the PTCA procedures in which diatrizoate was used. The difference was statistically not significant. Bradycardia occurred during 5.7%

of procedures in which iopamidol was used and during 5.1% of procedures in which diatrizoate was used. The difference was also not statistically significant. The overall incidence of ventricular tachycardia or ventricular fibrillation, or both, was 1% for iopamidol and 2.5% for diatrizoate. This difference was statistically significant. There were no differences between the 2 groups in allergic reactions, myocardial infarction, coronary artery bypass grafting surgery, or death.

Conclusion.—Iopamidol used as the contrast agent in patients undergoing PTCA reduces only the overall incidence of ventricular tachycardia or fibrillation, or both, compared with diatrizoate, but does not reduce the incidence of hypotension, bradycardia, or in-hospital complications.

▶ This is an important contribution to resolving the issue of the appropriate use of nonionic contrast, a much more expensive control agent. Use of nonionic contrast can be a major contributor to increasing costs of imaging procedures.—R.L. Frye, M.D.

The Dutch Experience in Percutaneous Transluminal Angioplasty of Narrowed Saphenous Veins Used for Aortocoronary Arterial Bypass
Thijs Plokker HW, Meester BH, Serruys PW (Interuniversity Cardiology Inst of The Netherlands, Utrecht; Erasmus Univ, Rotterdam, The Netherlands; St Antonius Hosp, Nieuwegein, The Netherlands)
Am J Cardiol 67.361–366, 1991   1–49

Background.—Percutaneous transluminal balloon angioplasty has been tried in patients with recurrence of angina pectoris after aortocoronary bypass surgery, but little is known about the long-term outcomes. Long-term clinical effects of balloon angioplasty in venous bypass grafts in 454 patients were evaluated.

Methods.—Over about 8½ years, 19,994 percutaneous transluminal coronary angioplasties were performed in The Netherlands. The 454 cases evaluated represented 2.7% of these procedures. Of these, sequential graft angioplasty was attempted in 54% and a single graft angioplasty was attempted in 46%. The patients' mean age was 60, and 81% were men. Reduction of the stenosis by 50% or more with no major complication was defined as a primary success.

Results.—The primary success rate was 90%, and in-hospital mortality was .7%. A procedural myocardial infarction was evident in 2.8% of patients, and emergency bypass surgery was done in 1.3%. At 5 years, 74% of patients were alive and 26% were alive with no myocardial infarction, repeat bypass surgery, or repeat angioplasty. Only 3% of patients whose initial angioplasty attempt was unsuccessful were event-free at 5 years, compared with 27% of patients whose initial angioplasty was successful. A significant predictor of 5-year event-free survival was time between the angioplasty attempt and previous surgery. Event-free survival rates were 45% for patients who had bypass surgery 1 year previously, 25% for those who had bypass surgery between 1 and 5 years previously, and 19% for those who had bypass surgery more than 5 years previously.

Conclusions.—It appears that 74% of patients who have angioplasty in a venous graft will survive for 5 years, and only 26% remain free of any major event. Long-term results are better in those who require angioplasty within 1 year of bypass surgery. In some patients with previous coronary artery bypass surgery, angioplasty of a venous graft stenosis may be an alternative to reoperation.

▶ The Dutch experience with this large group of patients provides a perspective of angioplasty of saphenous vein grafts used for aortocoronary bypass surgery. This is certainly an important clinical problem, considering the large number of patients throughout the world who have had coronary bypass surgery. One would like to avoid repeat sternotomies in such patients. The outcomes with angioplasty are not ideal, and selection of patients must be individualized on the basis of the characteristics of the demonstrated lesion in the setting of the specific clinical characteristics.—R.L. Frye, M.D.

Restenosis After Directional Coronary Atherectomy: Differences Between Primary Atheromatous and Restenosis Lesions and Influence of Subintimal Tissue Resection
Garratt KN, Holmes DR Jr, Bell MR, Bresnahan JF, Kaufmann UP, Vlietstra RE, Edwards WD (Mayo Clin and Found, Rochester, Minn)
J Am Coll Cardiol 16:1665–1671, 1990   1–50

Background.—Percutaneous coronary angioplasty is used to treat patients with ischemic coronary syndromes even though re-stenosis occurs in 45% of those having this procedure. Directional coronary atherectomy is a possible alternative to balloon angioplasty as a method of relieving coronary artery disease. The incidence of re-stenosis in patients 6 months after directional coronary atherectomy was examined.

Methods.—Angiography was performed with the Judkins technique and standard cardiac catheterization equipment. Atherectomy was performed with the directional AtheroCath device. All patients received aspirin and heparin before atherectomy, nifedipine and nitroglycerin during atherectomy, and aspirin throughout the follow-up period. Patients returned at 3 and 6 months after the atherectomy for an evaluation. Angiography was performed earlier than 6 months after atherectomy if symptoms of myocardial ischemia were noted. Re-stenosis was defined as greater than 50% severity of the lesion in the involved vessel or loss of more than half of the initial gain.

Results.—Seventy-six patients with 80 lesions had successful directional atherectomy during a 13-month period. Five patients were lost to follow-up. Thus, the 70 patients with 74 lesions participating in the follow-up examinations demonstrated a reduction in stenosis severity from 86% before atherectomy to 16% afterward. Re-stenosis occurred in half of the 74 treated lesions and in 36 of the 70 patients (51%). Individuals with re-stenosis were older and more likely to have diabetes mellitus than those without re-stenosis. Re-stenosis occurred in 42% of lesions with intimal resection only, in half of those with medial resection, and in 63% of those with adventitial resection. Subintimal resection of postballoon angioplasty re-stenosis lesions resulted in a significantly greater re-stenosis rate than that from intimal resection only. Re-stenosis rates were similar for the blockages in the various arteries examined. Microscopic analysis of re-stenosis lesion tissue from 8 patients showed loosely arranged hyperplastic smooth muscle cells in the neointimal layer after directional atherectomy.

Conclusions.—These findings indicate that intimal hyperplasia occurs after percutaneous directional atherectomy in a similar way as it does after balloon angioplasty. These results may be improved by careful patient selection and modification of the atherectomy instrumentation and operative method to better control the depth of tissue resection.

▶ The incremental value of atherectomy over balloon angioplasty has yet to be proven. These re-stenosis rates emphasize the need to document objectively the usefulness of new devices in the treatment of patients with coronary disease. Fortunately, a multicenter trial, CAVEAT, is under way and should provide important results for the practice community.—R.L. Frye, M.D.

Predictors of Long-Term Cardiac Survival in Patients With Multivessel Coronary Artery Disease Undergoing Percutaneous Transluminal Coronary Angioplasty

Vandormael M, Deligonul U, Taussig S, Kern MJ (St Louis Univ Hosp)
Am J Cardiol 67:1–6, 1991   1–51

Background.—Percutaneous transluminal coronary angioplasty (PTCA) is often used to treat patients with multivessel coronary artery disease (CAD). The procedure has a mortality rate of 2% and a nonfatal myocardial infarction rate of 2% to 3% after an average follow-up of 15–31 months. The long-term survival of patients undergoing PTCA for multivessel CAD was assessed so that guidelines could be established for better patient selection and follow-up.

Methods.—Between May 1983 and June 1988, 637 patients with multivessel CAD had the PTCA procedure. Multivessel CAD was defined as a diameter stenosis of ≥50% of 2 major coronary arteries, attained by averaging caliper measurements in 2 views. All patients were eligible for ≥1 year of follow-up evaluation. The patients' functional status and occurrence of cardiac events were prospectively measured by questionnaire, telephone interview, or a clinic visit at 6 months and 1 year after PTCA, and then at 1-year intervals thereafter.

Results.—Seventy-two percent had 2-vessel and 28% had 3-vessel CAD. The PTCA procedures resulted in angiographic success in 85% of narrowings and in clinical success in 83% of patients. Follow-up of ≥1 year was completed for 608 patients (95%). The 30-day mortality rate for these patients was 3.2%. A second revascularization after a successful first PTCA was required for 130 patients. Cardiac survival at 1–5 years was estimated to be 93%, 92%, 90%, 88%, and 86%, respectively. Clinical success was associated significantly with more favorable 5-year cardiac survival. The only significant independent predictor of cardiac mortality was a left ventricular contraction measurement of ≥12, with an estimated relative risk ratio of 6.2.

Conclusions.—These findings suggest that left ventricular function is the most important factor in cardiac survival for patients with multivessel CAD who undergo the PTCA procedure. Old age and diabetes mellitus are also risk factors for this procedure.

▶ This observational study of angioplasty in the setting of multivessel coronary disease is interesting. Fortunately, we have several international multicenter trials comparing angioplasty with bypass surgery, and these data will be crucial in evaluating the proper use of coronary angioplasty in the setting of multivessel coronary disease.—R.L. Frye, M.D.

Angiographic Follow-Up After Placement of a Self-Expanding Coronary-Artery Stent

Serruys PW, Strauss BH, Beatt KJ, Bertrand ME, Puel J, Rickards AF, Meier B, Goy J-J, Vogt P, Kappenberger L, Sigwart U (Erasmus Univ, Rotterdam, The Netherlands; Centre Hospitalier Universitaire Vaudois, Lausanne, Switzerland; Centre Hospitalier Universitaire, Rangueil, France; Natl Heart Inst, London; Univ Hosp, Geneva, et al)
N Engl J Med 324:13–17, 1991   1–52

Background.—Acute occlusion and late re-stenosis are the 2 main limitations on the use of coronary angioplasty. In May 1988, 5 European centers reported their experience with implanting an endoluminal stent in the coronary arteries of patients undergoing balloon dilation in an effort to avoid these 2 problems. The results of long-term angiographic follow-up of the patients receiving the original 117 stents were reported.

Methods.—Of the 105 patients included, 95 had 1 stent implanted and 10 patients received more than 1. Of the latter 10, 7 patients required 2 overlapping stents to cover long lesions. The endovascular prosthesis Wallstent was used. Anticoagulation protocols evolved throughout the trial, and different regimens were used at various centers. Two different criteria were used to define re-stenosis: a reduction of ≥.72 mm in the minimal luminal diameter of the narrowing vessel, or an increase in the percentage of stenosis from <50% after implanting the stent to ≥50% at the follow-up examination.

Results.—The total mortality for all patients after 1 year was 7.6% (8 deaths). The mean time to the angiographic follow-up visit was 5.7 months. Twenty angiograms were completed during the initial month after stent implantation, and all showed occlusions. For all patients, the minimal luminal diameter was increased from a mean 1.21 mm to 1.88

mm after percutaneous transluminal coronary angioplasty and then, significantly, to 2.48 mm immediately after insertion of the stent. At the follow-up evaluation, the mean diameter of these vessels had decreased to 1.68 mm. The percentage of stenosis had significantly changed from a mean 61% after percutaneous transluminal coronary angioplasty to 21% after stent insertion. At the follow-up visit, the percentage of stenosis had increased significantly to 48%. The incidence of re-stenosis, however, depended on the definition of stenosis. Using a change of ≥.72 mm in minimal luminal diameter, re-stenosis occurred in 32% of patients. With the definition of stenosis as an increase to ≥50%, re-stenosis was observed in 14% of patients.

Conclusions.—These findings indicate that occlusion and late re-stenosis remain important problems with the use of the coronary artery stent. Therefore, the clinical indications for the use of this type of vascular device remain undefined.

▶ This careful and objective evaluation of stenting after coronary artery balloon dilatation is important. It emphasizes the need for additional study of the basic biology involved in re-stenosis and early thrombotic occlusion. The investigators called for controlled clinical trials, and this seems to be again a critical area for additional investigation.—R.L. Frye, M.D.

Percutaneous Excimer Laser Coronary Angioplasty

Litvack F, Eigler NL, Margolis JR, Grundfest WS, Rothbaum D, Linnemeier T, Hestrin LB, Tsoi D, Cook SL, Krauthamer D, Goldenberg T, Laudenslager JR, Segalowitz J, Forrester JS (Cedars-Sinai Med Ctr, Los Angeles; Univ of California, Los Angeles; South Miami Hosp, Miami; St Vincent's Hosp, Indianapolis; Advanced Interventional Systems Inc, Irvine, Calif)
Am J Cardiol 66:1027–1032, 1990   1–53

Background.—There is a need for intravascular interventions that can reduce atheroma mass. A multiple fiberoptic bundle that can be passed over a conventional coronary angioplasty wire has been developed. The efficacy of this technique, as either an adjunct or an alternative to conventional balloon angioplasty, was studied in a multicenter trial of 55 patients.

Methods.—Percutaneous coronary excimer laser angioplasty was performed as a modification of conventional balloon angioplasty. The catheter was 1.6 mm in diameter and was constructed of 12 individual silica fibers arranged concentrically around a guidewire lumen. Catheter tip energy densities of 35 to 50 mJ/mm^2 and a mean of 1,272 pulses at 20 Hz were used. Sixty-seven lesions in 56 arteries were treated at 3 different hospitals. An increase in minimal stenotic diameter of at least 20% and a resulting lumen diameter of at least 1 mm after laser treatment were the parameters for acute success.

Results.—The acute success rate was 84%. Seventy-five percent of patients had adjunctive balloon angioplasty. As determined by quantitative angiography, the mean diameter stenosis was 83% at baseline, 49% after laser treatment, and 38% in patients who had adjunctive balloon angioplasty. The baseline mean minimal stenotic diameter was .5 mm; this improved to 1.6 mm after laser treatment and to 2.1 mm after balloon angioplasty. No patient died and none developed vascular perforation, although 1 required emergency coronary bypass surgery.

Conclusions.—Atheroma can safely be ablated and coronary stenosis can be reduced by percutaneously delivered excimer laser energy. More patients are required for complete analysis, and a randomized trial may be needed to compare this technique with balloon angioplasty.

▶ The place of laser therapy in percutaneous coronary interventions remains unsettled. As the investigators note, proper randomized trials are needed to determine incremental value of laser techniques over and above existing angioplasty and other new devices such as atherectomy.—R.L. Frye, M.D.

2 Noncoronary Heart Disease in Adults

Introduction

I have selected 6 articles for the section on valvular heart disease, 3 for infective endocarditis, 13 for myocardial diseases, 1 for pericardial disease, 12 for heart failure, and 19 for disturbances of cardiac rhythm and conduction. All have been selected to provide the cardiologist with information relative to patients who might be encountered in clinical practice. In each of these fields of cardiology, there have been important and significant advances, many of which should be promptly applied to patient management. As noted in the comments, some advances require confirmation.

In general, the rate of increase in our knowledge of the basic science of cardiovascular disease exceeds the rate of increase in our ability to prevent or to treat cardiovascular disease. Although the latter may sometimes appear to be slow, in actuality it also has been quite explosive if looked from a broad, historical viewpoint.

Robert C. Schlant, M.D.

Valvular Heart Disease

Correlation Between the Position of Transducers and Mitral Valve Gradient in Mitral Stenosis

Cha SD, Cha RI, Maranhao V (Deborah Heart and Lung Ctr, Browns Mills, NJ)
Cathet Cardiovasc Diag 24:6–9, 1991   2–1

Introduction.—A transducer must be positioned at the same level as the catheter tip to obtain a correct intracardiac pressure. The pressure reading will be low if the position of the transducer is higher than the level of the catheter, and high when the level of the transducer is lower than the catheter. To assess the severity of mitral stenosis related to the level of transducers, the mitral valve gradient was obtained from 15 patients using pulmonary wedge and left ventricle.

Methods.—The mitral valve gradient was recorded in the patients while both transducers were positioned at mid chest level. Using the level pointer and lateral cinefluoroscopy, the level of each transducer was adjusted to the level of its respective catheter tip and the gradient again obtained. Two gradients were calculated using the cardiac output obtained by Fick's principle.

Results.—When a catheter was in the wedge position, its level was lower than mid chest level in 14 of 15 patients. The position of the catheter in the left ventricle was at the same level or up to 6 cm higher than mid chest level. At mid chest level, the mean mitral valve gradient was 14 mm Hg with a mitral valve area of 1.3 cm^2. With the adjusted level of transducers, the mitral valve gradient was 18 mm Hg with a valve area of 1.0 cm^2. The mean level of the catheter tip in the wedge was 3.5 cm below the mid chest level, whereas the mean level in the left ventricle was 2.5 cm higher than the mid chest level. The latter was statistically insignificant.

Conclusion.—The mitral valve gradient obtained at mid chest level underestimates the severity of mitral stenosis. The difference of gradient and area may be more pronounced in patients with enlarged hearts or large anterior-posterior diameter.

▶ The error caused by catheter tips in the chest and transducers being at different levels was recognized many years ago by Dexter, Gorlin, and a number of other investigators. Whereas the errors caused by this phenomenon are usually small, it should be taken into account whenever comparisons are made with valve areas estimated from pressure differences by the Gorlin formula and other techniques. One should also consider this potential source of error whenever the calculated valve area at cardiac catheterization does not correlate well with other clinical features of the patient.—R.C. Schlant, M.D.

Percutaneous Balloon Versus Surgical Closed Commissurotomy for Mitral Stenosis: A Prospective, Randomized Trial

Turi ZG, Reyes VP, Raju BS, Raju AR, Kumar DN, Rajagopal P, Sathyanarayana PV, Rao DP, Srinath K, Peters P, Connors B, Fromm B, Farkas P, Wynne J (Harper Hosp, Wayne State Univ, Detroit; Nizam's Inst of Med Sciences, Hyderabad, India)

Circulation 83:1179–1185, 1991   2–2

Background.—The use of percutaneous balloon mitral commissurotomy as an alternative to surgery was first described in 1984. The 2 methods were compared prospectively in India, and charges were compared with patients hospitalized in the United States.

Method.—Thirty-nine patients with severe rheumatic mitral stenosis were randomized to either balloon or surgical commissurotomy. The data analysts were blinded to the treatment assignment or phase of the study.

Results.—Hemodynamics in the 2 groups were similar. Pulmonary artery wedge pressure, mitral valve gradient, pulmonary artery systolic pressures, and mitral valve area improved significantly in both groups 1 week after surgery and showed continued improvement during the average 8 months of follow-up. In patients receiving balloon commissurotomy, gradients and left atrial pressures were slightly higher at 1 week follow-up than immediately postprocedure. The cost of disposables may account for balloon commissurotomy costing 6 times as much in India as in the United States. On the other hand, the fee for surgical closed commissurotomy in the United States was nearly double the charge in India, probably because of physicians' fees and room charges.

Conclusion.—No significant differences occurred in hemodynamic results between balloon and surgical closed commissurotomy through 8 months of follow-up. There was no death, stroke, or myocardial infarction. The cost of balloon commissurotomy may exceed the cost of surgical commissurotomy in developing countries, but may represent a significant savings in industrialized nations.

▶ This is one of the few, large prospective randomized trials comparing balloon valvuloplasty with surgical closed commissurotomy for mitral stenosis. The good results obtained with balloon valvuloplasty are in agreement with several other recent reports (1–4). Mitral balloon valvuloplasty (or valvotomy) has been used in high-risk patients (5), during pregnancy (6), and to open a stenotic mitral bioprosthesis (7). Complications include mitral regurgitation (8), mitral valve disruption (9), and cardiac tamponade (11). A long-term follow-up of closed mitral commissurotomy provides a good comparison of what may be expected in long-term results from balloon valvotomy (12).—R.C. Schlant, M.D.

References

1. Casale PN, et al: Percutaneous balloon valvotomy for patients with mitral stenosis: Initial and follow-up results. *Am Heart J* 121:476–479, 1991.
2. Tuzcu EM, et al: Comparison of early versus late experience with percutaneous mitral balloon valvuloplasty. *J Am Coll Cardiol* 17:1121–1124, 1991.
3. Hung J-S, et al: Short- and long-term results of catheter balloon percutaneous transvenous mitral commissurotomy. *Am J Cardiol* 67:854–862, 1991.
4. Benit E, et al: Early and 3 months follow-up results in 22 adult patients undergoing percutaneous transvenous mitral valvuloplasty. *Acta Cardiologica* 45:425–440, 1990.
5. Lefevre T, et al: Percutaneous mitral valvuloplasty in surgical high risk patients. *J Am Coll Cardiol* 17:348–354, 1991.
6. Esteves CA, et al: Effectiveness of percutaneous balloon mitral valvotomy during pregnancy. *Am J Cardiol* 68:930–934, 1991.
7. Babic UU, et al: Balloon valvoplasty of mitral bioprosthesis. *Int J Cardiol* 30:230–232, 1991.
8. Pan J-P, et al: Frequency and severity of mitral regurgitation one year after balloon mitral valvuloplasty. *Am J Cardiol* 67:264–268, 1991.
9. Ramondo A, et al: Mitral valve disruption following percutaneous balloon valvuloplasty. *Cathet Cardiovasc Diagn* 21:239–244, 1990.
10. Pan M, et al: Cardiac tamponade complicating mitral balloon valvuloplasty. *Am J Cardiol* 68:802–805, 1991.
11. Hickey MS, et al: Outcome probabilities and life history after surgical mitral commissurotomy: Implications for balloon commissurotomy. *J Am Coll Cardiol* 17:29–42, 1991.

Effects of Aerobic Exercise Training on Symptomatic Women With Mitral Valve Prolapse
Scordo KA (Cardiology Consultants, Inc, Cincinnati)
Am J Cardiol 67:863–868, 1991   2–3

Introduction.—Symptomatic mitral valve prolapse (MVP) in women was treated with a 12-week aerobic exercise training program. The effects of such an exercise protocol have not been previously described in the literature.

Methods.—Thirty-two symptomatic women with a diagnosis of MVP were randomly assigned to a control or exercise group for 12 weeks. Before and after the training period patients were asked to complete the State Trait Anxiety Inventory and General Well-Being Schedule, and they also underwent maximal multistage treadmill testing and determinations of plasma levels of catecholamines at rest and during peak exercise. Patients kept a record of their symptoms during the 12-week period. The exercise program was based on the American Heart Association's phase II cardiac rehabilitation program.

Results.—In the exercise group most symptoms declined in frequency, with the greatest reported decline at week 6. Chest pain, palpitations, and dyspnea declined in frequency in both the exercise and control groups, possibly because of various physiological changes. The exercise group demonstrated a significant decrease in anxiety levels as shown by lower scores on inventories; functional capacities also increased in this group.

Discussion.—Aerobic training appears to be beneficial for patients with symptomatic MVP. An exercise training program of this type has the potential to improve feelings of well-being in patients and reduce the frequency of symptoms.

▶ This report confirms my own experience, as well as that of colleagues, who have often noted an improvement in symptomatology in females with MVP after exercise training. It is not known whether the apparent benefit is the result of changes in ventricular size and less valve-chamber size disproportion, of unknown beneficial effects of exercise training, or is just because the symptoms of MVP often vary considerably without any specific intervention. In selected patients with MVP, exercise training appears to be a useful modality of therapy.—R.C. Schlant, M.D.

Effects of Long-Term Vasodilator Therapy on Electrocardiographic Abnormalities in Chronic Aortic Regurgitation

Wilson R, Perlmutter N, Jacobson N, Siemienczuk D, Szlachcic J, Bristow JD, Cheitlin M, Massie B, Greenberg B (Oregon Health Sciences Univ, Portland; San Francisco VA Med Ctr; Univ of California, San Francisco)
Am J Cardiol 68:935–939, 1991   2–4

Introduction.—Vasodilator drugs acutely reduce regurgitant flow and improve cardiac performance in patients with chronic aortic regurgitation (AR). Recent studies have shown that chronic vasodilator therapy reduces volume overload in clinically stable patients with chronic AR. However, the effects of long-term vasodilator drug therapy on the ECG abnormalities of AR have not previously been studied. A double-blind, randomized clinical trial was undertaken to examine how oral hydralazine therapy affects the ECG abnormalities of chronic AR.

Patients.—Sixty patients with significant chronic AR but preserved ejection fraction were enrolled in the study. Thirty-two patients were initially randomized to receive 25 mg of hydralazine orally twice daily. The dose was titrated up to a total of 3 mg/kg of body weight daily; the average daily dose was 205 mg, with a range of 150 mg to 300 mg. The other 28 patients were randomized to receive matching placebo. In addition to standard 12-lead rest ECG, each patient underwent radionuclide angiography and M-mode echocardiography.

Results.—Both groups had similar ST-segment depression and left ventricular hypertrophy (LVH) at baseline. After a mean follow-up of 19 months, hydralazine-treated patients had a small but highly significant reduction in ST-segment depression and LVH scores compared with placebo-treated patients. Similarly, chronic hydralazine therapy significantly reduced LV end-diastolic and end-systolic volume indexes and improved LV ejection fraction compared with placebo. However, none of the patients showed a change in the presence or absence of LVH voltage or strain repolarization abnormalities during follow-up.

Conclusion.—Because ECG abnormalities in patients with chronic AR are considered prognostic of a poor outcome, long-term oral vasodilator drug therapy may have a beneficial effect on the natural history of this disorder.

► This report extends the previous report of this study (1), which demonstrated the overall benefits of vasodilator therapy by the objective improvement in electrocardiographic evidence of left ventricular hypertrophy, and by improvement in left ventricular volumes and function evaluated by echocardiography and radionuclide ventriculography. It is probable that the changes would be more impressive in a larger group of patients followed for a longer time. At present, we usually prefer to use an ACE inhibitor or a calcium channel antagonist such as nifedipine to decrease afterload in patients with aortic regurgitation.—R.C. Schlant, M.D.

Reference

1. Greenberg B, et al: Long-term vasodilator therapy of chronic aortic insufficiency: A randomized double-blinded, placebo-controlled clinical trial. *Circulation* 78:92–103, 1988.

Twelve-Year Comparison of a Bjork-Shiley Mechanical Heart Valve With Porcine Bioprostheses
Bloomfield P, Wheatley DJ, Prescott RJ, Miller HC (Royal Infirmary of Edinburgh)
N Engl J Med 324:573–579, 1991   2–5

Introduction.—Previously it was reported that there were no significant differences in survival rates for patients with a mechanical or a porcine prosthesis for heart valve replacement after 5.6 years. In the present study the survival, valve-related complications, and valve failures in the 2 types of replacement valves are examined after 12 years of use.

Materials.—The 541 patients who underwent valve replacement were randomly assigned to receive either a mechanical Bjork-Shiley 60-degree spherical tilting-disk valve or a porcine biosprosthetic valve. Two hundred sixty-one patients had mitral valve replacement, 211 had aortic valve replacement, and 61 had both replacements. No technical reasons precluded the use of either type of valve in any of the patients. All received warfarin for 2 months after surgery, and those who received a Bjork-Shiley prosthesis continued to take warfarin throughout the study. Follow-up data were collected at each postoperative visit.

Findings.—The mean duration of follow-up for all surviving patients, except 10 lost to follow-up, was 12 years. Forty-four of the 533 patients died in hospital and 235 died after leaving the hospital. The actuarial survival results for all patients demonstrated a trend toward better survival after 12 years for patients who received a Bjork-Shiley prosthesis. Eighty-five patients, 17 with the Bjork-Shiley device and 68 with the porcine valve (27 with the Hancock valve and 41 with the Carpentier-Edwards valve), had replacement of the prosthetic valve. The actuarial incidence of reoperation was the same for both valve type groups after 5 years, but significantly favored the Bjork-Shiley valve group after 12 years. Patients

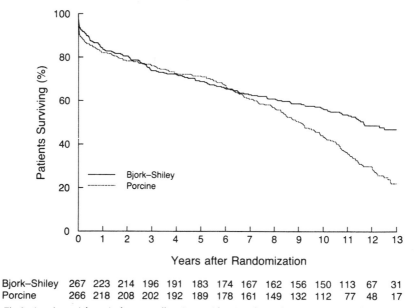

Bjork–Shiley	267	223	214	196	191	183	174	167	162	156	150	113	67	31
Porcine		266	218	208	202	192	189	178	161	149	132	112	77	48	17

Fig 2–1.—Actuarial survival among all patients with original prosthesis intact (survival without re-operation) after 12 years. Valve survival was significantly better in patients with Bjork-Shiley prostheses. Numbers of surviving patients with original prosthesis intact are shown at bottom of figure. (Courtesy of Bloomfield P, Wheatley DJ, Prescott RJ, et al: *N Engl J Med* 324:573–579, 1991.)

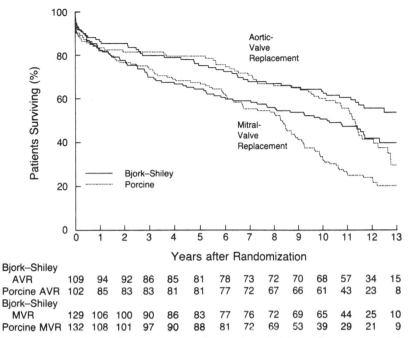

Bjork–Shiley
AVR	109	94	92	86	85	81	78	73	72	70	68	57	34	15
Porcine AVR	102	85	83	83	81	81	77	72	67	66	61	43	23	8

Bjork–Shiley
MVR	129	106	100	90	86	83	77	76	72	69	65	44	25	10
Porcine MVR	132	108	101	97	90	88	81	72	69	53	39	29	21	9

Fig 2–2.—Actuarial survival among patients with original prosthesis intact after 12 years, according to site of implantation (aortic vs. mitral valve). Valve survival among patients who had mitral valve replacement (MVR) was significantly better in those who received Bjork-Shiley prostheses than in those who received porcine prostheses, but valve survival among those with aortic valve replacement (AVR) did not differ significantly between these subgroups. Numbers of surviving patients with original prostheses intact are shown at bottom of figure. (Courtesy of Bloomfield P, Wheatley DJ, Prescott RJ, et al: *N Engl J Med* 324:573–579, 1991.)

receiving this valve also did significantly better for mechanical valve failure after 12 years (Fig 2–1) and for overall survival with the original prosthesis intact after 12 years (Fig 2–2). In nearly all reoperations for a porcine valve failure, the failure resulted from extreme regurgitation from the rupture of 1 or more of the cusps of the prosthesis. The actuarial incidence of all major events, including bleeding, embolism, endocarditis, reoperation, and death, demonstrated no significant differences between prostheses groups after 5 years, but there was a significant difference favoring the Bjork-Shiley prosthesis after 12 years.

Recommendations.—The results of this study suggest that patients who undergo mitral valve replacement should receive a mechanical prosthesis. Those for whom anticoagulant therapy is contraindicated can receive a bioprosthesis, with the knowledge that reoperation may be required at a later time.

▶ This report confirms the opinions of most cardiac surgeons that tissue valves are less durable than mechanical valves after 10 years and that they are best used in patients who have a contraindication to long-term anticoagulation or who are very elderly. In an editorial accompanying this article, Dr. Collins wrote,

"Every model of a heart valve ever marketed has suffered some mechanical failures resulting from thrombosis, wear, or structural fractures. Good valves have been succeeded by better valves, and the succession will continue unless the industry is so punished by the press and professional critics that innovation is stifled and the risk of failure becomes too great to continue. When that occurs, yet another form of technology pioneered and developed in the United States will disappear from these shores" (1).—R.C. Schlant, M.D.

Reference

1. Collins JJ, Jr: The evolution of artificial heart valves. *N Engl J Med* 324:624–626, 1991.

Predictors of Event-Free Survival After Balloon Aortic Valvuloplasty
Kuntz RE, Tosteson ANA, Berman AD, Goldman L, Gordon PC, Leonard BM, McKay RG, Diver DJ, Safian RD (Charles A Dana Research Inst; Beth Israel Hosp; Harvard Med School and School of Public Health, Boston)
N Engl J Med 325:17–23, 1991   2–6

Introduction.—Early reports suggested that balloon dilation of the stenosed aortic valve was safe and hemodynamically effective in elderly, symptomatic patients. Long-term hemodynamic improvement was, however, limited by a high rate of re-stenosis, approaching 50% within a year of valvuloplasty.

Series.—Valvuloplasty was carried out in 205 patients having symptomatic aortic stenosis in a 3.5-year period. Patients who were not candidates for surgery and those who refused operation were considered for valvuloplasty. The mean age was 78 years.

Outcome.—Valvuloplasty was completed successfully in all but 2 patients and lowered the peak transaortic pressure gradient from 67 to 33 mm Hg. Cardiac output rose from 4.4 to 4.8 L/min. Symptoms recurred in 82% of 189 patients followed up for an average of 2 years. More than 20% of the patients had repeat valvuloplasty. Event-free survival rates were 50% at 1 year and 25% at 2 years. Independent predictors of event-free survival included baseline aortic systolic pressure, baseline pulmonary capillary wedge pressure, and the percent reduction in peak aortic-valve gradient.

Conclusions.—The same patients who would be expected to have a good long-term outcome after aortic-valve replacement do relatively well after balloon valvuloplasty. Apart from patients who are not surgical candidates, valvuloplasty might be considered for those having severe left ventricular dysfunction as a "bridge" to valve replacement.

▶ This report confirms several studies noted in the YEAR BOOK OF CARDIOLOGY for the last 3 years and other more recent reports (1–9), which confirm previous conclusions that balloon valvuloplasty of the aortic valve is an effective, short-term palliative treatment for severely symptomatic patients who cannot tolerate aortic valve replacement and who have only minimal aortic regurgitation. Acute catastrophic complications include ventricular perforation, acute severe aortic regurgitation, fatal cardiac arrest, fatal cerebrovascular accident, and limb amputation (10).—R.C. Schlant, M.D.

References

1. NHLBI Balloon Valvuloplasty Registry Participants: Percutaneous balloon aortic valvuloplasty. Acute and 30-day follow-up results in 674 patients from the NHLBI balloon valvuloplasty registry. *Circulation* 84:2383–2397, 1991.
2. Holmes DR Jr, et al: In-hospital mortality after balloon aortic valvuloplasty: Frequency and associated factors. *J Am Coll Cardiol* 17:189–192, 1991.
3. McKay RG, et al: The Mansfield Scientific Aortic Valvuloplasty Registry: Overview of acute hemodynamic results and procedural complications. *J Am Coll Cardiol* 17:485–491, 1991.
4. Nishimura R, et al: Follow-up of patients with low output, low gradient hemodynamics after percutaneous balloon aortic valvuloplasty: The Mansfield Scientific Aortic Valvuloplasty Registry. *J Am Coll Cardiol* 17:828–833, 1991.
5. Ferguson JJ, et al: Efficacy of multiple balloon aortic valvuloplasty procedures. *J Am Coll Cardiol* 17:1430–1435, 1991.
6. Harrison JK, et al: Serial left ventricular performance evaluated by cardiac catheterization before, immediately after and at 6 months after balloon aortic valvuloplasty. *J Am Coll Cardiol* 16:1351–1358, 1990.
7. Geibel A, et al: Clinical and Doppler echocardiographic follow-up after percutaneous balloon valvuloplasty for aortic valve stenosis. *Am J Cardiol* 67:616–621, 1991.
8. Davidson CJ, et al: Determinants of one-year outcome from balloon aortic valvuloplasty. *Am J Cardiol* 68:75–80, 1991.
9. Cribier A: Emergency balloon valvuloplasty as initial treatment of patients with aortic stenosis and cardiogenic shock. *N Engl J Med* 326:646, 1992.
10. Isner JM, et al: Acute catastrophic complications of balloon aortic valvuloplasty. *J Am Coll Cardiol* 17:1436–1444, 1991.

Infective Endocarditis

Diagnostic Value of Transesophageal Compared With Transthoracic Echocardiography in Infective Endocarditis

Shively BK, Gurule FT, Roldan CA, Leggett JH, Schiller NB (Univ of New Mexico; Univ of California, San Francisco)

J Am Coll Cardiol 18:391–397, 1991   2–7

Introduction.—Transthoracic M-mode echocardiography is useful for documenting vegetative lesions and assessing the extent of valvular damage in patients with active infective endocarditis, but the technique has a low diagnostic sensitivity in patients with clinically suspected but unconfirmed endocarditis. The diagnostic accuracy of transesophageal echocardiography and that of transthoracic Doppler color flow echocardiography were compared in 62 patients with suspected infective endocarditis.

Patients.—Paired transesophageal and transthoracic echocardiograms were obtained in 62 patients during 66 episodes of suspected endocarditis. Four patients were examined twice. All echocardiograms were read by an experienced interpreter at another institution. The echocardiographic results were compared with the later confirmed clinical diagnoses. Sixteen healthy volunteers also had both examinations.

Results.—Sixteen patients eventually had a diagnosis of endocarditis, 14 of them by pathologic criteria at surgery or autopsy and 2 by clinical criteria, including new murmur and positive blood cultures. When an almost certain probability of endocarditis was considered positive, results of only 7 (44%) of the 16 transthoracic studies were positive, compared with 15 (94%) of the 16 transesophageal studies. Forty-nine of the 50 transthoracic studies in patients without endocarditis were normal, yielding a specificity of 98%. Results of all 50 transesophageal studies were normal, yielding a specificity of 100%.

Conclusion.—Transesophageal echocardiography is highly sensitive and highly specific for the diagnosis of infective endocarditis. Transesophageal echocardiography also appears to be useful in cases of an intermediate clinical suspicion of infective endocarditis when transthoracic studies are inconclusive.

▶ This study confirms previous articles noted in the YEAR BOOK OF CARDIOLOGY for the last several years and in many other reports that support the greater value of transesophageal echocardiography (TEE) in the evaluation of patients with infective endocarditis. The evaluation of prosthetic valve endocarditis (1) and perivalvular abscesses are also improved by the use of TEE (See Abstract 2–9), and TEE is also helpful in the evaluation of patients with stroke and in those who have a potential cardiac source of embolism (2).—R.C. Schlant, M.D.

References

1. Pederson WR, et al: Value of transesophageal echocardiography as an adjunct to transthoracic echocardiography in evaluation of native and prosthetic valve endocarditis. *Chest* 100:351–356, 1991.
2. Cujec B, et al: Transesophageal echocardiography in the detection of potential cardiac source of embolism in stroke patients. *Stroke* 22:727–753, 1991.

Emboli in Infective Endocarditis: The Prognostic Value of Echocardiography
Steckelberg JM, Murphy JG, Ballard D, Bailey K, Tajik AJ, Taliercio CP, Giuliani ER, Wilson WR (Mayo Clinic and Found, Rochester, Minn)
Ann Intern Med 114:635–640, 1991   2–8

Introduction.—Embolic events are a common complication of infective endocarditis and should be prevented when at all possible. Two-dimensional echocardiography is used to establish hemodynamic status and in 13% to 78% of cases of infective endocarditis valvular vegetations are visualized. The association between these vegetations and the development of subsequent emboli was evaluated.

Methods.—A total of 207 patients who had received 2-dimensional

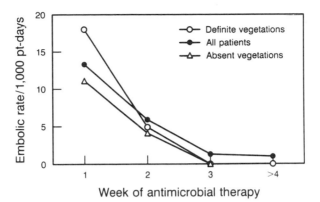

Week of antimicrobial therapy

Fig 2–3.—Incidence of embolic events in patients with infective endocarditis. *Abbreviation: PT*, patient. (Courtesy of Steckelberg JM, Murphy JG, Ballard D, et al: *Ann Intern Med* 114:635–640, 1991.)

echocardiography within 72 hours of beginning antimicrobial therapy were studied retrospectively. All study patients had native valve, left-sided infective endocarditis. Valvular vegetations were classified and embolic events were recorded.

Results.—The overall rate of first embolic event was not significantly associated with the presence of vegetations, and the echocardiographic findings overall did little to assist in predicting embolic events. Prevalence of emboli was significantly affected by the type of causative microorganism present, with relative risk rates increasing the most for viridans streptococcal and *Staphylococcus aureus* infections.

Conclusions.—After the initiation of antimicrobial treatment the rate of embolic events declined with time (Fig 2–3). The presence of vegetations on echocardiograms was not associated with increased risk of emboli, but the presence of certain microorganisms was associated with increased risk and should be further investigated.

▶ In this report the authors found the risk of embolus was more related to the organism involved rather than to the presence of vegetations on echocardiography. Their experience is different from our own and other published reports (1,2), which have found that the size, extent, mobility, and consistency of vegetations are independent markers of a future complication.—R.C. Schlant, M.D.

References

1. Mugge A, et al: Echocardiography in infective endocarditis: Reassessment of prognostic implications of vegetation size determined by the transthoracic and the transesophageal approach. *J Am Coll Cardiol* 14:631–638, 1989.
2. Sanfilippo AJ, et al: Echocardiographic assessment of patients with infectious endocarditis: Prediction of risk for complications. *J Am Coll Cardiol* 18:1191–1199, 1991.

Aortic Root Complications of Infective Endocarditis: Influence on Surgical Outcome

John RM, Pugsley W, Treasure T, Sturridge MF, Swanton RH (Middlesex Hosp, London)
Eur Heart J 12:241–248, 1991   2–9

Introduction.—In infective endocarditis, aortic root abscess or mycotic aneurysm formation occurs most commonly with aortic valve involvement, especially when a prosthetic valve in the aortic position is infected. The preoperative noninvasive detection of aortic root complications by using transesophageal echocardiography has emerged as a valuable diagnostic tool. The present retrospective study was done to examine the influence of aortic root complications on surgical outcome in patients operated on because of infective endocarditis.

Patients.—During a 6-year study period 41 men and 9 women aged 21 to 80 years were referred for the treatment of aortic valve endocarditis. All patients had severe aortic regurgitation at the time of referral, and 41 had ventricular failure. Twenty-three patients (46%) had an aortic root abscess (ARA) and 27 had a nonaortic root abscess (NARA). Twelve of the 23 patients with ARA and 4 of the 27 with NARA had prosthetic valve endocarditis. Thus, ARA was significantly associated with prosthetic valve endocarditis.

Results.—Forty-four patients were operated on, and 37 survived the operation. Seven patients (16%) died in the immediate postoperative period; 6 had an ARA and 1 had an NARA. Surgical mortality in the ARA group (13.6%) was significantly higher than in the NARA group (2.2%). Eight of the 14 surviving patients with ARA (57%) and 2 of the 23 surviving patients with NARA (9%) had postoperative aortic regurgitation. The difference was statistically significant.

Conclusion.—An aortic root abscess is a common occurrence in patients with aortic valve endocarditis. Its presence is associated with an increased surgical mortality and a high incidence of postoperative aortic regurgitation.

▶ The important diagnosis of perivalvular abscess is considerably improved by the use of transesophageal echocardiography (1), which should be performed in patients with persistent signs of infection and those who do not respond to therapy. It should be noted that transesophageal echocardiography is usually not possible in patients with fever unless the fever is lowered by medication because most esophageal transducers are automatically turned off by more than mild temperature elevations.—R.C. Schlant, M.D.

Reference

1. Daniel WG, et al: Improvement in the diagnosis of abscesses associated with endocarditis by transesophageal echocardiography. *N Engl J Med* 324:795–800, 1991.

Myocardial Diseases

Patterns of Myocardial Fibrosis in Idiopathic Cardiomyopathies and Chronic Chagasic Cardiopathy

Rossi MA (Univ of São Paulo, Brazil)
Can J Cardiol 7:287–294, 1991

2–10

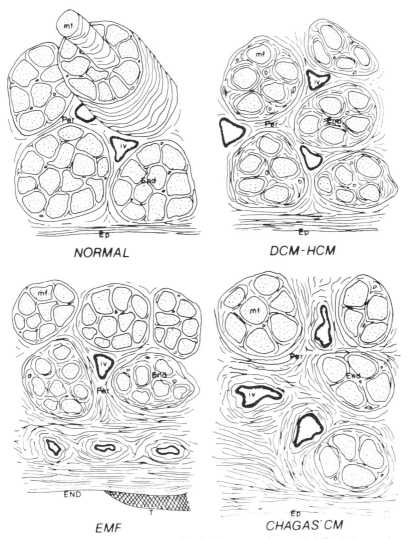

Fig 2–4.—Diagrammatic representation of the basic patterns of myocardial fibrosis in control myocardium *(NORMAL)*, dilated and hypertrophic cardiomyopathies *(DCM-HCM)*, endomyocardial fibrosis *(EMF)*, and chronic Chagasic cardiopathy *(CHAGAS' CM)*. *End* indicates endomysial collagen matrix; *END*, endocardium; *Ep*, epimysial collagen matrix; *iv*, intramural coronary vessel; *mf*, myofiber; *Per*, perimysial collagen matrix; *T*, thrombus. (Courtesy of Rossi MA: *Can J Cardiol* 7:287–294, 1991.)

Introduction.—The picrosirius red technique and polarization micros-copy were used to describe the fibrillar nature and structural features of the collagenous interstitium of the myocardium. Forty-six adult hearts obtained at autopsy were studied.

Methods.—There were 23 hearts with chronic Chagasic cardiomyopa-thy, 9 with dilated cardiomyopathy, 5 with hypertrophic cardiomyopa-thy, and 4 with endomyocardial fibrosis affecting the left ventricle. The remaining 5 hearts, which had no evidence of cardiac disease, served as controls. Fragments of myocardial tissue were obtained from the equator of the left ventricle free wall, fixed in formalin, dehydrated, and embed-ded in paraffin.

Results.—In both dilated and hypertrophic cardiomyopathies, the my-ocardium showed diffuse fibrosis. Both endomysial and perimysial colla-gen fibers appeared diffusely increased, particularly surrounding individ-ual myocytes. Muscle cells appeared hypertrophic. Microscopic study of hearts with endomyocardial fibrosis revealed a thickened fibrotic en-docardium. Interstitial and diffuse fibrosis was seen to a variable degree in all cases of Chagas' disease. Most cells within the muscle fiber bundles had a hypertrophic appearance. In all, there were 3 distinct patterns of myocardial fibrosis observed in cardiomyopathic human hearts compared with controls (Fig 2–4).

Conclusions.—The precise relationship between myocardial fibrosis and cardiac function in dilated and hypertrophic cardiomyopathies is not known. Further research into the patterns and mechanisms of the fibrotic process may aid in developing preventive or corrective therapy for these conditions.

► The results of this study suggest that it may be possible to get clues about the pathogenesis of various forms of heart muscle disease, including Chagas' heart disease (American trypanosomiasis), by careful analysis of the pattern of myocardial fibrosis. Two other reports summarized Chagas' heart disease in the United States (1) and the apparent benefit in patients with Chagas' cardio-neuropathy of therapy with Cronassial (mixed gangliosides), which may pos-sess reinnervation-stimulating activities in neuropathies of various causes (2).—R.C. Schlant, M.D.

References

1. Hagar JM, et al: Chagas' heart disease in the United States. *N Engl J Med* 325:763–768, 1991.
2. Iosa D, et al: Chagas' cardioneuropathy: Effect of ganglioside treatment in chronic dysautonomic patients—a randomized, double-blind, parallel, placebo-controlled study. *Am Heart J* 122:775–785, 1991.

Reversibility of Cardiac Abnormalities in Human Immunodeficiency Virus (HIV)-Infected Individuals: A Serial Echocardiographic Study

Blanchard DG, Hagenhoff C, Chow LC, McCann HA, Dittrich HC (Univ of California, San Diego)
J Am Coll Cardiol 17:1270–1276, 1991   2–11

Introduction.—The occurrence of cardiac abnormalities has been reported in patients infected with HIV. Patients with HIV were studied prospectively using serial echocardiography to follow the evolution of cardiac lesions in these patients.

Patients.—The study population consisted of 69 men and 1 woman aged 24 to 64 years who were enrolled between January 1987 and June 1989. Fifty of the 70 patients had AIDS or AIDS-related complex and 20 had HIV infection but were asymptomatic. None of the patients had symptomatic heart disease at the start of the study. Forty-seven patients with AIDS or AIDS-related complex were taking zidovudine; the other 3 patients died before 1988. Eleven of the 20 asymptomatic patients were taking zidovudine, 8 were taking zidovudine or placebo, and 1 patient was lost to follow-up. All patients underwent baseline and follow-up echocardiography examinations at regular intervals.

Results.—During the study 22 patients with AIDS (44%) and 1 with HIV infection (5%) died. Follow-up echocardiographic studies were obtained at a mean of 9 months after baseline in 52 patients (74%) and again at a mean of 15 months after baseline in 29 patients (41%). Twenty-six of the 50 AIDS patients (52%) and 8 of the 20 HIV patients (40%) had cardiac abnormalities at baseline or at follow-up. Seven patients with AIDS had an abnormal left ventricular ejection fraction or fractional shortening at baseline, but 3 of them had normal left ventricular function on a later echocardiogram. All AIDS patients with left ventricular dysfunction on 2 serial studies died within 1 year after the baseline echocardiogram. One patient with HIV infection had persistent left ventricular dysfunction. The ejection fraction did not change between baseline and 2 follow-up studies in either group. Right-sided cardiac enlargement resolved in 5 of 10 AIDS patients and in 3 of 8 HIV patients. Pericardial effusions resolved in 5 of 12 AIDS patients and in 2 of 4 HIV patients. There was no association between the presence of left ventricular dysfunction or right-sided cardiac enlargement and CD4 counts.

Conclusions.—Echocardiographic abnormalities are common in asymptomatic patients with HIV infection. The prognosis in AIDS patients with persistent left ventricular dysfunction is poor. Transient left ventricular dysfunction, right-sided cardiac enlargement, and pericardial effusion are not consistently associated with clinically apparent intercurrent illnesses.

▶ As noted in the last two editions of the YEAR BOOK OF CARDIOLOGY, evidence of cardiac involvement in patients who have AIDS is relatively common, although patients rarely die directly from cardiac causes. It is very important to note not only that patients with AIDS frequently have echocardiographic evidence of left ventricular dysfunction, but also that the abnormalities often resolve spontaneously. Hakas and Generalovich (1) reported the spontaneous regression of heart muscle dysfunction in a patient with AIDS.—R.C. Schlant, M.D.

Reference

1. Hakas JF, et al: Spontaneous regression of cardiomyopathy in a patient with the acquired immunodeficiency syndrome. *Chest* 99:770–772, 1991.

Effects of Abstinence on Alcoholic Heart Muscle Disease
Jacob AJ, McLaren KM, Boon NA (Royal Infirmary, Edinburgh; Edinburgh Med School)
Am J Cardiol 68:805–807, 1991   2–12

Introduction.—There is anecdotal evidence that cardiac failure resulting from chronic alcoholism can be reversed with abstinence. To determine whether alcoholism is the sole cause of left ventricular dysfunction in a group of patients, thereby showing conclusively that alcoholic heart muscle disease is a reversible condition, 6 patients with a history of chronic alcohol abuse and concomitant heart failure were studied prospectively.

Methods.—The evaluation included ECG, chest roentgenography, and analysis of blood samples for hematologic indexes and renal and hepatic function. Coronary angiography was used to exclude ischemic heart disease and ultrasonography was used to assess left ventricular function and exclude valvular heart disease. The patients underwent serial radionuclide ventriculography over a period of up to 32 months using technetium-99m-labeled human serum albumin.

Results.—In the 3 patients who abstained from alcohol, there was a significant increase in left ventricular ejection fractions. Chest roentgenograms showed significant accompanying reductions in the cardiothoracic ratio. No such changes were apparent in the patients who continued to drink (Fig 2–5).

Conclusion.—A number of human, animal, and in vitro studies have confirmed that alcohol can damage heart muscle, though the mechanisms underlying such damage remain to be established. Hereditary factors, associated behavior, and malnutrition may also be involved in the damage to cardiac muscle. Alcoholic heart muscle disease can be reversed and emphasizes the need to encourage abstinence in patients with the disorder.

▶ This excellent study clearly demonstrates the value of abstinence in patients with alcoholic heart muscle disease. Other pertinent studies have shown that preclinical alcoholic heart muscle disease is relatively rare in chronic alcoholics less than 40 years of age (1), that left ventricular mass is related to alcohol use (2), but that the amount of left ventricular hypertrophy and dysfunction are poorly related to the duration and severity of self-reported alcohol abuse (3).—R.C. Schlant, M.D.

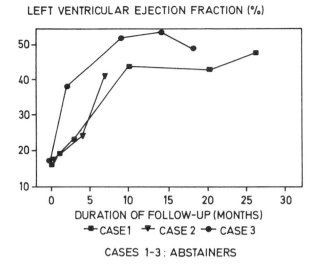

CASES 1-3 : ABSTAINERS

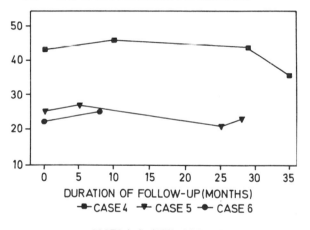

CASES 4-6 : NON-ABSTAINERS

Fig 2–5.—Left ventricular function in abstainers and nonabstainers. (Courtesy of Jacob AJ, McLaren KM, Boon NA: *Am J Cardiol* 68:805–807, 1991.)

References

1. Cerqueira MD, et al: Rarity of preclinical alcoholic cardiomyopathy in chronic alcoholics <40 years of age. *Am J Cardiol* 67:183–187, 1991.
2. Manolio TA, et al: Relation of alcohol intake to left ventricular mass: The Framingham Study. *J Am Coll Cardiol* 17:717–721, 1991.
3. Kupari M, et al: Left ventricular size, mass and function in relation to the duration and quantity of heavy drinking in alcoholics. *Am J Cardiol* 67:274–279, 1991.

Time of Onset of Supraventricular Tachyarrhythmia in Relation to Alcohol Consumption

Kupari M, Koskinen P (Helsinki Univ Central Hosp)
Am J Cardiol 67:718–722, 1991   2–13

Background.—Heavy alcohol consumption has been associated with supraventricular tachyarrhythmias. The onset of this condition was studied in 289 patients admitted to the emergency ward and its relation to alcohol use was evaluated.

Methods.—Each case was classified as disease-related or idiopathic on the basis of clinical examination, ECG, chest roentgenograms, laboratory tests, and previous cardiac studies. Alcohol consumption during the week preceding the event was also determined. Patients were screened for alcohol abuse.

Results.—Arrhythmias were idiopathic in 104 patients and disease-related in 185. There was an increased incidence of weekend arrhythmias in patients with idiopathic arrhythmias who had drunk alcohol during the last 7 days. In the disease-related arrhythmias group, there was no difference in the frequency of recent alcohol consumption and weekend or weekday episodes. Idiopathic arrhythmias on weekends were twice as likely to occur in heavy alcohol drinkers than in patients with weekday occurrences. The prevalence of postholiday arrhythmias was not significant.

Discussion.—Alcohol abuse was evident in more than double the number of patients who had idiopathic arrhythmias on the weekend, compared with those seen during the week. However, this finding may be of a relative rather than an absolute nature. Onset of arrhythmia was related to heavy alcohol consumption but not to most recent alcohol use.

▶ I have been impressed with several patients who have noted that they experience tachycardia (regular or irregular) approximately 5–8 hours after they begin moderate wine drinking (red or white) or about 3–6 hours after they finish, at a time well past when they would be expected to have their peak blood alcohol level. It is not known whether or not this delay in onset of tachycardia is related to levels of metabolites of ethyl alcohol, such as acetaldehyde or a delayed catecholamine release. In some patients who apparently are very sensitive to this effect of alcohol, the episodes of tachycardia can be prevented by the prophylactic use of a β-blocker.

During the Korean conflict, it was relatively common to see a number of Army recruits with acute atrial fibrillation on Sunday evening after their first weekend of leave from boot camp. In most instances, they had had little or no alcohol for at least the preceding 3–4 weeks; in most instances their atrial fibrillation resolved overnight with the help of digoxin.

Koskinen (1) found chronic alcohol intake in Finland, which is often moderately high, did not correlate with either recurrent atrial fibrillation or chronic atrial fibrillation. In my experience, I have had the impression that alcohol was a frequent cause of recurrent atrial fibrillation and probably contributed to the persistence of chronic atrial fibrillation in a significant number of patients.—R.C. Schlant, M.D.

Reference

1. Koskinen P: A 4-year prospective follow-up study of the role of alcohol in recurrences of atrial fibrillation. *J Intern Med* 230:423–426, 1991.

Echocardiographic Evidence for the Existence of a Distinct Diabetic Cardiomyopathy (The Framingham Heart Study)

Galderisi M, Anderson KM, Wilson PWF, Levy D (Framingham Heart Study, Framingham, Mass; National Heart, Lung, and Blood Inst, Bethesda, Md)
Am J Cardiol 68:85–89, 1991   2–14

Introduction.—Epidemiologic evidence indicates that persons with diabetes are at increased risk of cardiovascular morbidity and death, and there is some evidence that a diabetic cardiomyopathy exists that may be independent of coronary atherosclerosis. Left ventricular (LV) morphology and systolic function in relation to glucose intolerance were examined in subjects from the Framingham Study population.

Findings.—Glucose intolerance was demonstrated in 243 men (12.2% of those assessed) and 138 women (5.5%). In both sexes, diabetes was associated with higher heart rates. Women with diabetes had an increased LV wall thickness, LV end-diastolic dimension, and LV mass. Men with glucose intolerance exhibited increases in LV end-diastolic and end-systolic dimensions. Multivariate analysis suggested that LV mass increased disproportionately with advancing age in women with diabetes.

Conclusions.—Whereas many of the echocardiographic findings in persons with diabetes can be explained by concomitant factors (e.g., obesity, smoking, and hypertension), the study findings support an independent association between both LV mass and LV wall thickness and diabetes in women. Women with diabetes may have a distinctive cardiomyopathy.

▶ This study adds further epidemiologic support to the concept that diabetes mellitus is sometimes associated with a specific type of heart muscle disease even in patients without hypertension or significant coronary artery disease on coronary arteriography.—R.C. Schlant, M.D.

Left Ventricular Diastolic Filling Abnormalities Identified by Doppler Echocardiography in Asymptomatic Patients With Sickle Cell Anemia

Lewis JF, Maron BJ, Castro O, Moosa YA (Howard Univ, Washington, DC; Natl Heart, Lung, and Blood Inst, Natl Inst of Health, Bethesda, Md)
J Am Coll Cardiol 17:1473–1478, 1991   2–15

Introduction.—Patients with sickle cell anemia often have signs or symptoms of congestive heart failure. However, there is controversy over whether cardiomyopathy is part of the disease spectrum of sickle cell anemia because previous investigations of left ventricular (LV) function in patients with sickle cell anemia failed to demonstrate abnormalities in LV systolic performance. Whether or not these patients might have LV diastolic abnormalities that could serve as early subclinical markers of subsequent cardiac disease was investigated in an echocardiographic study.

Patients.—Two-dimensional Doppler echocardiographic studies were obtained in 15 men and 15 women aged 19–39 years with sickle cell anemia, and in 30 age-matched healthy volunteers without sickle cell anemia. Twenty-three patients (77%) had homozygous sickle cell anemia and 7 had the heterozygous form of the disease. None of the patients had experienced symptoms of heart failure and all had normal LV systolic function.

Results.—Seventeen patients (57%) had evidence of abnormal LV diastolic filling. Six of those 17 patients had a Doppler pattern consistent with restrictive filling characterized by abrupt and premature decrease in early diastolic flow velocity. The other 11 patients with restrictive filling showed a Doppler pattern consistent with impaired LV relaxation characterized by abnormally delayed early diastolic filling. The 13 patients without restrictive filling patterns showed normal transmitral flow velocity waveforms.

Conclusion.—Many patients with sickle cell anemia have abnormal LV filling patterns on Doppler echocardiographic studies, even in the absence of symptoms of heart failure or LV systolic dysfunction. However, the prognostic implications of abnormal Doppler diastolic indexes in sickle cell anemia remain to be determined.

▶ The clinical significance of the echocardiographic abnormalities of left ventricular diastolic function found in this study, which were not thought to be related to heart rate or loading conditions, must await a long-term follow-up.—R.C. Schlant, M.D.

Cardiomyopathy of the Aging Human Heart: Myocyte Loss and Reactive Cellular Hypertrophy
Olivetti G, Melissari M, Capasso JM, Anversa P (Univ of Parma, Italy; New York Med College, Valhalla)
Circ Res 68:1560–1568, 1991   2–16

Background.—It is well established that growth of the heart is controlled by hypertrophy of myocytes and hyperplasia of capillary endothelial cells and interstitial fibroblasts. The number of muscle cells or muscle cell nuclei in the tissue are not altered by DNA synthesis with ploidy formation in adult human cardiac myocytes. Therefore, the total number of myocytes or nuclei can be used as a marker for evaluation of the effects of aging on the myocardium. Myocyte cell loss throughout the human life span was studied to determine possible links to the occurrence of congestive heart failure in the elderly.

Method.—Sixty-seven human cadaver hearts were obtained from individuals aged 17–90 years who died of causes other than cardiovascular disease.

Findings.—Regression analysis determined that, in humans, 38 million myocyte nuclei from the left ventricle and 14 million myocyte nuclei from the right ventricle are lost during each year of life beyond sexual maturity. The myocyte cell volume per nucleus increased in both ventricles as a function of age, but the cellular hypertrophy was inadequate to preserve ventricular weight.

Conclusion.—Aging of the human heart is characterized by myocyte loss, reactive myocyte cellular hypertrophy, and reduction in ventricular mass. Alterations of the myocyte compartment of the myocardium are greater on the left side of the heart. These processes may be the underlying cause of the onset of myocardial dysfunction and failure in the elderly.

▶ The changes that occur in the heart of the aged were referred to as "presbycardia" by William Dock in an analogy with presbyopia. Whereas the aged heart changes significantly in structure and function as well as in reserve function, it is not well established that such changes, by themselves, result in heart failure in the absence of precipitating factors such as tachycardia, ischemia, or changes in afterload. Age-related alterations of left ventricular filling have again been noted in echocardiographic studies of apparently healthy elderly subjects (1).—R.C. Schlant, M.D.

Reference

1. Kitzman DW, et al: Age-related alterations of Doppler left ventricular filling indexes in normal subjects are independent of left ventricular mass, heart rate, contractility and loading conditions. *J Am Coll Cardiol* 18:1243–1250, 1991.

The Upper Limit of Physiologic Cardiac Hypertrophy in Highly Trained Elite Athletes

Pelliccia A, Maron BJ, Spataro A, Proschan MA, Spirito P (Comitato Olimpico Nazionale Italiano, Rome; Natl Heart, Lung, and Blood Inst, Bethesda, Md)
N Engl J Med 324:295–301, 1991   2–17

Background.—The "athlete's heart" is recognizable by increases in the diastolic dimension of the LV cavity, in the thickness of the LV mass, and in the calculated LV mass. The thickness of the LV wall may resemble cardiac disease such as hypertrophic cardiomyopathy. Differential diagnosis must distinguish between physiologic and pathologic hypertrophy.

Methods.—To study the upper limit of LV wall hypertrophy, echocardiographic measurements were taken of LV dimensions in 947 elite athletes.

Findings.—Left ventricular wall thickness of 13 mm or more is compatible with the diagnosis of hypertrophic cardiomyopathy. This thickness was found in 15 rowers or canoeists and 1 cyclist among 947 athletes. The group with a wall thickness of at least 13 mm represented only 7% of the 219 rowers, canoeists, and cyclists included in the total group of 947 athletes. The athletes with walls of at least 13 mm thickness also had enlarged LV end-diastolic cavities. The upper limit for wall thickness increased by athletic training was 16 mm.

Conclusion.—Although the recognized "athlete's heart" may have increased thickness of the LV wall, a thickness of 13 mm or more was found in only 16 of 947 elite athletes. An LV wall thickness of 16 mm was the upper limit found in these athletes. An athlete with a wall thickness of more than 16 mm and a nondilated LV cavity is likely to have primary pathologic hypertrophy (e.g., hypertrophic cardiomyopathy).

▶ An echocardiographic study of elite athletes in Scotland found an increase in the thickness of the ventricular septum, posterior LV wall, and LV mass index in association with normal left diastolic function (1). Another study found increased LV diastolic compliance and distensibility in athletes (2). These changes were suggested as being a mechanical, nonautonomic cause of the orthostatic hypotension that is occasionally noted in trained athletes.—R.C. Schlant, M.D.

References

1. McFarlane N, et al: A comparative study of left ventricular structure and function in elite athletes. *Br J Sports Med* 25:45–48, 1991.
2. Levine BD, et al: Left ventricular pressure-volume and Frank-Starling relations in endurance athletes. Implications for orthostatic tolerance and exercise performance. *Circulation* 84:1016–1023, 1991.

Preclinical Diagnosis of Familial Hypertrophic Cardiomyopathy by Genetic Analysis of Blood Lymphocytes

Rosenzweig A, Watkins H, Hwang D-S, Miri M, McKenna W, Traill TA, Seidman JG, Seidman CE (Massachusetts Gen Hosp, Boston; Harvard Med School; Brigham and Women's Hosp, Boston; St George's Hosp Med School, London; Taichung Veterans Gen Hosp, Taichung, Taiwan; et al)
N Engl J Med 325:1753–1760, 1991   2–18

Background.—It may be difficult to diagnose familial hypertrophic cardiomyopathy in childhood, because the characteristic clinical and echographic findings may not be present until adulthood. However, it is important to identify young individuals who are affected because sudden death may be the initial manifestation.

Method.—Mutations in the cardiac myosin heavy-chain genes cause familial hypertrophic cardiomyopathy in some families; therefore, a test was developed to detect mutations in the β myosin heavy-chain gene. The polymerase chain reaction technique was used to amplify β cardiac myosin heavy-chain messenger RNA (mRNA) from blood lymphocytes. The amplified base sequences were then analyzed with a ribonuclease protection assay to detect small deletions, abnormal splicing, and missense mutations.

Observations.—A novel missense mutation was found in a patient with familial hypertrophic cardiomyopathy. Fifteen adult relatives of the patient were evaluated; of these, 8 exhibited the mutation, whereas 7 did not. Only 1 of the 14 children in the family had typical echocardiographic findings, 7 of the 14 were found to have inherited the missense mutation.

Implications.—Transcripts of β cardiac myosin may be detected in blood lymphocytes and used to screen for the mutations causing familial hypertrophic cardiomyopathy. Preclinical diagnosis is now a possibility, and longitudinal studies may help identify factors that promote aberrant growth of the heart.

▶ The widespread availability of the diagnostic test used in this study will represent a major advance in our ability to identify subjects with very early, asymptomatic hypertrophic cardiomyopathy. As noted in last year's YEAR BOOK OF CARDIOLOGY, familial hypertrophic cardiomyopathy is a genetically heterogeneous disease. One recent study has provided additional evidence that many persons with hypertrophic cardiomyopathy have a locus in chromosome 14q1 (1).—R.C. Schlant, M.D.

Reference

1. Hejtmancik F, et al: Localization of gene for familial hypertrophic cardiomyopathy to chromosome 14q1 in a diverse US population. *Circulation* 83:1592–1597, 1991.

Quantitative Assessment of Ultrasonic Myocardial Reflectivity in Hypertrophic Cardiomyopathy

Lattanzi F, Spirito P, Picano E, Mazzarisi A, Landini L, Distante A, Vecchio C, L'Abbate A (Univ of Pisa; Ente Ospedaliero Ospedali Galliera, Genoa, Italy)
J Am Coll Cardiol 17:1085–1090, 1991   2–19

Introduction.—Conventional echocardiography in patients with hypertrophic cardiomyopathy often shows increased ultrasonic (US) reflectivity of the left ventricular (LV) wall. However, interpretation of this US feature has been hampered by the operator-dependent measures of individual echocardiographic instruments. The relation between the acoustic properties of the myocardium and the magnitude of LV hypertrophy in patients with hypertrophic cardiomyopathy was investigated.

Patients.—M-mode echocardiographic studies were obtained in 25 patients ages 17–60 years with confirmed hypertrophic cardiomyopathy and in 25 normal age-matched controls. Twenty patients were asymptomatic or had only mild cardiac symptoms and 5 patients had moderate-to-severe symptoms. An online radio frequency analysis system was used to obtain quantitative operator-independent measurements of the integrated backscatter signal of the ventricular septum and of the posterior free wall. The backscatter signal was acquired at end diastole. Integrated radio frequency signal values were expressed in percent of normal pericardial interface values.

Results.—Technically satisfactory conventional echocardiographic images and radio frequency US signals were obtained in all 50 studies. The mean thickness of hypertrophied LV septum was 20 mm compared with a 9-mm LV septum thickness in normal controls. Patients and controls both had a mean posterior free wall thickness of 9 mm. Compared with control values, tissue reflectivity values for both hypertrophied LV septum and nonhypertrophied posterior free wall were significantly increased in patients with hypertrophic cardiomyopathy, even in the 5 patients with only mild and localized LV hypertrophy. Thus, most patients with hypertrophic cardiomyopathy will have abnormal myocardial reflectivity that is largely independent of the degree of LV hypertrophy.

Conclusion.—Quantitative measurement of US myocardial reflectivity can be used to differentiate patients with hypertrophic cardiomyopathy from normal controls.

▶ This interesting technique will be of great diagnostic value when it is confirmed in larger studies. At present, the echocardiographic diagnosis of hypertrophic cardiomyopathy can be very difficult in many patients with early or milder forms of the disease. The technique described in Abstract 2–18 will also add significantly to our diagnostic capabilities.—R.C. Schlant, M.D.

Sudden Death During Empiric Amiodarone Therapy in Symptomatic Hypertrophic Cardiomyopathy
Fananapazir L, Leon MB, Bonow RO, Tracy CM, Cannon RO III, Epstein SE (Natl Heart, Lung, and Blood Inst, Bethesda, Md)
Am J Cardiol 67:169–174, 1991   2–20

Background.—Patients with hypertrophic cardiomyopathy using amiodarone for ventricular tachycardia (VT) reported symptomatic improvement unrelated to control of arrhythmias. Symptomatic relief of refractory symptoms was assessed prospectively in patients using amiodarone, and the effect of amiodarone on VT as detected by Holter monitoring was evaluated. Reportedly, empiric amiodarone therapy entirely prevents sudden death in patients with VT and hypertrophic cardiomyopathy.

Methods.—Amiodarone treatment was initiated in 50 patients with hypertrophic cardiomyopathy for symptoms refractory to calcium antagonists and β-adrenergic blocking drugs. Treatment includes a loading period of 38 days and a maintenance dose of 400 mg/day. Dosage was adjusted by symptomatology and blood level. Twenty-one of the patients (42%) had VT during Holter monitoring.

Results.—Amiodarone significantly improved the patients' symptoms and exercise capacity. Left ventricular diastolic filling was favorably influenced by amiodarone in most patients, and the incidence of nonsustained VT during Holter monitoring was reduced. However, 6 sudden deaths occurred within 5 months (mean, 2.5 months) of initiation of treatment, and a total of 8 deaths occurred during a mean follow-up of 2 years. The 6-month mortality rate was higher (38%) in patients with VT than in patients without VT (3%) on ambulatory monitoring. A decrease in the peak left ventricular filling rate within 10 days of starting amiodarone therapy was associated with sudden death.

Conclusion.—Amiodarone significantly improved refractory symptoms in patients with hypertrophic cardiomyopathy. However, contrary to earlier reports, amiodarone was implicated as contributing to the unexpectedly high frequency of early sudden death. The occurrence of sudden death clustered around 5–20 weeks from initiation of amiodarone treatment, and the survival rate was significantly worse in patients with VT. Amiodarone may provoke malignant arrhythmias or conduction abnormalities, particularly in patients with reduced left ventricular diastolic filling associated with exposure to the drug.

Arrhythmias in Hypertrophic Cardiomyopathy
Stewart JT, McKenna WJ (St George's Hosp Med School, London)
J Cardiovasc Electrophysiol 2:516–524, 1991   2–21

Introduction.—Various arrhythmias, especially atrial fibrillation and nonsustained ventricular tachycardia (VT), are common in adults with hypertrophic cardiomyopathy. The annual mortality rate of sudden cardiac death is 2% to 3%. In children and adolescents, sudden death may be the first indication of the disease.

Types of Arrhythmia.—Paroxysmal supraventricular tachycardia occurs in up to half of all adults with hypertrophic cardiomyopathy. Atrial fibrillation is the most frequent type of supraventricular arrhythmia. Patients who have this arrhythmia and whose left ventricular function is impaired may deteriorate symptomatically. Sustained clinical monomorphic VT is rare in hypertrophic cardiomyopathy, but nonsustained VT occurs frequently. The latter arrhythmia is always asymptomatic and appears to be benign. The factors associated with sudden death include a diagnosis in childhood or adolescence; a positive family history of the disease and of sudden death; and syncopal episodes.

Management.—Atrial fibrillation commonly has little effect on functional status if the ventricular rate is controlled. Digoxin is usually an appropriate treatment. Amiodarone may be helpful if paroxysmal fibrillation is present. Low-dose amiodarone improves short- and medium-term survival in patients with nonsustained VT. Use of the automatic implantable cardioverter-defibrillator is reasonable if sustained tachyarrhythmia is documented in a treatment-resistant patient.

▶ In the study of Fananapazir et al. (Abstract 2–20), a disturbing number of patients died suddenly while on empiric amiodarone therapy despite careful monitoring. Of the 7 patients who died suddenly, 3 had a history of syncope, but none had VT on ambulatory electrocardiographic monitoring after 10 days and 2 months of amiodarone treatment. Two closely related papers from the same institute describe the value of electrophysiologic studies (EPS) in such patients, especially those who survive cardiac arrest (1,2). They found amiodarone to cause important conduction abnormalities in about 20% of patients and to facilitate the induction of VT in about half of patients (1). These reports and a subsequent case report (3) raise serious implications for the safety and cost-benefit ratio of empiric amiodarone therapy in these patients. It would appear prudent to perform careful EPS when initiating amiodarone therapy in patients with hypertrophic cardiomyopathy to identify those who should receive a pacemaker and those in whom such therapy should be discontinued. Although Stewart and McKenna (Abstract 2–21) advised empiric treatment with low-dose amiodarone in patients in whom nonsustained VT is found on ambulatory ECG recording, such therapy may be associated with a high incidence of sudden death. Thus, a more complete evaluation, including EPS and cardiac catheterization and, at times, treadmill exercise testing, echocardiography, signal-averaged electrocardiography, radionuclide angiography, and thallium scintigraphy, would appear to be appropriate for such patients (4).—R.C. Schlant, M.D.

References

1. Fananapazir L, et al: Value of electrophysiologic studies in hypertrophic cardiomyopathy treated with amiodarone. *Am J Cardiol* 67:175–182, 1991.
2. Fananapazir L, et al: Hemodynamic and electrophysiologic evaluation of patients with hypertrophic cardiomyopathy surviving cardiac arrest. *Am J Cardiol* 67:280–287, 1991.
3. Gilligan DM, et al: Sudden death due to ventricular tachycardia during amiodarone therapy in familial hypertrophic cardiomyopathy. *Am J Cardiol* 68:971–973, 1991.
4. Fananapazir L, et al: Investigation and clinical significance of arrhythmias in patients with hypertrophic cardiomyopathy. *J Cardiovasc Electrophysiol* 2:525–530, 1991.

Primary Restrictive Cardiomyopathy: Clinical and Pathologic Characteristics

Katritsis D, Wilmshurst PT, Wendon JA, Davies MJ, Webb-Peploe MM (St Thomas' Hosp, London; St George's Hosp, London)

J Am Coll Cardiol 18:1230–1235, 1991   2–22

Case Definition.—Among more than 11,000 patients having diagnostic cardiac catheterization in a 17-year period were 24 who received a diagnosis of restrictive cardiomyopathy. The patients had a history of cardiac failure and increased ventricular filling pressures, but the left ventricular end-diastolic volume index was normal and there was no coronary artery or valvular disease. In addition, hypertrophic cardiomyopathy was excluded.

Histologic Findings.—Ten of the 24 patients had primary restrictive cardiomyopathy with findings of myocyte hypertrophy and/or interstitial fibrosis. Seven other patients had amyloidosis, and 1 each had findings of hemochromatosis and systemic sclerosis. Two patients had nonspecific abnormalities associated with clinical and serologic features of acute viral myocarditis.

Outcome.—Patients with amyloid changes had a worse outlook than those with primary restrictive cardiomyopathy. Four of the latter patients had permanent complete heart block and 2 of those had skeletal myopathy, features not found in patients with amyloidosis. Hemodynamic abnormalities were comparable in the 2 groups of patients. In each group, survival was related to the cardiac index but not to filling pressures.

Implications.—Patients with primary restrictive cardiomyopathy have a better prognosis than those with amyloid changes. All patients with restrictive cardiomyopathy should undergo endomyocardial biopsy. Family surveillance is appropriate when amyloidosis and other specific cardiac muscle disorders are ruled out.

▶ It should be noted that it may be impossible to distinguish between primary restrictive cardiomyopathy and cardiac amyloidosis on either clinical and echocardiographic findings. In general, an endomyocardial biopsy is appropriate in most patients with restrictive cardiomyopathy. In patients with cardiac amyloidosis, the strongest echocardiographic predictors of cardiac death were the Doppler variables of shortened deceleration time and an increased ratio of early diastolic filling velocity to atrial filling velocity (1). Early idiopathic hemochromatosis may also produce a clinical and echocardiographic syndrome of restrictive cardiomyopathy, whereas in its more advanced state with increased iron overload, hemochromatosis results in a heart muscle disease that clinically resembles primary, idiopathic dilated cardiomyopathy (2).—R.C. Schlant, M.D.

References

1. Klein AL, et al: Prognostic significance of Doppler measures of diastolic function in cardiac amyloidosis. A Doppler echocardiography study. *Circulation* 83:808–816, 1991.
2. Cecchetti G, et al: Cardiac alterations in 36 consecutive patients with idiopathic haemochromatosis: Polygraphic and echocardiographic evaluation. *Eur Heart J* 12:224–230, 1991.

Pericardial Diseases

Tuberculous Pericarditis
Fowler NO (Univ of Cincinnati)
JAMA 266:99–103, 1991   2–23

Introduction.—Tuberculosis is an infrequent cause of pericarditis in the United States today, but cases do continue to be seen, especially in AIDS patients. Pericarditis develops in an estimated 1% to 2% of patients with pulmonary tuberculosis. In addition to constrictive or effusive-constrictive pericarditis, complications include myocarditis, spread to other organs, and cardiac tamponade.

Clinical Features.—Patients are seen most often with dyspnea, cough, and weight loss. Hepatic congestion may produce right upper-quadrant pain. Cardiomegaly and fever are frequently noted; tachycardia, pulsus paradoxus, and hepatomegaly are also seen, but less frequently. Patients with constrictive pericarditis may have inspiratory swelling of the neck veins. The echographic findings are nonspecific. The ECG characteristically exhibits low-voltage QRS and inverted T waves. Hemodynamic findings may be normal in the phase of fibrinous pericarditis or in pericardial effusion without cardiac tamponade.

Management.—Triple drug therapy is recommended for at least 9 months, and for 6 months or longer after culture conversion. Prednisone may be added if pericardial effusion persists or recurs despite antituberculosis drug therapy. Some have recommended pericardiectomy for all patients having tuberculous pericarditis.

AIDS Patients.—Tuberculous pericarditis may be an initial manifestation of AIDS. However, AIDS appears to limit the inflammatory response to tubercle bacilli, and cardiac tamponade or constrictive pericarditis may be less frequent in patients who have both AIDS and tuberculosis.

▶ Tuberculous pericarditis is increasingly important because of the current epidemic of AIDS and because of the more recent increased prevalence of tuberculosis. Part of the increase in the number of cases of tuberculosis is caused by drug-resistant organisms. It should be emphasized that about half of patients with AIDS and tuberculous pericarditis have a negative PPD skin test. Frequently, the diagnosis of tuberculous pericarditis is greatly enhanced by histologic examination of a pericardial biopsy. In one series, an increase in the concentration of adenosine desaminase in pericardial fluid to above 60 μ/L was found to have 100% sensitivity and 80% specificity for the diagnosis of tuberculous pericarditis (1). Some of the other causes of elevation in its concentration include neoplasia, lymphoma, bacterial infection, sarcoidosis, and collagen vascular disease.—R.C. Schlant, M.D.

Reference

1. Telenti M, et al: Pericardite tuberculeuse: Valeur diagnostique de l'adenosine desaminase. *La Presse Med* 20:637–640, 1991.

Heart Failure

Current Role of Digitalis Therapy in Patients With Congestive Heart Failure

Kulick DL, Rahimtoola SH (Univ of Southern California School of Medicine, Los Angeles)

JAMA 265:2995–2997, 1991
                                                                    2–24

Clinical Effects.—A great majority of studies have shown digitalis to have considerable clinical advantage in patients with congestive heart failure of varying severity. Hemodynamic and symptomatic improvement are documented both at rest and on exercise. Digitalis can improve left ventricular (LV) systolic performance in patients with congestive heart failure. Functional exercise capacity has improved in most, but not all, studies.

Treatment Policy.—Patients with class III or class IV congestive heart failure are logically treated initially with digitalis, diuretics, and vasodilators. Single-drug treatment generally is less than optimal, even in patients with less severe congestive heart failure. Digitalis alone probably will not control the sodium and water retention associated with severe LV dysfunction. Digitalis has the advantages of being both well tolerated and effective in a single daily dose.

Asymptomatic Patients.—Digitalis reduces LV end-diastolic pressure and increases LV systolic performance in patients recovering from acute myocardial infarction. Reduced LV volume has been reported in patients with severe coronary artery disease but no symptoms of congestive heart failure. The clinical importance of digitalis administration to asymptomatic patients remains to be determined. Careful dosing will limit the potential arrhythmogenic, neurologic, and gastrointestinal side effects of digitalis.

▶ This is an excellent, balanced review of the current state of knowledge regarding the use of digitalis in heart failure. Digitalis remains an important component of the therapy of patients with moderate or severe heart failure with systolic ventricular dysfunction, whether or not the patient is in sinus rhythm. On the other hand, patients who have diastolic left ventricular dysfunction but have normal systolic function and normal sinus rhythm are unlikely to benefit from digitalis or any other currently available predominantly inotropic agent.— R.C. Schlant, M.D.

Effect of Oral Milrinone on Mortality in Severe Chronic Heart Failure

The PROMISE Study Research Group (Mt Sinai School of Medicine, New York)
N Engl J Med 325:1468–1475, 1991   2–25

Background.—Milrinone is a phosphodiesterase inhibitor, which enhances cardiac contractility by increasing intracellular levels of cyclic adenosine monophosphate. In a double-blind, placebo-controlled trial, 1,088 patients with severe chronic heart failure were studied to determine the long-term effect of milrinone on patient survival. The median period of follow-up was 6 months.

Results.—Milrinone treatment was associated with a 28% increase in mortality from all causes (Fig 2–6) and a 34% increase in cardiovascular mortality, as compared with placebo treatment. The adverse effect of milrinone was greatest in those patients with the most severe symptoms. Milrinone had no beneficial effects on the survival of any subgroup within the study. Patients treated with milrinone had significantly more

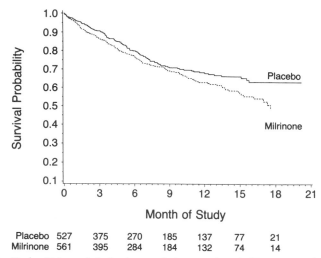

Fig 2–6.—Kaplan-Meier analysis showing cumulative rates of survival in patients with chronic heart failure treated with milrinone or placebo. Mortality was 28% higher in the milrinone group than in the placebo group (*P* = .038). The numbers of patients at risk are shown at the bottom of the figure. (Courtesy of PROMISE Study Research Group: *N Engl J Med* 325:1468–1475, 1991.)

hospitalizations, withdrawal from therapy, and adverse reactions than those treated with placebo.

Conclusion.—Long-term therapy with the positive inotropic drug, milrinone, increases morbidity and mortality in patients with severe chronic heart failure. The mechanisms of the adverse effects of this drug remain unknown.

► This is an important negative study. The negative results in patients with chronic heart failure in this study resemble the results of previous studies of the chronic use of other phosphodiesterase inhibitors. On the other hand, some phosphodiesterase inhibitors can be of significant benefit when given acutely for short periods of time to patients with systolic ventricular dysfunction.— R.C. Schlant, M.D.

Effect of Enalapril on Survival in Patients With Reduced Left Ventricular Ejection Fractions and Congestive Heart Failure
Studies of Left Ventricular Dysfunction (SOLVD) investigators (Natl Heart, Lung and Blood Inst, Bethesda, Md)
N Engl J Med 325:293–302, 1991   2–26

Background.—Because congestive heart failure is frequent, often requires hospitalization, and has a high mortality, even a moderately effective agent could prevent thousands of hospitalizations and premature deaths each year. The angiotensin-converting-enzyme inhibitor enalapril in patients receiving conventional treatment for heart failure was evaluated.

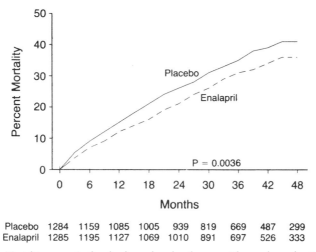

Fig 2–7.—Mortality curves in the placebo and enalapril groups. The numbers of patients alive in each group at the end of each period are shown at the bottom of the figure. $P = .0036$ for the comparison between groups by the log-rank test. (Courtesy of Studies of Left Ventricular Dysfunction investigators: *N Engl J Med* 325:293–302, 1991.)

Randomization.—A placebo-controlled trial was carried out in 2,569 patients who initially had an ejection fraction of .35 or less and were already taking drugs other than an angiotensin-converting-enzyme inhibitor. Patients randomized to receive enalapril took 2.5 or 5 mg twice daily. If there were no side effects, the dose was titrated up to a maximum of 10 mg twice daily. Follow-up averaged 41 months.

Results.—Mortality was 16% lower in enalapril-treated patients (Fig 2–7). The difference was most marked in the first 2 years of follow-up. The chief difference in mortality involved deaths caused by progressive heart failure (Fig 2–8). Hospitalization for heart failure was 26% less frequent in the enalapril group than in placebo recipients. Blood pressure was significantly lower in patients given enalapril, and there were small but significant increases in serum potassium and creatinine levels in this group.

Conclusions.—Enalapril significantly lowered mortality and hospitalization for congestive heart failure in this trial. The results are encouraging, but cannot be extrapolated to asymptomatic patients having only a low ejection fraction. Most treatments probably will not lower overall mortality by more than 10% to 20% unless they influence more than 1 mechanism of death.

▶ It is important to note the characteristics of the patients who received enalapril in this study. At baseline, 11.4% were in New York Heart Association functional class I, 56.8% were in class II, 30.1% in class III, and only 1.5% in class IV. Their other therapy included digitalis (65.7%), diuretics (85.6%), nitrates (39.6%), calcium-channel blockers (29.4%), anticoagulants (15.8%), and antiplatelet agents (32.9%). It would appear reasonable today to use triple ther-

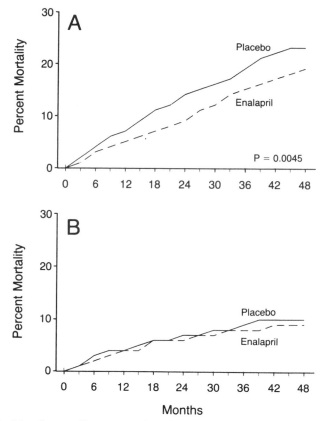

Fig 2–8.—Mortality caused by progressive heart failure (**A**) (P = .0045) and presumed to be a result of an arrhythmia but not preceded by worsening congestive heart failure (**B**) (P is not significant). (Courtesy of Studies of Left Ventricular Dysfunction investigators: *N Engl J Med* 325:293–302, 1991.)

apy (digitalis, diuretic and angiotensin-converting-enzyme inhibitor) as standard therapy for patients with moderate-to-severe heart failure associated with decreased systolic left ventricular function.—R.C. Schlant, M.D.

A Comparison of Enalapril With Hydralazine-Isosorbide Dinitrate in the Treatment of Chronic Congestive Heart Failure

Cohn JN, Johnson G, Ziesche S, Cobb F, Francis G, Tristani F, Smith R, Dunkman WB, Loeb H, Wong M, Bhat G, Goldman S, Fletcher RD, Doherty J, Hughes CV, Carson P, Cintron G, Shabetai R, Haakenson C (Univ of Minnesota Med School, Minneapolis)
N Engl J Med 325:303–310, 1991   2–27

Objective.—The efficacy of vasodilator therapy for chronic congestive heart failure was examined in 804 men receiving digoxin and

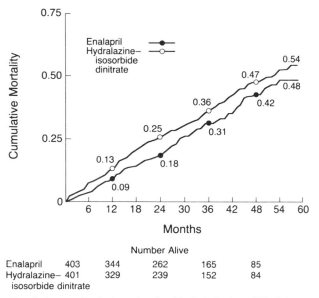

Fig 2–9.—Cumulative mortality in the enalapril and hydralazine-isosorbide dinitrate treatment arms over the entire follow-up period. Cumulative mortality rates are shown after each 12-month period. For the comparison of the treatment arms after 2 years and overall, $P = .016$ and $P = .08$, respectively (log-rank test). The number of patients alive after each year is shown below the graph. (Courtesy of Cohn JN, Johnson G, Ziesche S, et al: *N Engl J Med* 325:303–310, 1991.)

diuretic therapy. The patients, aged 18–75 years, had chronic heart failure and were seen at 13 Veterans Affairs medical centers. They were assigned to receive either 20 mg of enalapril or 300 mg of hydralazine plus 160 mg of isosorbide dinitrate daily. The average follow-up was 2½ years.

Findings.—Enalapril-treated patients had significantly lower mortality 2 years after randomization (Fig 2–9). Sudden deaths in particular were less frequent in the enalapril group, especially in patients with less marked symptoms. The left ventricular ejection fraction increased earlier in the study in patients given hydralazine-isosorbide dinitrate. Exercise tolerance increased only in these patients; but after 1 year, it declined in both groups. Azotemia was more frequent in enalapril-treated patients.

Discussion.—Enalapril and hydralazine-isosorbide dinitrate have independent beneficial effects in patients with chronic heart failure. Both their combined use and earlier intervention should be considered.

▶ In this study, the reduction in mortality with enalapril was significantly greater than with hydralazine-isosorbide dinitrate, although the latter produced more improvement in exercise performance and left ventricular function. It is hoped that future studies will evaluate the potential benefit of using both therapies in addition to digitalis and diuretics. In the meantime, it would be appropriate to treat most patients with moderate or severe heart failure caused bysystolic dysfunction with triple therapy (including digoxin, diuretic and an angiotensin-converting-enzyme inhibitor) as noted above.— R.C. Schlant, M.D.

Increased Plasma Level of Substance P in Patients With Severe Congestive Heart Failure Treated With ACE Inhibitors
Valdemarsson S, Edvinsson L, Ekman R, Hedner P, Sjöholm A (Univ Hosp, Lund, Sweden)
J Intern Med 230:325–331, 1991   2–28

Introduction.—With the identification of the detrimental effects resulting from increased conversion of angiotensinogen to angiotensin II (AII) in patients with congestive heart failure, some of these patients are now treated with angiotensin-converting-enzyme (ACE) inhibitors. The extent to which the addition of ACE inhibitors to conventional digoxin and diuretic therapy might affect the vasoregulatory systems known to be activated in congestive heart failure was investigated in 42 patients.

Methods.—Of the patients, 10 were in New York Heart Association (NYHA) class I or II and 32 were in NYHA class III or IV. Most had been conventionally treated for congestive heart failure, and 15 of those in NYHA class III or IV were also receiving ACE inhibitors at the time that they were first seen. The variables studied were compared with those for 31 healthy controls.

Results.—Catecholamines and neuropeptide Y-like immunoreactivity (NPY-LI) were increased to the same extent in patients with severe congestive heart failure with or without ACE inhibition. Calcitonin gene-related peptide (CGRP-LI) was not affected by ACE inhibitors and showed no changes relative to controls in any of the patient groups. All patient groups had a significant increase in the substance P level. In patients with severe congestive heart failure on ACE inhibition, the mean substance P level was 4.05 pmol I^{-1}; the mean concentration was 2.28 pmol I^{-1} in patients with a comparable degree of congestive heart failure but without ACE inhibition. These 2 groups had similar increases in the atrial natriuretic peptide level, but patients receiving ACE inhibitors had significantly lower vasopressin levels (Fig 2–10).

Conclusion.—Patients with congestive heart failure show increased activity of the nerve fiber system as well as of the sympathetic and renin-angiotensin systems. These findings suggest that there are additional mechanisms in the beneficial effect of ACE inhibitors in congestive heart failure.

► This study adds to the important information about the many mechanisms by which ACE inhibitors benefit patients with heart failure. The addition of ACE inhibitors to the treatment of patients with heart failure has been a major therapeutic advance. It is likely that future studies will add even more mechanisms by which such therapy is of benefit.— R.C. Schlant, M.D.

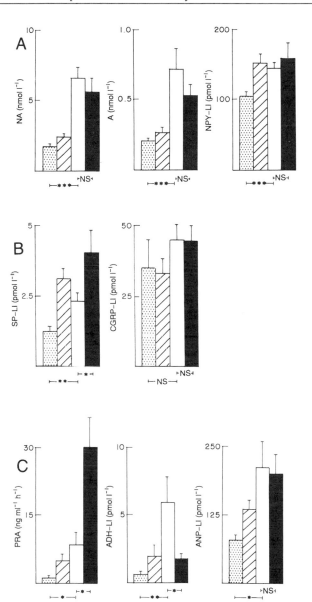

Fig 2–10.—Plasma levels of (**A**) noradrenaline *(NA)*, adrenaline *(A)*, and neuropeptide Y (NPY-LI–like immunoreactivity), (**B**) substance P *(SP-LI)* and calcitonin gene-related peptide *(CGRP-LI)*, and (**C**) renin activity *(PRA)*, arginine-vasopressin *(ADH-LI)* and h-α-atrial natriuretic peptide *(ANP-LI)* in healthy persons (n = 31, *dotted bars*), patients with mild congestive heart failure (NYHA I–II, n = 10, *hatched bars*), patients with severe congestive heart failure (NYHA III–IV, n = 17, *open bars*) and patients with severe congestive heart failure on ACE inhibition (NYHA III–IV, n = 15, *closed bars*). *Asterisk* indicates P < .05; *double asterisk,* P < .01; *triple asterisk,* P < .0001. (Courtesy of Valdemarsson S, Edvinsson L, Ekman R, et al: *J Intern Med* 230:325–331, 1991.)

Usefulness of OPC-8212, a Quinolinone Derivative, for Chronic Congestive Heart Failure in Patients With Ischemic Heart Disease or Idiopathic Dilated Cardiomyopathy

Feldman AM, Baughman KL, Lee WK, Gottlieb SH, Weiss JL, Becker LC, Strobeck JE (Johns Hopkins Univ; The Valley Hosp, Ridgewood, NJ)
Am J Cardiol 68:1203–1210, 1991   2–29

Background.—Attempts to treat chronic congestive heart failure caused by left ventricular systolic dysfunction with inotropic agents have not provided clear cut results. A placebo-controlled, randomized trial of the inotropic drug OPC-8212 was undertaken in 76 patients with chronic congestive heart failure to examine its safety and efficacy.

Procedure.—Patients were randomly allocated to receive 12 weeks of double-blind therapy with either OPC-8212 or placebo in addition to their normal medication. The primary study outcome was the time to mortality or substantial worsening of heart failure.

Results.—Over the 12 weeks of therapy, treatment with OPC-8212 significantly decreased major morbidity and mortality (Fig 2–11). Quality of life was also significantly improved in those receiving the drug. Ventricular premature contractions were not increased by OPC-8212 therapy.

Conclusion.—The inotropic agent, OPC-8212, can be useful in the treatment of patients with chronic congestive heart failure. Further

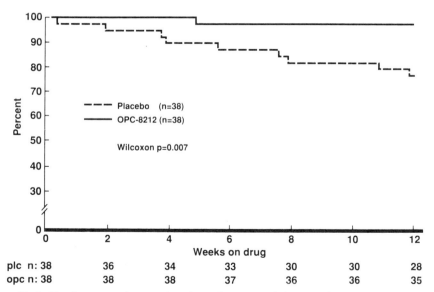

Fig 2–11.—Percentage of patients free of mortality or a morbid event in the OPC-8212 *(opc)* and placebo *(plc)* group during treatment period. The statistical difference between the curves was analyzed with the Peto-Prentice Wilcoxon test. (Courtesy of Feldman AM, Baughman KL, Lee WK, et al: *Am J Cardiol* 68:1203–1210, 1991.)

studies of this drug in a larger patient population should be undertaken.

▶ The drug OPC-8212 is an interesting new inotropic agent for the treatment of patients with heart failure. Unfortunately, it is not possible to determine the number of patients in each group in this report who were also receiving digoxin, although the dosage was routinely adjusted to .125 mg/day, and the mean blood digoxin level was .84 in patients receiving OPC-8212. It is to be hoped that ongoing studies of OPC-8212 will show that the incidence of neutropenia is not excessive, and that OPC-8212 will prove to be a useful additional agent for the treatment of patients with heart failure.—R.C. Schlant, M.D.

Long-Term (2 Year) Beneficial Effects of Beta-Adrenergic Blockade With Bucindolol in Patients With Idiopathic Dilated Cardiomyopathy

Anderson JL, Gilbert EM, O'Connell JB, Renlund D, Yanowitz F, Murray M, Roskelley M, Mealey P, Volkman K, Deitchman D, Bristow M (Univ of Utah, Salt Lake City)
J Am Coll Cardiol 17:1373–1381, 1991   2–30

Background.—Idiopathic dilated cardiomyopathy affects a greater proportion of patients under age 50 than ischemic heart disease. Beta-adrenergic blocking agents are an effective, but still unconventional, therapy. Bucindolol, a nonselective β-blocking agent with "nonspecific" vasodilator properties, is well tolerated in small, gradually ascending doses in patients with idiopathic dilated cardiomyopathy. In an earlier study, the short-term effects of bucindolol versus placebo were measured over 90 days. In this study, the short-term response was compared with response during 2-year long-term maintenance therapy.

Methods.—The long-term assessment was made in 20 patients who completed the 90-day study. The hypothesis was that the initial beneficial results would be maintained or augmented over the long term.

Results.—The beneficial effects of β-blockade with bucindolol observed during the short-term 90-day trial persisted during long-term maintenance therapy. Left ventricular ejection fraction and functional class were maintained or improved in most patients. Stable exercise performance and maximal oxygen uptake were maintained. Concurrent therapy included diuretics (90%), digoxin (75%), angiotensin-converting-enzyme inhibitor drugs (65%), warfarin (45%), and anti-arrhythmic agents (25%).

Conclusions.—Beta-blocker therapy provided both short- and long-term benefit in patients with idiopathic dilated cardiomyopathy. Bucindolol provided excellent drug tolerance, survival rate, and functional efficacy. Left ventricular ejection fraction and functional class were maintained or improved in most patients. Beta-blocker therapy merits further evaluation, especially in patients with idiopathic dilated cardiomyopathy, functional classes II and III.

Exercise Hemodynamics and Myocardial Metabolism During Long-Term Beta-Adrenergic Blockade in Severe Heart Failure

Andersson B, Blomström-Lundqvist C, Hedner T, Waagstein F (Sahlgren's Univ Hosp, Göteborg, Sweden)
J Am Coll Cardiol 18:1059–1066, 1991   2–31

Introduction.—Recent long-term trials in patients with congestive heart failure showed that β-blocker therapy protects the failing heart by reducing adrenergic overstimulation. However, the precise mechanism responsible for this improvement is still poorly understood. Whether the beneficial effects of long-term β-blockade on hemodynamics and myocardial metabolism seen in patients with severe congestive heart failure at rest are maintained during exercise was examined in 21 patients.

Methods.—The patients, aged 24–67 years, were investigated by 2-dimensional echocardiography or radionuclide angiocardiography at rest and during maximal exercise on a sitting bicycle before and after long-term metoprolol therapy. Thirteen patients had congestive heart failure resulting from idiopathic dilated cardiomyopathy, 6 as a result of ischemic cardiomyopathy, 1 had congestive heart failure after valve replacement, and 1 had rheumatic cardiomyopathy. Metoprolol was slowly titrated up to a final mean dose of 127 mg/day; the final dose was determined by clinical status and adverse effects.

Results.—The mean functional capacity increased during long-term metoprolol therapy. The maximal working capacity increased by 25%. That increment was comparable with the increment achieved by treatment with angiotensin-converting-enzyme inhibitors. Cardiac output and filling pressures improved at rest. After β-blocker therapy, arterial pressure, cardiac output, and stroke work were increased during exercise, but heart rate and filling pressures remained unchanged. Metoprolol reduced the number of lactate producers and did not change myocardial oxygen consumption or total coronary sinus flow. Patients with nonischemic cardiomyopathy appeared to benefit more from metoprolol than did patients with coronary artery disease. Whereas some patients with nonischemic cardiomyopathy showed remarkable clinical improvement, those with ischemic cardiomyopathy showed no obvious improvement. Patients with very severe heart failure and extensive myocardial damage did not appear to improve with long-term β-blockade. These patients may not have enough viable myocardium and thus blockade of the few remaining β-receptors would lead to inotropic failure.

Conclusion.—Long-term β-blocker therapy in patients with congestive heart failure improves working capacity, filling pressures, and cardiac output. Circulating arterial norepinephrine levels decrease and myocardial energetics improve, allowing increased myocardial work load without higher metabolic costs.

▶ These two studies (Abstracts 2–30 and 2–31) lend further support to the very careful use of β-blockers in the therapy of highly selected patients with heart failure. In the first study (Abstract 2–30), bucindolol was initiated at a dose of 12.5 mg twice daily. The dose was slowly increased at no less than 1 week intervals to 25, 50, and finally 100 mg twice daily during careful monitoring. Most patients in this trial were maintained on traditional triple therapy for heart failure. In the second study (Abstract 2–31), metoprolol was begun at a dose of 5 mg twice a day and the dosage was increased very slowly up to a mean total daily dose of 127 mg. Details of concurrent therapy were not provided in the second study. It is noteworthy that in the second study, which was done in Sweden, patients with ischemic heart muscle disease ("cardiomyopathy") showed no obvious improvement. That group reported an impression that patients with "very severe heart failure and extensive myocardial damage represent a group that does not improve with long-term β-blockade."

These two studies add further support for an ongoing large clinical trial evaluating the use of β-blocker therapy to up-regulate the β-receptors of different groups of patients with heart failure. In the meantime, such therapy should probably be used only when the patients are followed on a very careful clinical trial protocol.— R.C. Schlant, M.D.

Congestive Heart Failure Symptoms in Patients With Preserved Left Ventricular Systolic Function: Analysis of the CASS Registry
Judge KW, Pawitan Y, Caldwell J, Gersh BJ, Kennedy JW, and CASS Participants (Univ of Washington; Seattle VA Med Ctr; Mayo Clin and Found, Rochester, Minn; CASS Coordinating Ctr, Seattle)
J Am Coll Cardiol 18:377–382, 1991   2–32

Introduction.— Although most patients with congestive heart failure have systolic dysfunction of the left ventricle, a subgroup of patients have left ventricular diastolic dysfunction. To characterize those with congestive heart failure symptoms and a left ventricular ejection fraction of .45 or greater, data on 284 patients in the Coronary Artery Surgery Study (CASS) registry were reviewed.

Methods.— The CASS registry contains data on 24,959 patients studied at 15 centers in 1975–1979. Patients identified for this study had symptoms of moderate-to-severe congestive heart failure ≤2 months before enrollment in CASS together with well preserved left ventricular systolic function (ejection fraction ≥.45). A control group used for comparison included 13,071 registry patients without symptoms of heart failure and with an ejection fraction ≥.45.

Results.— Patients and controls differed markedly in a number of clinical variables. Those with congestive heart failure were older and were more likely to be female than those without heart failure. Heart failure in the absence of left ventricular systolic dysfunction was associated with the presence of hypertension, diabetes, chronic lung disease, severe angina, and prior myocardial infarction. At 6-year follow-up, survival was 82% in the heart failure group and 91% in the control group (Fig 2–12). The additional presence of coronary artery disease significantly reduced survival among the patients with heart failure: the 6-year survival rate

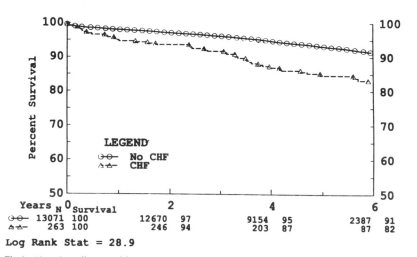

Log Rank Stat = 28.9

Fig 2–12.—Overall survival by congestive heart failure *(CHF)* status. The 6-year survival of CASS registry patients with an ejection fraction of .45 or greater and congestive heart failure *(triangles)* is compared with that of registry patients with an ejection fraction of .45 or greater without congestive heart failure *(circles)* (P < .0001). (Courtesy of Judge WK, Pawitan Y, Caldwell J, et al: *J Am Coll Cardiol* 18:377–382, 1991.)

was 68% for those with 3-vessel disease and 92% for those without coronary artery disease (Fig 2–13).

Conclusion.—Patients with suspected coronary artery disease and significant congestive heart failure symptoms, but without global left ventricular systolic dysfunction, are quite different from patients without

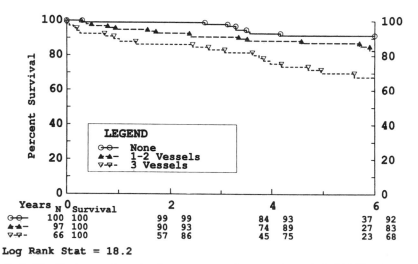

Log Rank Stat = 18.2

Fig 2–13.—The impact of severity of coronary artery disease on the survival of CASS registry patients with congestive heart failure and an ejection fraction of .45 or greater. The 6-year survival curves are shown for registry patients with no significant coronary disease *(circles)*, patients with 1- and 2-vessel coronary disease *(closed triangles)*, and patients with 3-vessel coronary disease *(open triangles)* (P < .0001). (Courtesy of Judge WK, Pawitan Y, Caldwell J, et al: *J Am Coll Cardiol* 18:377–382, 1991.)

clinical heart failure. In this CASS registry subgroup of patients with heart failure but ejection fraction ≥.45, surgical revascularization did not improve survival over a 6-year follow-up period.

▶ The patients in this retrospective study had symptoms of congestive heart failure ≤2 months before enrollment in CASS despite a left ventricular ejection fraction of ≥.45. In view of the rather low diagnostic accuracy of symptoms of heart failure, one must question the accuracy of the diagnosis of heart failure. The fact that revascularization failed to improve survival in these patients may be related to the small number of patients studied, although it is in accord with early CASS reports that show no advantage to surgical revascularization in patients with intact left ventricular systolic function unless the left main coronary artery was involved (1). On the other hand, a later CASS registry study demonstrated a benefit to surgical treatment in patients with severe angina and 3-vessel disease (2).— R.C. Schlant, M.D.

References

1. CASS Principal Investigators and Associates. Coronary Artery Surgery Study (CASS): A randomized trial of coronary artery bypass surgery: Survival data. *Circulation* 68:939–950, 1983.
2. Myers WO, et al: Improved survival of surgically treated patients with triple vessel coronary artery disease and severe angina pectoris; A report from the Coronary Artery Surgery Study (CASS) registry. *J Thorac Cardiovasc Surg* 97:487–495, 1989.

Prevention of High-Altitude Pulmonary Edema by Nifedipine
Bärtsch P, Maggiorini M, Ritter M, Noti C, Vock P, Oelz O (Swiss School of Sports; Univ Hosp, Zurich; Inselspital, Bern, Switzerland)
N Engl J Med 325:1284–1289, 1991   2–33

Introduction.—High-altitude pulmonary edema, which develops in some individuals after rapid ascent to altitudes above 2,500–3,000 meters, can be resolved readily with a return to sea level or the administration of supplemental oxygen. An important pathogenic factor in the condition appears to be high pulmonary-artery pressure resulting from hypoxic vasoconstriction.

Methods.—To determine whether nifedipine, an agent known to lower pulmonary-artery pressure, might prevent high-altitude pulmonary edema in susceptible mountaineers, 21 mountaineers with a mean age of 42 years were studied. All had experienced radiographically documented episodes of high-altitude pulmonary edema. Patients were randomly assigned to receive either nifedipine or placebo every 8 hours while ascending rapidly (within 22 hours) from a low altitude to 4,559 meters. Treatment continued during the next 3 days at this altitude. Outcome was assessed by means of chest radiography, Doppler echocardiography, and arterial blood sampling.

Results.—Pulmonary edema developed in 7 of 11 patients given pla-

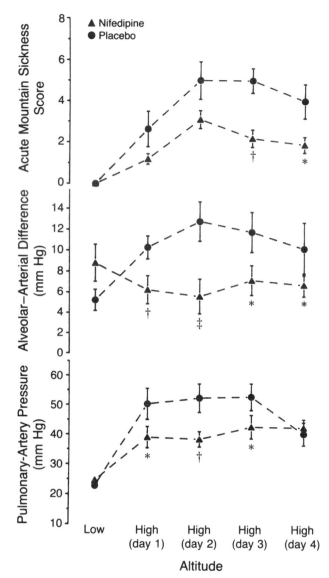

Fig 2–14.—Mean (± SE) acute mountain sickness scores, differences between alveolar and arterial oxygen pressure, and systolic pulmonary-artery pressure in 11 persons who received placebo and 10 who received nifedipine. Measurements were made at 490 m (low altitude) and 4,559 m (high altitude). The number of persons who received placebo was reduced on day 2 (n = 10), day 3 (n = 9), and day 4 (n = 5) at 4,559 m because of premature termination of the study. The *asterisk* denotes $P < .05$; *dagger*, $P < .01$; and *double dagger*, $P < .001$ for the comparison of changes from baseline between the study groups. (Courtesy of Bärtsch P, Maggiorini M, Ritter M, et al: *N Engl J Med* 325:1284–1289, 1991.)

cebo, but in only 1 of 10 given nifedipine. The single affected patient given nifedipine felt well enough to continue mountaineering activities, whereas 5 patients in the placebo group had to terminate the study prematurely. The nifedipine group had a significantly lower acute mountain sickness score than the placebo group (Fig 2–14).

Conclusion.—Slow-release nifedipine (20 mg every 8 hours) significantly reduced the incidence of high-altitude pulmonary edema in subjects with a history of this condition. The drug caused no side effects that interfered with mountaineering performance at a high altitude. The use of nifedipine is only recommended, however, when the most important preventive measure, a slow ascent to high altitude, has failed.

▶ It should be noted that the nifedipine was begun prophylactically before the ascent. The same investigators have previously reported the improvement in high altitude pulmonary edema when nifedipine is given as treatment (1). Nifedipine may attenuate the nonhomogeneous, exaggerated hypoxic pulmonary arteriolar vasoconstriction in patients who are susceptible to high-altitude pulmonary edema. It may also decrease an increase in pulmonary capillary permeability (2).—R.C. Schlant, M.D.

References

1. Oelz O, et al: Nifedipine for high altitude pulmonary oedema. *Lancet* 2:1241–1244, 1989.
2. Reeves JT, et al: When lungs on mountains leak. Studying pulmonary edema at high altitudes. *N Engl J Med* 325:1306–1307, 1991.

Depression in Elderly Patients With Congestive Heart Failure
Freedland KE, Carney RM, Rich MW, Caracciolo A, Krotenberg JA, Smith LJ, Sperry J (Washington Univ, St Louis)
J Geriatr Psychiatry 24:59–71, 1991   2–34

Introduction.—Congestive heart failure is a major cause of disability and death in the elderly. Prevalence estimates of depression in the elderly vary widely, but major depression is known to increase the risk of medical morbidity and mortality in younger patients with coronary artery disease.

Study.—The prevalence of major depression was determined in hospitalized patients, aged 70 years or older, with congestive heart failure. Sixty such patients were administered a modified version of the Diagnostic Interview Schedule. Survivors were followed up by phone 3 months after the index admission.

Findings.—Ten of the 60 patients evaluated (17%) met DSM-III-R criteria for current depressive disorder. Fatigue and insomnia are symptoms of both major depression and congestive heart failure, but all 10 patients met more stringent criteria for depression. Two nondepressed patients and none of the depressed patients died during the index admission. Survivors showed no clinical differences at follow-up according to whether or not depression was diagnosed. Major depression occurred in one fourth of white persons in the series and in no black persons.

Discussion.—Major depression was more frequent in these elderly patients with congestive heart failure than in the general geriatric population, and surprisingly occurred only in white persons. Further work is needed on how depression influences the course of congestive heart failure.

▶ This important aspect of elderly patients with acute congestive heart failure is often not well recognized. The fact that none of the elderly black patients in this study had evidence of depression is not readily explained and is different from my own experience.—R.C. Schlant, M.D.

Cholesterol: A Useful Parameter for Distinguishing Between Pleural Exudates and Transudates
Valdés L, Pose A, Suàrez J, Gonzalez-Juanatey JR, Sarandeses A, San José E, Alvarez Dobaña JM, Salgueiro M, Rodríguez Suárez JR (Hosp Provincial, Hosp General de Galicia, La Coruña, Spain)
Chest 99:1097–1102, 1991   2–35

Background.—Distinguishing between pleural exudates and transudates requires careful and sometimes exhaustive testing. In the present study the use of pleural fluid cholesterol (PCHOL) and the pleural cholesterol-serum cholesterol ratio (P/SCHOL) in distinguishing between transudates and exudates was evaluated in cases of pleuritis of different causes.

Methods.—Classification of pleural effusions as transudates, neoplastic exudates, tuberculous exudates, or miscellaneous exudates was done in 253 pleural effusions. Distinguishing between pleural exudates and transudates was done by using the parameters of pleural fluid lactic dehydrogenase (PLDH), pleural LDH-serum LDH ratio (P/SLDH), and pleural protein-serum protein ratio (P/SPROT) as compared with PCHOL and P/SCHOL findings.

Results.—Sensitivity of PCHOL for exudates was 91% and specificity was 100%; PCHOL had the fewest errors in distinguishing between exudates and transudates, with a misclassification rate significantly different from that of PLDH and P/SLDH but not from that of P/SCHOL and P/SPROT (Fig 2–15). Biochemical criteria previously used to differentiate between exudates and transudates had lower rates than PCHOL in distinguishing between the 2.

Conclusions.—It is suggested that determination of PCHOL and P/SCHOL be included routinely in pleural effusion cases because their success rates in distinguishing between exudates and transudates exceed those from any previously used methods.

▶ If the results of this study are confirmed by future studies, the measurement of cholesterol in pleural fluid will be very useful clinically. It will be particularly

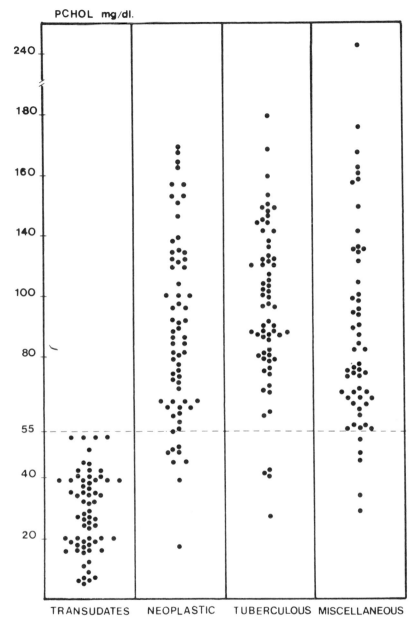

PCHOL mg/dl.

TRANSUDATES   NEOPLASTIC   TUBERCULOUS MISCELLANEOUS

Fig 2–15.—Pleural fluid cholesterol levels (mg/dL) in different groups studied. (Courtesy of Valdés L, Pose A, Suàrez J, et al: *Chest* 99:1097–1102, 1991.)

useful if the distinction between transudates and exudates remains accurate for chronic, long-standing transudates. One also wonders whether or not measurement of cholesterol concentration would be useful in the analysis of pericardial fluid.—R.C. Schlant, M.D.

Disturbances of Cardiac Rhythm and Conduction

Evidence of a Selective Increase in Cardiac Sympathetic Activity in Patients With Sustained Ventricular Arrhythmias
Meredith IT, Broughton A, Jennings GL, Esler MD (Baker Med Research Inst; Alfred Hosp, Melbourne, Australia)
N Engl J Med 325:618–624, 1991   2–36

Introduction.—In most sudden cardiac deaths resulting from ventricular tachyarrhythmia, the patient has had a history of coronary artery disease and poor left ventricular function. One important factor in the genesis of ventricular arrhythmias and sudden cardiac death appears to be an enhanced efferent cardiac sympathetic nervous activity. Using radiotracer kinetic techniques, this activity was quantified in patients at high risk for spontaneous, life-threatening ventricular arrhythmias.

Methods.—The 12 patients had recovered from a spontaneous, sustained episode of ventricular tachycardia or ventricular fibrillation outside the hospital at a mean of 13 days earlier. In 9 patients, there was a history of myocardial infarction and 4 had previous ventricular arrhythmias. Data on this group were compared with data on 18 patients with coronary artery disease, 6 patients with atypical chest pain, and 12 normal volunteers. Cardiac sympathetic nervous activity was obtained by measuring the rates of total and cardiac norepinephrine spillover into the plasma.

Results.—The 4 groups were similar in age, sex distribution, weight, heart rate at rest, and blood pressure. Those in the group with ventricular arrhythmias, however, had reduced left ventricular ejection fractions and increased end-systolic-volume indexes. The rates of total norepinephrine spillover into the plasma were similar in the 3 reference groups but were

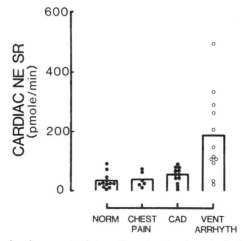

Fig 2–16.—Rates of cardiac norepinephrine spillover into the plasma in the 3 reference groups *(solid circles)* and the patients with ventricular arrhythmias *(open circles)*. Bars indicate mean values. (Courtesy of Meredith IT, Broughton A, Jennings GL, et al: *N Engl J Med* 325:618–624, 1991.)

80% higher in the study group. The mean rate of cardiac norepinephrine spillover was 32 pmol/minute in normal volunteers and 176 pmol/minute in patients with ventricular arrhythmias (Fig 2–16). Analysis of covariance revealed that left ventricular ejection fraction was the main determinant of the higher levels of cardiac norepinephrine spillover in the latter group.

Conclusion.—Patients who recovered from a life-threatening arrhythmia clearly showed an increase in cardiac sympathetic nervous activation. It is unlikely that the extent of this activation was simply a consequence of that episode of arrhythmia. Measurements of cardiac sympathetic nervous activity may aid in predicting the risk of major ventricular arrhythmias.

▶ It is important to note in this study that β-blockers, anti-arrhythmic agents, anti-anginal drugs, calcium antagonists, angiotensin-converting-enzyme inhibitors, and diuretics were all discontinued for at least 12 hours and that tea, coffee, cigarettes, and alcohol were withheld for at least 24 hours before samples were obtained. The results of this study may help to explain some of the benefits of β-blockers as effective anti-arrhythmic agents, especially in patients with coronary artery disease and diminished left ventricular ejection fraction.

Zipes has found that myocardial ischemia and infarction can result in regional sympathetic denervation and possibly denervation supersensitivity with autonomic and electrical heterogeneity (1,2). In the presence of increased catecholamines, these changes could set the stage for a tachyarrhythmia (1). See also Abstract 2–37.—R.C. Schlant, M.D.

References

1. Zipes DP: Sympathetic stimulation and arrhythmias. *N Engl J Med* 325:656–657, 1991.
2. Zipes DP: Influence of myocardial ischemia and infarction on autonomic innervation of the heart. *Circulation* 82:1095–1105, 1990.

Macroreentry in the Infarcted Human Heart: The Mechanism of Ventricular Tachycardias With a "Focal" Activation Pattern
de Bakker JMT, van Capelle FJL, Janse MJ, van Hemel NM, Hauer RNW, Defauw JJAM, Vermeulen FEE, Bakker de Wekker PFA (Interuniversity Cardiology Inst of The Netherlands, Academic Med Ctr, Amsterdam; Antonius Hosp, Nieuwegein; Univ Hosp, Utrecht, The Netherlands)
J Am Coll Cardiol 18:1005–1014, 1991   2–37

Background.—Human endocardial and epicardial activation mapping studies have associated the macroreentry around scar tissue from a myocardial infarction with ventricular tachycardia. Intraoperative mappings demonstrate that most tachycardias produce a focal activation form. Electrical activity was measured by endocardial mapping in 150 patients with chronic myocardial infarction.

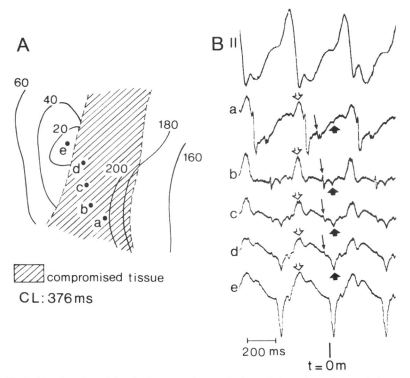

Fig 2–17.—**A**, endocardial activation map of a sustained ventricular tachycardia recorded in a patient during anti-arrhythmic surgery for infarct-related ventricular tachycardia. The isochrones in the endocardial border zone of the infarct are drawn at 20-ms intervals and are timed with respect to the onset of endocardial activation (t = 0 ms in **B**). **B**, surface ECG lead II and 5 unipolar signals recorded during tachycardia from sites located in the area of compromised tissue between the site of latest activation of 1 cycle *(site a)* and the site of earliest activation of the next cycle *(site e)*. The configuration of the signals demonstrates the characteristics of unipolar records. CL indicates cycle length of the tachycardia. (Courtesy of de Bakker JMT, van Capelle FJL, Janse MJ, et al: *J Am Coll Cardiol* 18:1005–1014, 1991.)

Methods.—Endocardial mapping of electrical activity was performed as a determinant of anti-arrhythmic surgery. All of the patients had drug-resistant ventricular tachycardia related to chronic myocardial infarction. Mapping was accomplished with a 64-channel data acquisition system, with recordings made in a unipolar mode. Figure 2–17 presents a map of a recording during anti-arrhythmic surgery for ventricular tachycardia.

Results.—In 20 chosen patients, 46 induced monomorphic sustained ventricular tachycardias resulted in different configurations. Three patients with an inferior infarction had epicardial activation after endocardial activation onset. The earliest diastolic potentials were recorded at a mean of 91 ms before the earliest endocardial activation. In 27 of the tachycardias, diastolic potentials occurred at 3 or more sites. In 26 of the 27 tachycardias, the activation sequence for the diastolic potentials moved along toward the exit point. The first endocardial activation arose at the base of the septum near the area of compromised tissue. In no patient did the diastolic potential sites from 2 or more inducible tachycardias match. Endocardial mapping was conducted during the sinus rhythm in 11 of the 20 selected patients, and in 4 late potentials occurred at the same sites where the diastolic potentials were observed during tachycardia.

Implications.—The mechanism(s) of ventricular tachycardias do relate to reentry in the macrocircuit of the postinfarct surviving tissue. The lack of late potetials during a sinus rhythm does not preclude arrhythmogenic pathways.

▶ The mechanism of macroreentry described in this paper likely explains the failure of localized catheter ablation to eliminate episodes of recurrent ventricular tachycardia in some patients. In patients in whom this mechanism is identified, more extensive ablative or extensive resection may be necessary.—R.C. Schlant, M.D.

Routine Programmed Electrical Stimulation in Survivors of Acute Myocardial Infarction for Prediction of Spontaneous Ventricular Tachyarrhythmias During Follow-Up: Results, Optimal Stimulation Protocol and Cost-Effective Screening
Bourke JP, Richards DAB, Ross DL, Wallace EM, McGuire MA, Uther JB (Westmead Hosp, Westmead, New South Wales, Australia)
J Am Coll Cardiol 18:780–788, 1991   2–38

Introduction.—Ventricular tachyarrhythmias are the major cause of death in the first year after acute myocardial infarction. Programmed electrical stimulation, the single best test for predicting arrhythmic death, is invasive and has a low yield. The results of 9 years of routine electrophysiologic testing in a large group of survivors of myocardial infarction were reviewed to determine the means of improving the cost-benefit ratio of such testing.

Methods.—At the study institution, programmed electrical stimulation has been routinely offered since 1980 to all survivors of myocardial infarction. Of 3,286 consecutive patients, 1,209 (37%) met the study criteria and agreed to the programmed electrical stimulation protocols. These patients were making an uncomplicated recovery and underwent testing at a mean of 11 days after infarction.

Results.—Sustained monomorphic ventricular tachycardia was inducible in 75 (6.2%) patients. Regardless of the test results, anti-arrhythmic therapy was not routinely prescribed. During the first year of follow-up, 14 (19%) infarct survivors with and 34 (2.9%) without inducible ventricular tachycardia experienced spontaneous ventricular tachycardia or fibrillation. At later follow-up (median 28 months), 19 patients with inducible ventricular tachycardia had a spontaneous electrical event. More than one third (37%) of these first events were fatal (table).

Conclusions.—Patients who underwent electrophysiologic testing were considered a low-risk group. Excluded were those with uncontrolled ischemia, heart failure, or who had experienced ventricular tachycardia or fi-

Comparison of Clinical Outcome During the First Year
of Follow-up Among 75 Infarct Survivors With and
1,134 Without Inducible Sustained Ventricular Tachycardia
at the Time of Hospital Discharge

	Ventricular Tachycardia		
	Inducible (n = 75)	Not Inducible (n = 1,134)	p Value
Reinfarction	5 (7%)	60 (5%)	0.6
Electrical event	14 (19%)	35 (3%)	<0.0005
Spontaneous VT/VF	10 (13%)	20 (2%)	<0.0005
Instantaneous death	5 (7%)	16 (1%)	<0.0005
Other death	10 (13%)	46 (4%)	<0.0005
After reinfarction	3 (4%)	0 (0%)	<0.0005
Other	7 (9%)	46 (4%)	<0.0005
Alive	60 (80%)	1,072 (95%)	<0.0005

Abbreviations: *Electrical event,* witnessed instantaneous death or documented sustained ventricular tachycardia or fibrillation without new ischemia; *instantaneous death,* witnessed instantaneous death in the absence of new ischemic symptoms; *VF,* ventricular fibrillation; *VT,* ventricular tachycardia.
(Courtesy of Bourke JP Richard DAB, Ross DL, et al: *J Am Coll Cardiol* 18:780–788, 1991.)

brillation more than 48 hours after infarction. The most cost-effective strategy for predicting arrhythmia involves restricting testing to infarct survivors whose left ventricular ejection fraction is less than 40% and using a stimulation protocol containing 4 extra stimuli.

▶ The results of this study, which provide data that the routine use of electrophysiologic testing (EPS) in survivors of myocardial infarction is not cost-effective, are not unexpected. It still remains to be demonstrated that the use of EPS in survivors of infarction whose ejection fraction is less than 40% is cost-effective, particularly given the limited number of anti-arrhythmic drugs available (1). The presence of late potentials on a signal-averaged ECG appears to be a useful technique to identify patients at higher risk for ventricular arrhythmias. Perhaps the combination of both low ejection fraction and the presence of late potentials would better identify a group of postinfarct patients to consider EPS.

Richards et al. (2) concluded that inducible ventricular tachycardia (VT) at EPS was the single best predictor of spontaneous VT and sudden death after myocardial infarction.—R.C. Schlant, M.D.

References

1. Goldman L: Electrophysiological testing after myocardial infarction. A paradigm for assessing the incremental value of a diagnostic test. *Circulation* 83:1090–1092, 1991.
2. Richards DAB, et al: What is the best predictor of spontaneous ventricular tachycardia and sudden death after myocardial infarction? *Circulation* 83:756–763, 1991.

The Arrhythmogenicity of Theophylline: A Multivariate Analysis of Clinical Determinants

Bittar G, Friedman HS (State Univ of New York Health Science Ctr, Brooklyn, NY)

Chest 99:1415–1420, 1991

2–39

Introduction.—The occurrence of cardiac arrhythmias with theophylline toxicity is well recognized. However, there is controversy over whether cardiac arrhythmias can occur at therapeutic serum theophylline concentrations (STCs). The relation between STCs and the occurrence of cardiac arrhythmias was examined in 100 patients hospitalized for acute respiratory insufficiency from asthma or obstructive pulmonary disease.

Patients.—All patients had concurrent ECG and STC examinations. The patients were selected for inclusion in this analysis only on the basis of STC. Twenty-five patients had STCs of less than 2.5 mg/L, 25 had STCs ranging from 2.5 mg/L to 10 mg/L, 25 had STCs ranging from 10 mg/L to 20 mg/L, and 25 had STCs greater than 20 mg/L. Sixty-seven patients received theophylline orally and 33, intravenously, with similar distribution over the 4 groups. The groups also did not differ with respect to age, gender, clinical diagnoses, ECG patterns, arterial pH or gases, serum calcium, or β-agonists.

Results.—Cardiac arrhythmias were more common in patients with STCs above 10 mg/L than in patients with subtherapeutic STCs. Multivariate analysis performed to determine the contribution of individual variables to the occurrence of arrhythmias identified STC as the most important clinical determinant of arrhythmia, with age and gender following in importance. Serum potassium was not an independent predictor of arrhythmia. Treatment with steroids or digoxin was at most only weakly associated with arrhythmia. After logistic regression analysis, digoxin was not an independent predictor for arrhythmia. Heart rate was directly related to STC. Multifocal atrial tachycardia was found in 8% of patients with therapeutic STCs and in 16% of patients whose STCs were above the therapeutic range. Two patients died suddenly within 24 hours of the discovery of multifocal atrial tachycardia. Neither patient had concomitant ventricular arrhythmias.

Conclusion.—Theophylline can cause tachycardia and serious arrhythmias, even at STCs considered to be therapeutic. Multifocal atrial tachycardia may herald sudden cardiac death. The role of theophylline as a therapeutic agent may require reassessment.

▶ This paper indirectly addresses a daily dilemma in the management of patients with both chronic obstructive pulmonary disease and coronary artery disease. In such patients, the therapy of the chronic obstructive pulmonary disease with theophylline and β-adrenergic agents often results in tachycardia and, occasionally, evidence of myocardial ischemia. In general, it is preferable to use both of these agents in the lowest dose that is clinically effective. Part of the increase in mortality in patients with attacks of acute asthma, which has been noted in some countries in the last decade or so (1), may be related to tachycardia and other effects of β-antagonists and theophylline. There is some evidence that terbutaline enhances digitalis-induced arrhythmia (2). On the other hand, in one group of 10 patients who survived respiratory arrest, severe respiratory acidosis was noted, but serious cardiac arrhythmias were not (3). Thus, some asthma patients may die from overtreatment, whereas others die from undertreatment.— R.C. Schlant, M.D.

References

1. Robin ED: Death from bronchial asthma. *Chest* 93:614–618, 1988.
2. Zavecz JH: The bronchodilator terbutaline enhances digitalis-induced arrhythmia. *Am J Med Sci* 302:148–151, 1991.
3. Molfino NA, et al: Respiratory arrest in near fatal asthma. *N Engl J Med* 324:285–288, 1991.

The Diagnostic Performance of Computer Programs for the Interpretation of Electrocardiograms

Willems JL, Abreu-Lima C, Arnaud P, van Bemmel JH, Brohet C, Degani R, Denis B, Gehring J, Graham I, van Herpen G, Machado H, Macfarlane PW, Michaelis J, Moulopoulos SD, Rubel P, Zywietz C (Univ of Leuven, Belgium; Univ of Porto, Portugal; INSERM, Lyon, France; Erasmus Univ, Rotterdam; Univ of Louvain, Brussels; et al)
N Engl J Med 325:1767–1773, 1991   2–40

Introduction.—Although more than half of the 100 million ECGs recorded each year in the United States are probably interpreted using a computer, the quality of these computer programs has not been assessed systematically. The diagnostic results achieved using 9 computer programs were compared with the interpretations of 8 cardiologists who analyzed the same ECGs. Records were obtained from 1,220 patients who had ventricular hypertrophy or myocardial infarction at various sites.

Results.—Computer programs made a median of 91% correct diagnoses, compared with 96% made by the cardiologists. The programs were significantly less sensitive than the cardiologists were in diagnosing both ventricular hypertrophy and myocardial infarction. However, the best of the computer programs performed nearly as well as the most accurate of the cardiologists.

Conclusions.—Although some computer programs for interpreting ECGs are nearly as accurate as cardiologists in diagnosing major cardiac disorders, others perform substantially less well and need to be improved.

▶ The important message from this and similar studies is that computer ECG interpretations must be overread by a physician with special competence in electrocardiography. This is particularly important in the diagnosis of acute myocardial ischemia and the diagnosis of many cardiac arrhythmias.— R.C. Schlant, M.D.

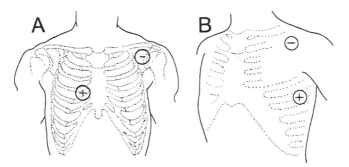

Fig 2–18.—Electrode positions for obtaining the bipolar or modified precordial leads MCL$_1$ (**A**) and MCL$_6$ (**B**). (Courtesy of Drew BJ, Scheinman MM: *J Am Coll Cardiol* 18:1025–1033, 1991.)

Value of Electrocardiographic Leads MCL$_1$, MCL$_6$ and Other Selected Leads in the Diagnosis of Wide QRS Complex Tachycardia

Drew BJ, Scheinman MM (Univ of California, San Francisco Med Ctr)
J Am Coll Cardiol 18:1025–1033, 1991   2–41

Introduction.—The common 12-lead ECG can be used to distinguish a supraventricular tachycardia with aberrant conduction from a ventricular tachycardia, with the 2 unipolar precordial leads V$_1$ and V$_6$ proving valuable in diagnosing the wide QRS tachycardia in particular. The bipolar precordial leads MCL$_1$ and MCL$_6$ have been substituted for the V$_1$ and V$_6$ leads (Fig 2–18). The 2 sets of leads and other selected leads were compared for diagnostic accuracy in continuous bedside ECG recording.

Methods.—One hundred twenty-one wide QRS complex tachycardias from 92 patients were analyzed prospectively. A Marquette instrument recorded the conventional 12-lead ECGs for both leads MCL$_1$ and V$_1$ and for MCL$_6$ and V$_6$. New criteria were developed for ECG assessment.

Findings.—Of the 121 wide QRS complex tachycardias analyzed, 86 were ventricular tachycardia and 35 were supraventricular tachycardia with aberrant conduction. The 2 observers made 424 comparisons be-

Right Bundle Branch Block Patterns			Aberrant (%)	Ventricular Tachycardia (%)	P
Monophasic R		MCL$_1$	20	6	NS
		V$_1$	14	17	NS
Taller left peak		MCL$_1$	0	11	< .05
		V$_1$	0	14	< .025
Biphasic qR, or Rs		MCL$_1$	0	21	< .005
		V$_1$	0	11	< .05
Bimodal rR′ or triphasic rsR′		MCL$_1$	31	7	< .005
		V$_1$	46	8	< .0001

Fig 2–19.—Presence of the well-established morphologic criteria in lead MCL$_1$ compared with those in lead V$_1$ during tachycardias with a right bundle branch block pattern. (Courtesy of Drew BJ, Scheinman MM: *J Am Coll Cardiol* 18:1025–1033, 1991.)

Left Bundle Branch Block Patterns		Aberrant (%)	Ventricular Tachycardia (%)	P
Biphasic rS with one or more of the following: (a) R > 30 ms (b) Notched S descent (c) Late nadir > 60 ms	MCL₁	0	32	< .0001
	V₁	0	36	< .0001
Biphasic rS or Q with all of the following: (a) R ≤ 30 ms (b) Straight S descent (c) Early nadir ≤ 60 ms	MCL₁	34	9	< .005
	V₁	37	5	< .0001

Fig 2–20.—Presence of the well-established morphologic criteria in lead MCL_1 compared with those in lead V_1 during tachycardias with a left bundle branch block pattern. (Courtesy of Drew BJ, Scheinman MM: *J Am Coll Cardiol* 18:1025–1033, 1991.)

tween the leads with a >88% agreement between them in rating the similarity between the modified and the conventional precordial leads. A monophasic R wave pattern did not relate to ventricular tachycardia in either lead V_1 or MCL_1 (Fig 2–19). The QRS patterns that aided in defining tachycardias with a left bundle branch block contour included a prolonged R wave, a notched S downstroke, or a late nadir (Fig 2–20). For those tachycardias with a right bundle branch block pattern, a biphasic rS pattern with an R/S ratio <1 in lead V_6 usually indicated tachycardia (Fig 2–21). Most (77%) of the tachycardias produced QRS configurations in leads V_1 and MCL_1 that aided diagnosis, whereas 47% of the tachycardias using the leads V_6 and MCL_6 in this same configuration helped diagnosis. The combination of precordial lead MCL_1 plus MCL_6 or lead V_1 plus V_6 produced a correct identification in 90% of the tachycardias.

Conclusions.—The diagnostic accuracy of a single MCL_1, V_1, MCL_6, or VPV_6PV lead appears superior to that of a single lead II. In addition, the combination of leads is better than a single lead in diagnosing wide complex tachycardia.

Right Bundle Branch Block Patterns		Aberrant (%)	Ventricular Tachycardia (%)	P
Biphasic rS with R:S ratio < 1.0	MCL₆	3	9	NS
	V₆	3	19	< .05
Triphasic qRs with R:S ratio > 1.0	MCL₆	23	1	< .001
	V₆	23	3	< .005

Right or Left Bundle Branch Block Patterns

Monophasic or notched QS	MCL₆	0	38	< .0001
	V₆	0	31	< .0001
Biphasic qR	MCL₆	0	7	NS
	V₆	0	2	NS

Fig 2–21.—Presence of the well-established morphologic criteria in lead MCL_6 compared with those in lead V_6. (Courtesy of Drew BJ, Scheinman MM: *J Am Coll Cardiol* 18:1025–1033, 1991.)

A New Approach to the Differential Diagnosis of a Regular Tachycardia With a Wide QRS Complex

Brugada P, Brugada J, Mont L, Smeets J, Andries EW (OLV Hosp, Aalst, Belgium; Univ of Limburg, Maastricht, The Netherlands)
Circulation 83:1649–1659, 1991

2–42

Introduction.—It is difficult to distinguish between supraventricular tachycardia (SVT) with aberrant conduction and ventricular tachycardia (VT) because both tachycardias show a wide QRS complex on the 12-lead electrocardiogram. The reasons that the presently available differential criteria so often result in diagnostic error were examined, and 4 new criteria were incorporated into an easy-to-use algorithm.

Methods.—For the first part of the study, the presently used criteria were applied to 236 wide-complex tachycardias, of which 172 were VTs and 64 were SVTs with electrophysiologically confirmed aberrant conduction. Several current criteria for suggesting a diagnosis of VT, such as a left axis of the QRS complex in the frontal plane or a duration of the QRS complex of .14 second or more, were often present in SVT with aberrant conduction. Further analysis revealed that the absence of an RS complex in all precordial leads, or an RS interval of more than 100 ms in any precordial lead when an RS complex was present in one or more precordial leads, were each 100% specific for the diagnosis of VT. When the RS interval was shorter than 100 ms, the presence of atrioventricular (AV) dissociation was 100% specific for the diagnosis of VT. When AV dissociation was absent, a diagnosis of VT was made if the tachycardia fulfilled the morphologic criteria for VT in leads V_1 and V_6. When all 4 criteria for a diagnosis of VT were absent, a diagnosis of SVT with aberrant conduction was made by exclusion. The new criteria were prospectively applied to 554 wide-complex tachycardias, of which 384 were VTs and 170 were SVTs with aberrant conduction.

Results.—Using the 4 new criteria, 379 VTs (98.7%) and 164 SVTs with aberrant conduction (96.5%) were correctly classified. Re-analysis of the 11 misclassified tachycardias using both the currently used and the new criteria did not correctly classify any of them.

Conclusion.—Four new criteria are used to diagnose SVT with aberrant conduction by excluding a diagnosis of VT. This new approach may prevent diagnostic errors that could have potentially serious or even fatal consequences.

▶ Both of these studies (Abstracts 2–41 and 2–42) provide additional useful criteria for the differential diagnosis of a wide QRS complex tachycardia. It should be emphasized that in the study of Brugada et al. (Abstract 2–42), only an RS complex or its absence in all precordial leads are valuable for the diagnosis and that complexes with QR, QRS, QS, monophasic R, or rSR morphology are not considered RS complexes. Only when an RS interval is measurable can the complex be considered an RS complex.

Griffith et al. (1) performed a multivariate analysis of broad complex tachycardia in 102 patients and found the most useful indicators to be a history of myocardial infarction, the QRS waveforms in aVF and V_1, and a change in mean QRS axis from sinus rhythm of more than 40 degrees. If none of the criteria was met, the diagnosis was almost certainly supraventricular tachycardia. If one criteria was met, the diagnosis was probably ventricular tachycardia. Hayes et al. (2) reviewed the criteria for the diagnosis of narrow QRS ventricular tachycardia.—R.C. Schlant, M.D.

References

1. Griffith MJ, et al: Multivariate analysis to simplify the differential diagnosis of broad complex tachycardias. *Br Heart J* 66:166–174, 1991.
2. Hayes JJ, et al: Narrow QRS ventricular tachycardia. *Ann Intern Med* 114:458–463, 1991.

Propafenone Treatment of Symptomatic Paroxysmal Supraventricular Arrhythmias: A Randomized, Placebo-Controlled, Crossover Trial in Patients Tolerating Oral Therapy
Pritchett ELC, McCarthy EA, Wilkinson WE (Duke Univ)
Ann Intern Med 114:539–544, 1991   2–43

Background.—Propafenone is a new oral anti-arrhythmic agent in the treatment of ventricular arrhythmia. Several uncontrolled trials have suggested that propafenone may also be useful in the treatment of paroxysmal supraventricular arrhythmia. The present carefully controlled 2-phase trial was carried out to assess the prophylactic efficacy of propafenone against symptomatic recurrent arrhythmia in patients with paroxysmal supraventricular tachycardia or paroxysmal atrial fibrillation.

Patients.—Thirty-three patients were entered into a 6-month, open-label, dose-finding phase. Sixteen patients had supraventricular tachycardia and 17 had atrial fibrillation. All arrhythmias were confirmed by ECG before enrollment. Fourteen patients with tachycardia and 9 with fibrillation completed the dose-finding phase and were then entered into a randomized, double-blind, placebo-controlled, crossover phase. Nineteen of the 23 patients received propafenone, 300 mg 3 times daily; 3 were given 300 mg twice daily; and 1 received 150 mg twice daily. Each placebo or drug treatment period lasted 60 days, for a maximum study duration of 4 months. Symptomatic arrhythmia was documented by telephone transmission of the ECG.

Results.—Propafenone increased the time to the first recurrence of arrhythmia when compared with placebo. The recurrence rate of arrhythmia during propafenone therapy was estimated to be .21 times or approximately one fifth of the recurrence rate during treatment with placebo. The most common noncardiac adverse effects were bitter taste, nausea, anorexia, and weakness. Cardiac adverse experiences resulted in 11 premature discontinuations, 9 of them by patients with fibrillation and 2 by patients with tachycardia.

Conclusions.—Propafenone appears to be effective in reducing the rate of recurrence of arrhythmia in patients with paroxysmal supraventricular tachycardia or atrial fibrillation who can tolerate the drug. The rate of premature withdrawals among patients with paroxysmal atrial fibrillation was high. However, it was not established whether the high withdrawal rate was caused by the effects of the drug itself or by the type of patient who has this disorder.

▶ Propafenone is a new class I anti-arrhythmic drug that has been approved by the Food and Drug Administration for the treatment of patients with life-threatening ventricular arrhythmias (1) and appears also to be effective in decreasing recurrent episodes of supraventricular tachycardia or atrial fibrillation. Of the 33 patients with paroxysmal atrial fibrillation in this study, 11 discontinued participation in the study, mostly because of arrhythmias, including prolongation of their attacks of atrial fibrillation, tachycardia, and bradycardia. It is also noteworthy that flecainide, which also decreases the recurrence of paroxysmal supraventricular tachycardia, has been approved by the Food and Drug Administration for this indication.—R.C. Schlant, M.D.

Reference

1. Hernandez M, et al: Propafenone for malignant ventricular arrhythmia: An analysis of the literature. *Am Heart J* 121:1178–1184, 1991.

A Placebo-Controlled Trial of Continuous Intravenous Diltiazem Infusion for 24-Hour Heart Rate Control During Atrial Fibrillation and Atrial Flutter: A Multicenter Study
Ellenbogen KA, Dias VC, Plumb VJ, Heywood JT, Mirvis DM (Med College of Virginia, Richmond; Marion Merrell Dow, Inc, Kansas City, Mo; Univ of Alabama, Birmingham; Loma Linda Univ; Univ of Tennessee, Memphis)
J Am Coll Cardiol 18:891–897, 1991   2–44

Introduction.—Atrial arrhythmias are frequent in patients with cardiopulmonary disease and may be associated with worsening angina or heart failure. It would be very helpful to be able to reduce the ventricular response rapidly and safely before cardioversion or the institution of definitive anti-arrhythmic therapy.

Study Design.—The calcium channel blocker diltiazem was evaluated in 44 patients who initially responded to a 20-mg bolus dose of intravenous diltiazem. Forty-four such patients who had established atrial fibrillation or flutter were randomly assigned under double-blind conditions to receive 10–15 mg/hour of infused diltiazem or placebo for up to 24 hours.

Observations.—Three fourths of the 23 patients given diltiazem but none of 21 given a placebo infusion maintained a therapeutic response for 24 hours. When those who failed to respond to the bolus injection received a 24-hour open-label infusion, 83% of all patients maintained a response to diltiazem. The response was independent of age, body weight, and previous digoxin therapy. Treatment was, however, more effective against atrial fibrillation than against atrial flutter. No serious adverse effects occurred, although 2 patients became hypotensive.

Conclusions.— The use of intravenous infusion of diltiazem is a safe and rapidly effective approach in patients having atrial fibrillation or flutter. It appears to be a useful "bridge" for those awaiting cardioversion or the onset of anti-arrhythmic drug action.

▶ Intravenous diltiazem appears to be an effective and safe agent to rapidly slow the ventricular response of patients with atrial fibrillation or flutter. In additional clinical situations, there also may be contraindications to the use of alternatives such as digoxin, β-adrenergic blocking agents, or verapamil. Intravenous digoxin may take several hours to slow the ventricular response in some patients, whereas β-blockers and verapamil can significantly depress left ventricular function more than diltiazem. Intravenous diltiazem appears to be a very useful addition to our anti-arrhythmic armamentarium.— R.C. Schlant, M.D.

Usefulness of d,l Sotalol for Suppression of Chronic Ventricular Arrhythmias

Anastasiou-Nana MI, Gilbert EM, Miller RH, Singh S, Freedman RA, Keefe DL, Saksena S, MacNeil DJ, Anderson JL (Univ of Utah; LDS Hosp, Salt Lake City)
Am J Cardiol 67:511–516, 1991   2–45

Background.— Sotalol is a nonselective β-adrenergic receptor antagonist with some class III anti-arrhythmic activity reported to be effective in treatment of sustained or life-threatening ventricular arrhythmias. A trial was undertaken to quantify the degree of sotalol's ventricular anti-arrhythmic effects and assess its safety and tolerance.

Methods.— A low dose of sotalol (320 mg/day) and a high dose (640 mg/day) were compared to placebo in a 6-week, randomized, double-blind study of 114 patients. Patients had chronic ventricular premature complexes (VPCs) at frequencies of at least 30/hour.

Results.— In 38 patients given the low dose and 39 patients given the high dose, sotalol significantly reduced VPCs compared with placebo use in 37 patients. The individual efficacy criterion was achieved in 34% of low-dose and 71% of high-dose groups compared with only 6% of placebo-treated patients. The response was dose dependent for total VPCs, with 88% suppression in the group given high-dose sotalol and 75% suppression in those given the low dose. The frequency of repetitive VPCs was reduced comparably by low and high doses (Fig 2–22). Sotalol decreased the heart rate, increased the PR interval, and corrected the JT interval, but it did not change the ejection fraction. The effect of sotalol was almost completely achieved within the first 2–3 days of dosing. Nonfatal pro-arrhythmia occurred in 3 patients given sotalol and in 2 given placebo.

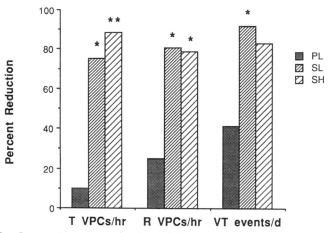

Fig 2–22.—Comparative responses of total ventricular premature complexes (T VPCs) and repetitive VPCs (R VPCs) per hour and ventricular tachycardia (VTC) events per day to sotalol and placebo. *Left column,* percent reduction in average hourly T VPCs in placebo (PL), low-dose sotalol (SL), and high-dose sotalol (SH) groups. *Middle* and *right columns,* percent reduction in average hourly R VPCs and daily VT events, respectively, in the same groups. $*P < .05$ vs. PL; $**P < .05$ vs. SL and PL. (Courtesy of Anastasiou-Nana MI, Gilbert EM, Miller RH, et al: *Am J Cardiol* 67:511–516, 1991.)

Conclusion.—Sotalol provides significant class III anti-arrhythmic activity and is an efficacious anti-arrhythmic drug for complex ventricular arrhythmias. The response was dose dependent for total VPCs but not for repetitive VPCs. In lower doses the drug is somewhat less effective but better tolerated. Pro-arrhythmia was infrequent, but this finding needs further assessment in a larger group.

▶ This study demonstrates that d,1 sotalol decreases the frequency of total VPCs, repetitive VPCs, and ventricular tachycardia. It is important to note that patients with myocardial infarction were excluded from this study. Adverse effects related to treatment occurred in 39% of low-dose and 51% of high-dose sotalol patients, compared with 11% of placebo patients. These effects included dyspnea, fatigue, and bradycardia. In this study, a small risk of pro-arrhythmia was observed. Others have noted a higher incidence in a more diseased population (1). Torsade de pointes may occur in 1.1% of patients treated for nonsustained ventricular tachycardia or VPCs, according to the manufacturers data base referred to in this article.

In view of the results from CAST in the last few years, it would not appear to be appropriate to use sotalol in patients with a recent myocardial infarction until the safety of such therapy is established by an appropriate large clinical trial.—R.C. Schlant, M.D.

Reference

1. Ruder MA, et al: Clinical experience with sotalol in patients with drug-refractory ventricular arrhythmias. *J Am Coll Cardiol* 13:145–152, 1989.

Catheter Modification of the Atrioventricular Junction With Radiofrequency Energy for Control of Atrioventricular Nodal Reentry Tachycardia
Lee MA, Morady F, Kadish A, Schamp DJ, Chin MC, Scheinman MM, Griffin JC, Lesh MD, Pederson D, Goldberger J, Calkins H, de Buitleir M, Kou WH, Rosenheck S, Sousa J, Langberg JJ (Univ of California, San Francisco; Univ of Michigan, Ann Arbor)
Circulation 83:827–835, 1991   2–46

Background.—Atrioventricular (AV) nodal re-entrant tachycardia (AVNRT) is a common indication for ablation of the AV junction. Cryodestruction and guided dissection of perinodal atrial tissue effectively eliminate AVNRT with a low incidence of inadvertent complete AV block, but both techniques require open heart surgery. The efficacy of transcatheter radiofrequency (RF) ablation for eliminating AVNRT was assessed.

Patients.—Thirty-nine patients aged 14 to 86 years with refractory AVNRT that had not responded to therapy with a mean of 3.7 anti-arrhythmic drugs made up the study group. All patients underwent baseline electrophysiologic study to confirm the diagnosis and inducibility of the AVNRT. A custom-designed 6 F ablation catheter with a large distal electrode was used to deliver RF energy. The catheter was positioned across the tricuspid anulus to several millimeters proximal to the site of the maximal His bundle electrogram, then withdrawn to obtain the largest atrial-to-ventricular electrogram ratio with a small His bundle electrogram. Each RF energy application lasted about 60 seconds. The endpoint was noninducibility of AVNRT before and during isoproterenol administration.

Results.—Radiofrequency energy was applied 289 times, for a mean of 6.8 applications per session, at a mean power level of 16.2 W, and a mean application duration of 48.1 seconds. Patients reported no significant pain during RF current application and additional analgesia or anesthesia was never required. Of the 39 patients, 30 (77%) had no inducible AVNRT with intact AV conduction after ablation, 3 (8%) had inadvertent complete AV block and required permanent pacemakers, and 6 (15%) continued to have AVNRT. Three of the 6 unimproved patients had repeat ablations with successful outcome and an additional patient later improved with medication. None of the patients with good outcomes had a recurrence before hospital discharge. After a mean follow-up of 8 months, 28 of 34 successfully treated patients had no recurrence of AVNRT, 2 patients were withdrawn from the study, and 4 had recurrences, 2 of whom underwent successful repeat ablation. In all, 32 of the 39 patients (82%) have remained free of AVNRT without sustaining a complete AV block.

Conclusion.—Radiofrequency ablation of the perinodal right atrium appears to be safe and effective for the treatment of AVNRT.

Catheter Ablation of Accessory Atrioventricular Pathways (Wolff-Parkinson-White Syndrome) by Radiofrequency Current

Jackman WM, Wang X, Friday KJ, Roman CA, Moulton KP, Beckman KJ, Mc-Clelland JH, Twidale N, Hazlitt HA, Prior MI, Margolis PD, Calame JD, Overholt ED, Lazzara R (Univ of Oklahoma; VA Med Ctr, Oklahoma City)
N Engl J Med 324:1605–1611, 1991   2–47

Background.—Surgical or catheter ablation of the accessory pathway has been used therapeutically for more than 20 years in patients with Wolff-Parkinson-White syndrome. High morbidity and mortality associated with accessory-pathway ablation has led to exploration of high-energy shock and nonsurgical alternatives for ablation. Radiofrequency current delivered by catheter provides an alternative energy source for ablation with less morbidity and mortality.

Methods.—Catheter techniques for applying radiofrequency ablation were tested and evaluated in 166 patients with 177 accessory pathways. Radiofrequency current was delivered through a catheter electrode positioned against the mitral or tricuspid annulus or a branch of the coronary sinus. The placement ensured that the radiofrequency current produced lesions potentially effective for accessory-pathway ablation. Accessory pathways were localized by recording accessory-pathway activation potentials.

Results.—Ventricular pre-excitation and atrioventricular re-entrant tachycardia were eliminated in 164 of 166 patients. A single procedure was required in 148 patients; in the remaining 16 patients, 2 procedures were required. In 166 patients, there were no deaths and only 6 complications. The recurrence of pre-excitation or atrioventricular re-entrant tachycardia in 15 patients was successfully treated by a second, successful ablation.

Conclusion.—Catheter delivery of radiofrequency current guided by direct recordings of accessory-pathway activation was highly effective in ablating accessory pathways. There was no mortality and lower morbidity in the patients treated with radiofrequency current compared with therapy by surgical or catheter ablation with high-energy shocks.

Diagnosis and Cure of the Wolff-Parkinson-White Syndrome or Paroxysmal Supraventricular Tachycardias During a Single Electrophysiologic Test

Calkins H, Sousa J, El-Atassi R, Rosenheck S, de Buitleir M, Kou WH, Kadish AH, Langberg JJ, Morady F (Univ of Michigan, Ann Arbor)
N Engl J Med 324:1612–1618, 1991   2–48

Purpose.—Radiofrequency current delivered through an electrode catheter has been used to either eliminate atrioventricular nodal re-entry or to ablate accessory pathways in the Wolff-Parkinson-White syndrome or paroxysmal supraventricular tachycardia. The approach has usually been staged with diagnosis followed by catheter ablation of the tachycardia or accessory pathway during a second procedure. The feasibility of establishing the diagnosis and performing radiofrequency ablation during a single electrophysiologic test was investigated.

Method.—A diagnostic electrophysiologic test and catheter ablation with radiofrequency current was performed on 106 patients. The patients had documented, symptomatic paroxysmal supraventricular tachycardia or the Wolff-Parkinson-White syndrome.

Results.—Among the 62 patients with paroxysmal supraventricular tachycardia, more than 90% had atrioventricular nodal re-entrant or atrioventricular reciprocating tachycardia that was amenable to ablation with radiofrequency current. A successful long-term outcome was also achieved in more than 90% of patients with the Wolff-Parkinson-White syndrome. Only 2 complications were reported. The mean duration of the procedure was under 2 hours.

Conclusion.—This abbreviated approach to diagnosis and cure of paroxysmal supraventricular tachycardia or the Wolff-Parkinson-White syndrome condenses the entire diagnostic and treatment process into a single procedure, eliminating the expense and inconvenience of the staged procedure. The abbreviated therapeutic approach using a single electrophysiologic test is feasible, practical, and has a favorable risk-benefit ratio. The abbreviated approach may eliminate the need for expensive testing, drug therapy, pacemakers, or surgical ablation.

Radiofrequency Current Catheter Ablation of Accessory Atrioventricular Pathways
Kuck K-H, Schlüter M, Geiger M, Siebels J, Duckeck W (Univ Hosp Eppendorf, Hamburg, Germany)
Lancet 337:1557–1561, 1991   2–49

Introduction.—Catheter ablation is an alternative to surgical treatment of refractory tachyarrhythmias mediated by an accessory atrioventricular (AV) pathway. Early reports of direct current ablation were encouraging, but general anesthesia was necessary and complications such as barotrauma were a problem.

Methods.—Of 105 consecutive patients seen with symptomatic tachyarrhythmia related to an accessory AV pathway, 83 had the Wolff-Parkinson-White syndrome, and 22 had a concealed accessory path with retrograde conduction only. After mapping of both AV rings, ablation was carried out using a generator supplying 300-kHz alternating current.

Results.—A total of 131 ablation procedures was directed at 111 accessory pathways. Only 31% of 18 attempts made using a standard-tip electrode catheter succeeded, but 93% of attempts made with a large-tip electrode catheter were successful. In 86% of patients, accessory-pathway conduction was interrupted in a single session. Complications included thrombotic occlusion of the femoral artery; AV fistula formation at the site of groin puncture; and left ventricular rupture with cardiac tamponade after direct-current shock. There were no deaths.

Conclusions.—Accessory AV paths at any site can be ablated using catheter-induced radiofrequency (RF) current. The chief advantage of RF over direct current is that the delivery of energy may be controlled according to the electrophysiologic changes achieved. Eventually RF-current catheter ablation may be considered as a preventive measure.

▶ Catheter ablation of the atrioventricular junction to control supraventricular arrhythmias has been performed since 1982 (1, 2). In recent years, interest has turned to radiofrequency energy (30 kHz–300 MHZ) rather than high-voltage defibrillator discharges to produce lesions to prevent tachyarrhythmias. The 4 papers in this series (Abstracts 2–46, 2–47, 2–48, and 2–49) reflect the rapid advances in the successful application of radiofrequency energy to control cardiac arrhythmias. The first paper by Lee et al. (Abstract 2–46) reviews their excellent results in the treatment of 39 patients with atrioventricular (AV) nodal re-entry tachycardia (AVNRT).

Jackson et al. (Abstract 2–47) describe their experience treating 166 patients with accessory AV pathways (Wolff-Parkinson-White syndrome). Calkins et al. (Abstract 2–48) describe their experience using radiofrequency ablation to treat 106 patients with Wolff-Parkinson-White syndrome or supraventricular tachycardia during a single, condensed session. Kuck et al. (Abstract 2–49) also used the technique with generally good results in 105 patients with symptomatic tachyarrhythmias, of whom 83 had the Wolff-Parkinson-White syndrome and 22 had a concealed accessory AV pathway with only retrograde conduction.

In all 4 series the results were very good, there was a low morbidity, and there was no mortality. Complications were unusual but included elevation of creatine kinase MB fraction, pericarditis or cardiac tamponade, complete AV block, and thrombotic occlusion of a coronary artery. Radiofrequency ablation of accessory pathways is likely to replace both surgery and catheter ablation using high energy in the treatment of many supraventricular tachyarrhythmias. The procedure is not easy to perform, and catheter ablation does require specialized training.— R.C. Schlant, M.D.

References

1. Scheinman MM, et al: Catheter-induced ablation of the atrioventricular junction to control refractory supraventricular arrhythmias. *JAMA* 248:851–855, 1982.
2. Gallagher JJ, et al: Catheter technique for closed-chest ablation of the atrioventricular conduction system: A therapeutic alternative for the treatment of refractory supraventricular tachycardia. *N Engl J Med* 306:194–200, 1982.

Left Cardiac Sympathetic Denervation in the Therapy of Congenital Long QT Syndrome: A Worldwide Report
Schwartz PJ, Locati EH, Moss AJ, Crampton RS, Trazzi R, Ruberti U (Univ of Pavia, Italy; Univ of Milan, Italy; Univ of Rochester, NY; Univ of Virgina, Charlottesville)
Circulation 84:503–511, 1991   2–50

Background.—Long QT syndrome (LQTS), a congenital disorder, is associated with a high incidence of sudden cardiac death. The treatment of first choice is β-adrenergic blockade, which is successful in 75% to 80% of patients. In patients in whom β-blockade does not prevent cardiac events, such as syncope or cardiac arrest, left cardiac sympathetic denervation (LCSD) may be beneficial.

Methods.—Eighty-five patients with LQTS worldwide who had LCSD were identified. The mean period between the first cardiac event and LCSD and the follow-up period after LCSD were similar at 5.6 and 5.9 years, respectively. Mean age of patients at surgery was 20 years.

Results.—A highly significant reduction (99% to 45%) in the number of patients with cardiac events followed LCSD. The mean number of cardiac events per patient fell from 22 to 1 after LCSD. In addition, the number of patients with 5 or more cardiac events dropped from 71% to 10%. Seven patients (8%) died suddenly. The 5-year survival rate was 94%.

Conclusions.—Left cardiac sympathetic denervation is an effective treatment for patients with LQTS who continue to have syncope or cardiac arrest despite β-blockade. The substantial decrease in the incidence of tachyarrhythmic syncope suggests that LCSD also reduces the risk for sudden death in these patients.

▶ This worldwide registry study over 15 years was necessary to obtain a large enough number of patients with the relatively rare condition of LQTS to assess adequately the benefit of LCSD. This study provides firm data that LCSD is very effective in patients with LQTS who continue to have syncope or cardiac arrest despite β-blocker therapy, and it should be offered to such patients in preference to permanent pacing (1).

Recently, LQTS has been found to have a structural defect, congenital myocardial sympathetic dysinnervation (CMSD) (2), an abnormal ventricular contraction pattern detectable by echocardiography (3), and abnormal dispersion of ventricular repolarization detectable by body surface maps (4).—R.C. Schlant, M.D.

References

1. Moss AJ, et al: Efficacy of permanent pacing in the management of high-risk patients with long QT syndrome. *Circulation* 84:1524–1529, 1991.
2. Kohl K, et al: Congenital myocardial sympathetic dysinnervation (CMSD)—A structural defect of idiopathic long QT syndrome. *PACE* 14:1544–1553, 1991.
3. Flippo N, et al: Unsuspected echocardiographic abnormality in the long QT syndrome. Diagnostic, prognostic, and pathogenetic implications. *Circulation* 84:1530–1542, 1991.
4. De Ambroggi L, et al: Dispersion of ventricular repolarization in the long QT syndrome.

Identification of False Positive Exercise Tests With Use of Electrocardiographic Criteria: A Possible Role for Atrial Repolarization Waves
Sapin PM, Koch G, Blauwet MB, McCarthy JJ, Hinds SW, Gettes LS (Univ of North Carolina, Chapel Hill)
J Am Coll Cardiol 18:127–135, 1991   2–51

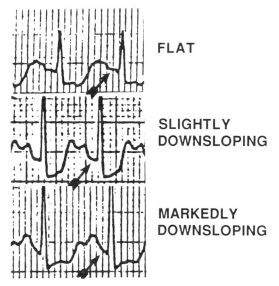

FLAT

SLIGHTLY
DOWNSLOPING

MARKEDLY
DOWNSLOPING

Fig 2–23.—Examples of the 3 PR segment slope classifications taken from actual ECG tracings. *Arrow* indicates PR segment. (Courtesy of Sapin PM, Koch G, Blauwet MB, et al: *J Am Coll Cardiol* 18:127–135, 1991.)

Introduction.—The exercise ECG is an important first step in evaluating patients with suspected ischemic heart disease, but its specificity was approximately 77% in a recent meta-analysis. A false positive exercise test, defined as ST segment depression in the absence of myocardial ischemia, may be associated with a number of factors. Exaggerated atrial repolarization waves may produce depression of the ST segment in the absence of myocardial ischemia (Fig 2–23). The P wave, PR segment, and ST segment in patients with false positive exercise tests were compared with results in a true positive test.

Methods.—The P waves, PR segments, and ST segments were studied in leads II, III, aVF, and V_4–V_6 in 69 patients with ECG findings suggesting ischemia. All patients had a normal ECG at rest. The true positive group was 44 patients selected retrospectively and at random.

Findings.—The false positive group showed markedly down-sloping PR segments at peak exercise, a significantly higher heart rate than the true positive group, and an absence of exercise-induced chest pain (Fig 2–24). The combination of downsloping PR segments in 2 of 3 inferior leads plus either exercise duration of ≥4 minutes or peak heart rate of ≥125 beats/minute identified false positive tests with a sensitivity and specificity of more than 80%.

Conclusions.—Exaggerated atrial repolarization waves may be a cause of a false positive exercise test. This study suggests some simple clinical and ECG criteria to predict a false positive exercise test. The finding of short, steeply down-sloping PR segments, particularly in the inferior ECG leads, is an independent marker of a false positive exercise test even in the presence of significant horizontal ST segment depression. Other non-

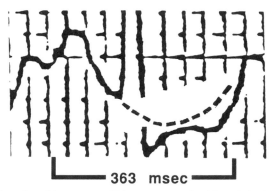

363 msec

Fig 2–24.—Illustration of the extent to which an exaggerated atrial repolarization wave might influence the ST segment. The lead II ECG complex is from a false positive test at a heart rate of 134 beats/minute. The *dotted line* indicates the hypothetical atrial repolarization wave. The duration of the P wave plus the atrial repolarization wave (363 ms) represents the 95% upper confidence limit above the mean P wave and atrial repolarization wave duration at that heart rate, derived from the data of Kesselman RH, Berkun MA, Donoso E, et al: *Am Heart J* 51:900–905, 1956. (Courtesy of Sapin PM, Koch G, Blauwet MB, et al: *J Am Coll Cardiol* 18:127–135, 1991.)

invasive procedures should be used to prove the presence of stress-induced myocardial ischemia before invasive procedures are recommended.

▶ It has been known for several decades that the Ta wave might affect the ST segment, especially in inferior leads. As noted in this study, it is important to recognize this potential cause of a false positive exercise test to avoid patient anxiety and inappropriate patient management.

Ellestad (1) emphasized the need for further study of the Ta wave, especially during ischemia or exercise.—R.C. Schlant, M.D.

Reference

1. Ellestad MH: Role of atrial repolarization in false positive exercise tests. *J Am Coll Cardiol* 18:136–137, 1991.

Stroke Prevention in Atrial Fibrillation Study: Final Results
Stroke Prevention in Atrial Fibrillation Investigators
Circulation 84:527–539, 1991   2–52

Background.—The Stroke Prevention in Atrial Fibrillation (SPAF) Study was begun in 1985 to determine the efficacy and safety of warfarin and aspirin compared with placebo in preventing ischemic stroke and systemic embolism. Late in 1989 the placebo arm was terminated because the superiority of both warfarin and aspirin has been established. The preliminary results of this study have already been published, and in the present report the final results in the entire population are presented.

Methods.—This multicenter, randomized trial compared the use of 325 mg/day of aspirin or warfarin with placebo in 1,330 inpatients and outpatients with constant or intermittent atrial fibrillation. The mean follow-up was 1.3 years.

Results.—The rate of primary events in patients given placebo was 6.3% per year, which was reduced by 42% in those given aspirin. In the subgroup of patients eligible for warfarin, most of whom were younger than age 76 years, warfarin dose adjusted to prolong prothrombin time to 1.3-fold to 1.8-fold that of controls decreased the risk of primary events by 67%. Warfarin reduced primary events or death by 58%, and aspirin reduced them by 32%. Patients given warfarin, aspirin, or placebo had a risk of significant bleeding of 1.5%, 1.4%, and 1.6% per year, respectively.

Conclusions.—Both aspirin and warfarin effectively reduce ischemic stroke and systemic embolism in patients with atrial fibrillation. Because patients who are eligible to receive warfarin comprise a subset of aspirin-eligible patients, the magnitude of reduction in events by warfarin and aspirin cannot be compared. Warfarin-eligible patients had too few events to directly evaluate the relative benefit of aspirin compared with warfarin. Patients with nonrheumatic atrial fibrillation who can safely take either warfarin or aspirin should be given prophylactic antithrombotic treatment to decrease their risk of stroke.

Canadian Atrial Fibrillation Anticoagulation (CAFA) Study
Connolly SJ, Laupacis A, Gent M, Roberts RS, Cairns JA, Joyner C for CAFA
Study Coinvestigators (Hamilton Gen Hosp, Hamilton, Ontario, Canada)
J Am Coll Cardiol 18:349–355, 1991   2–53

Background.—Patients with both atrial fibrillation and mitral stenosis are frequently treated with anticoagulants to decrease the risk of stroke. There is no consensus on the use of anticoagulants in patients with atrial fibrillation when mitral stenosis is not present. The Canadian Atrial Fibrillation Anticoagulation Study (CAFA) was a randomized double-blind, placebo-controlled trial designed to assess the potential of warfarin to reduce systemic thromboembolism and its inherent risk of hemorrhage.

Patients.—The protocol called for recruitment of 630 patients to be followed for an average of 2.5 years. However, because 2 similar trials published positive results, the CAFA was terminated early after randomizing 383 patients. One-hundred eighty-seven patients were randomized to warfarin and 191 to placebo. A primary outcome event was defined as any ischemic stroke except lacunar; other systemic embolism to the gut, kidney, arms, or legs; or intracranial or fatal hemorrhage. Secondary outcome events were transient ischemic attack, lacunar infarction, major or minor bleeding, or death.

Results.—Anticoagulation was of benefit in patients with nonrheumatic valvular atrial fibrillation in the prevention of systemic thromboembolism. The undesirable side effects were not prohibitive. Sixteen percent of the patients who received warfarin anticoagulation experienced minor bleeding and 9% of patients who received placebo also experienced bleeding. The relative risk reduction of a primary outcome cluster in patients treated with warfarin was 37%.

Conclusion.—The "positive" results of 2 similar studies led to termination of this trial after randomization of only 383 of a projected 630 patients. All studies support the use of warfarin in patients with nonrheumatic valvular atrial fibrillation for the prevention of systemic thromboembolism.

▶ Two other large studies on the prevention of stroke in patients with atrial fibrillation have recently been reported: the Copenhagen AFASAK study, in which warfarin and aspirin were compared (1), and the Boston Area Anticoagulation Trial for Atrial Fibrillation (BATAF) (2).

From the results of the SPAF and the CAFA studies summarized above and the AFASAK and the BATAF studies, it is clear that long-term warfarin therapy is indicated in patients with nonvalvular atrial fibrillation. Aspirin was also found to be effective at a dose of 325 mg/day in patients who were younger than 75 years in the SPAF study, but aspirin was not found to be effective at a dose of 75 mg/day in the AFASAK trial (1). In the BATAF trial, aspirin was taken in a nonrandomized fashion by some of the patients in the control group, and the investigators did not believe that it produced a beneficial effect.

The results of additional, ongoing studies comparing aspirin vs. warfarin treatment are awaited with great interest, particularly because many physicians are reluctant to use anticoagulant drugs for the prevention of strokes in elderly patients with atrial fibrillation (3). At present, it appears likely that aspirin is less effective than warfarin (4, 5), although it may be safer. Currently, I often use aspirin (325 mg/day) in younger patients with minimal or no associated heart disease or in patients who are poor candidates for warfarin therapy (6, 7).—R.C. Schlant, M.D.

References

1. Petersen P: Placebo-controlled randomized trial of warfarin and aspirin for prevention of thromboembolic complications in chronic atrial fibrillation: The Copenhagen AFASAK study. *Lancet* 1:175–179, 1989.
2. The Boston Area Anticoagulation Trial for Atrial Fibrillation Investigators. The effect of low-dose warfarin on the risk of stroke in patients with nonrheumatic atrial fibrillation. *N Engl J Med* 323:1505–1511, 1990.
3. Kutner et al: Physicians' attitudes toward oral anticoagulants and antiplatelet agents for stroke prevention in elderly patients with atrial fibrillation. *Arch Intern Med* 151:1950–1953, 1991.
4. Cairns JA, et al: Nonrheumatic atrial fibrillation. Risk of stroke and role of antithrombotic therapy. *Circulation* 84:469–481, 1991.
5. Albers G, moderator: Stroke prevention in nonvalvular atrial fibrillation. *Ann Intern Med* 115:727–736, 1991.
6. The Stroke Prevention in Atrial Fibrillation Investigators: Predictors of thromboembolism in atrial fibrillation: I. Clinical features of patients at risk. *Ann Intern Med* 116:1–5, 1992.
7. The Stroke Prevention in Atrial Fibrillation Investigators: Predictors of thromboembolism in atrial fibrillation: II. Echocardiographic features of patients at risk. *Ann Intern Med* 116:6–12, 1992.

A Standard Heparin Nomogram for the Management of Heparin Therapy

Cruickshank MK, Levine MN, Hirsh J, Roberts R, Siguenza M (McMaster Univ, Hamilton, Ont; Hamilton Civic Hosps Research Ctr)
Arch Intern Med 151:333–337, 1991   2–54

Background.—A nomogram for the adjustment of heparin dosage was developed to standardize heparin therapy and to reduce delays in achieving and maintaining a therapeutic activated partial thromboplastin time (APTT) result. Results of a first nomogram that was tested on 20 patients were analyzed and used to modify that nomogram. Further testing made it possible to refine and modify a nomogram for use in this test. Fifty consecutive patients were selected to have their continuous intravenous heparin therapy adjusted according to this nomogram. A control group of 53 patients similar in pre-heparin therapy characteristics was also chosen.

Methods.—Subjects received an intravenous bolus of heparin followed by continuous infusion of calcium heparin. The nomogram (table) was used to adjust the heparin dose 6 hours after the bolus injection and throughout the therapy. Heparin therapy was discontinued after an International Normalized Ratio of 2 was reached. Control patients received the same initial bolus and subsequent heparin dosage, with all dosage adjustments ordered by the physician. Adequacy of therapy in both groups was evaluated on a time-to-event and success-rate analysis.

Results.—Sixty-six percent of study patients reached therapeutic APTT 24 hours after the start of therapy. This proportion increased to 81% after 48 hours, compared with 37% and 58% for control patients, respectively. The mean time to reach targeted APTT was 24.3 hours in study patients and 56.9 hours in control patients. Additionally, correction of

| | | | Final Nomogram | |
APTT, s	Bolus, U	Hold, min	Rate Change, mL/h†	Repeat APTT
‹ 50††	5000	0	+3	6 h
50–59	0	0	+3	6 h
60–85	0	0	0	Next morning
86–95	0	0	−2	Next morning
96–120	0	30	−2	6 h
› 120	0	60	−4	6 h

Abbreviation: APTT, activated partial thromboplastin time.
*1 mL/hr = 40 units/hr.
†If APTT was subtherapeutic despite heparin dose of 1,440 units/hr (36 mL/hr) or greater at any time during first 48 hours of therapy, response to APTT of less than 50 seconds was heparin bolus of 5,000 units and rate increase of 5 mL/hr.
(Courtesy of Cruickshank MK, Levine MN, Hirsh J, et al: *Arch Intern Med* 151:333–337, 1991.)

APTT values that had drifted outside the therapeutic range after it was reached was more rapid in study patients.

Conclusions.—This nomogram, developed for a specific thromboplastin with a therapeutic range based on an APTT equivalent to a heparin level of .2 to .4 unit/mL as measured by protamine neutralization, is not likely to be generalizable to other APTT reagents. However, comparison of test reagents or the test reagent to the heparin assay could make the nomogram adaptable.

▶ The use of this nomogram should significantly improve the efficacy and safety of intravenous heparin therapy. It should be noted that the nomogram was developed for a specific thromboplastin (Actin FS) and that the therapeutic range (60–85 sec) was based on an APTT that is equivalent to a heparin level of .2–.4 units/mL measured by protamine neutralization. Hospitals using other reagents may need to adjust the nomogram accordingly.—R.C. Schlant, M.D.

3 Hypertension

Introduction

In 1991, significant advances were made in our understanding of the two extremes of hypertension, its beginnings in young people with borderline elevations of blood pressure, and its later manifestations in elderly patients with either combined or isolated systolic hypertension. In addition, important new information became available about the monitoring of blood pressure, the effects of multiple environmental factors and endothelium-derived substances on blood pressure, the benefits of various nondrug and drug therapies, and the management of various secondary causes. Particularly useful data were published relating to 2 groups of patients who are at significant risk from hypertension: those with diabetes and pregnant women.

Before going through these individual articles in an orderly manner, the results of 2 major long-term studies that reveal insights into the beginnings of hypertension will be considered: one (the Framingham Heart Study) (Abstract 3–1) is already well known; the other (the Tecumseh Blood Pressure Study, Abstract 3–3) promises to be equally as informative.

Norman M. Kaplan, M.D.

High-Normal Blood Pressure Progression to Hypertension in the Framingham Heart Study
Leitschuh M, Cupples LA, Kannel W, Gagnon D, Chobanian A (Boston Univ)
Hypertension 17:22–27, 1991   3–1

Background.—Persons with high-normal blood pressure, defined as a diastolic pressure of 85–89 mm Hg, may progress to hypertension more rapidly than those with normal blood pressure. Follow-up data from the Framingham Heart Study were analyzed to determine the rate of such progression.

Methods.—Individuals from the Framingham Heart Study were classified as either normal or high-normal and were followed up for 26 years. Hypertension was defined as a diastolic blood pressure of 95 mm Hg or greater or the initiation of antihypertensive treatment.

Results.—Among those with strictly normal blood pressure, 23.6% of the men and 36.2% of the women developed hypertension, compared with 54.2% of the men and 60.6% of the women with high-normal blood pressure. The relative risks for developing hypertension associated with high-normal blood pressure were 2.25 and 1.89 for men and women, respectively. When estimated by the proportional hazards model, the age-adjusted relative risks for men and women were 3.36 and 3.37, respectively. Of the risk factors studied, baseline systolic and diastolic blood pressure, Metropolitan relative weight, and change in weight over time significantly predicted future hypertension in men and women whose initial blood pressure was normal. Systolic blood pressure and weight change were risk factors for future hypertension in men with high-normal blood pressure.

Conclusions.—The probability of individuals with high-normal blood pressure developing hypertension is 2- to 3-fold higher than in those individuals with strictly normal blood pressure. Therefore, those with high-normal blood pressure should undergo frequent blood pressure testing and receive counseling on the modification of risk factors.

▶ Most of these subjects were between 30 and 50 years of age on entry into the Framingham study. The findings that higher initial blood pressures and increasing body weight predicted the development of hypertension come as no surprise. The findings were confirmed further in a 10-year follow-up of a large group of Swedish middle-aged men who also had an assessment of glucose tolerance and insulin resistance.—N. Kaplan, M.D.

Risk Factors for the Development of Hypertension: A 10-Year Longitudinal Study in Middle-Aged Men
Skarfors ET, Lithell HO, Selinus I (Uppsala, Sweden)
J Hypertens 9:217–223, 1991   3–2

Background.—A sample of 2,322 middle-aged men living in Uppsala, Sweden, was followed for 10 years to identify risk factors predisposing to the development of hypertension and assess their relative importance.

Methods.—The subjects, age about 50 years at the time of examination, attended a health examination survey in the years 1970–1973. This examination included a self-administered health questionnaire, blood pressure measurements, anthropometric measurements, serum lipid level analysis, and an intravenous glucose tolerance test with insulin determinations. One thousand eight hundred sixty men underwent the same examination 10 years later. All subjects who had a diastolic blood pressure of 90 mm Hg or less in the first survey were classified at the second survey as being either still normotensive or as hypertensive.

Results.—In the initial survey, a diastolic blood pressure of 95 mm Hg or greater or drug treatment for hypertension was found in 19.6% of participants. This figure increased to 34.7% at the second survey. Of the patients who were normotensive in the first survey, about one quarter were hypertensive at the second survey. The strongest predictor of future hypertension was baseline blood pressure; otherwise, the significant risk factors were fasting and late insulin levels during an intravenous glucose tolerance test, difference in body mass index during the 10-year interval between surveys, and a family history of hypertension. Body mass index was the only significant risk factor when a difference in diastolic blood pressure was used as an independent variable.

Conclusions.—The development of hypertension appears to be related to insulin resistance, as reflected by fasting, late insulin levels, and body mass index. Obesity, which aggravates insulin insensitivity, appears to be the most important life-style variable in the risk of hypertension.

▶ In addition to higher baseline blood pressure and increased body weight, the development of hypertension in these somewhat older subjects was shown to correlate with abnormal glucose tolerance and insulin resistance, associations that will recur throughout this review of the recent literature.

Even more informative data about the very beginnings of hypertension have come from the Tecumseh Blood Pressure Study, which last year (1) showed that even younger people (average age of 31) who had borderline hypertension tended to be overweight and to have higher blood insulin and lipid levels. In 1991, additional hemodynamic data from these patients with borderline hypertension in the Tecumseh study were presented.—N. Kaplan, M.D.

Reference

1. Julius S, et al: The association of borderline hypertension with target organ changes and higher coronary risk. Techumseh Blood Pressure Study. *JAMA* 264:354–358, 1990.

Hyperkinetic Borderline Hypertension in Tecumseh, Michigan

Julius S, Krause L, Schork NJ, Mejia AD, Jones KA, van de Ven C, Johnson EH, Sekkarie MA, Kjeldsen SE, Petrin J, Schmouder R, Gupta R, Ferraro J, Nazzaro P, Weissfeld J (Univ of Michigan, Ann Arbor)
J Hypertens 9:77–84, 1991   3–3

Background.—Hemodynamic and biochemical measurements of young, healthy subjects were obtained for a research study on precursors of hypertension. In particular, evidence was sought for a hyperkinetic state reflecting excessive autonomic drive.

Methods.—The subjects were 691 healthy residents of Tecumseh, Michigan, site of the ongoing blood pressure study. There were 364 men and 327 women, average age 32.3 years, all of whom had blood pressure records from previous examinations. Individuals being treated for hypertension were excluded. Subjects were taught to measure their blood pressure at home and reported to the clinic with records of the twice-daily measurements. They also underwent echocardiographic and Doppler examinations, forearm phlethysmography, and catecholamine determination.

Results.—Clinical blood pressure exceeded 140/90 mm Hg in 99 subjects, who were considered borderline hypertensive. Of this group, 37% had a heart rate of 7 beats/min and a cardiac index of 760 mL/min, along with increased forearm blood flow and plasma norepinephrine. Home blood pressure measurements were also elevated in those subjects. Blood pressure was elevated at 5, 8, 21, and 23 years of age in those with hyperkinetic borderline hypertension, and their parents' blood pressures were also elevated.

Conclusions.—The hyperkinetic state in borderline hypertension appears to be a significant clinical condition. Sympathetic hyperactivity appears to be present in a large proportion of unselected subjects with mild blood pressure elevation on the basis of the elevated norepinephrine levels found in this study.

▶ These data document the common presence of a hyperdynamic circulation in young people with borderline hypertension, likely reflecting an excessive autonomic drive. Such autonomic overactivity could reflect effects from weight gain (1) or psychological stress (2).

In all of these observational studies, weight gain and increased body mass keep appearing as critical determinants of the development of hypertension. The role of increased weight has been further documented in cross-sectional examinations of large numbers of Israeli 17-year-olds (3) and in a representative sample of over 7,000 Americans examined in the National Health and Nutrition Examination (4). Perhaps psychological stress leads to increased food intake, setting up a vicious cycle that eventuates in hypertension and includes insulin resistance as an aggravating factor.

Whatever initiates a rise in blood pressure in those who are genetically susceptible, the presence of even slightly elevated pressure over a long period of time will eventuate in structural changes that lead to the permanence of hypertension and all of the cardiovascular sequelae that accompany its presence. The sequence may go either way: cardiac hypertrophy may initiate the subsequent rise in pressure rather than follow it.—N. Kaplan, M.D.

References

1. Suurküla MB, et al: Body weight is more important than family history of hypertension for left ventricular function. *Hypertension* 17:661–668, 1991.
2. Perini C, et al: Suppressed aggression accelerates early development of essential hypertension. *J Hypertens* 9:499–503, 1991.
3. Seidman DS, et al: Birth weight, current body weight, and blood pressure in late adolescence. *BMJ* 302:1235–1237, 1991.
4. Ford ES, Cooper RS: Risk factors for hypertension in a National Cohort Study. *Hypertension* 18:598–606, 1991.

Echocardiographic Left Ventricular Mass and Electrolyte Intake Predict Arterial Hypertension

de Simone G, Devereux RB, Roman MJ, Schlussel Y, Alderman MH, Laragh JH (New York Hosp-Cornell Med Ctr, New York)
Ann Intern Med 114:202–209, 1991   3–4

Background.—Normotensive patients who will subsequently develop hypertension are difficult to identify. A longitudinal study of 132 normotensive adults was performed to determine whether left ventricular

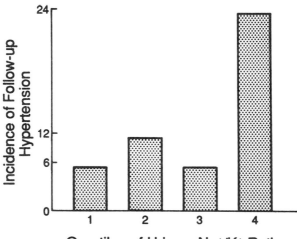

Fig 3–1.—Incidence of arterial hypertension during 4-year follow-up in relation to quartiles of urinary sodium/potassium ratio (Na^+/K^+). The relation is less evident than for left ventricular mass index for the first 3 quartiles but becomes evident for the highest quartile ($P < .04$). (Courtesy of de Simone G, Devereux RB, Roman MJ, et al: *Ann Intern Med* 114:202–209, 1991.)

mass is a predictor of hypertension regardless of demographic variables or risk factors.

Methods.—Subjects underwent echocardiography, standard blood tests, and a 24-hour urine collection initially and at annual intervals for 3 to 6 years.

Results.—Eleven percent (7 men, 8 women) had a systolic blood pressure greater than 140 mm Hg or a diastolic blood pressure greater than 90 mm Hg or both at follow-up. At baseline, those 15 subjects had a greater left ventricular mass index (LVMI) than the 117 who remained normotensive. They also had a higher 24-hour urinary sodium/potassium excretion ratio. No differences appeared in race, initial age, systolic or diastolic blood pressure, coronary risk factors, or plasma renin activity. The likelihood of developing hypertension rose from 3% in those with the lowest LVMI to 24% in those with the highest LVMI (Fig 3–1). A less regular parallel trend occurred in the sodium/potassium excretion ratio. Follow-up systolic pressures in all 132 subjects were predicted by initial age, systolic blood pressure, race, and sex-adjusted left ventricular mass index. Final diastolic blood pressure predictors were its initial value, plasma triglyceride levels, urinary sodium/potassium ratio, low renin activity, race, and plasma glucose level.

Conclusions.—The size of left ventricular mass by echocardiography predicts the development of elevated systolic pressure in normotensive subjects. Diastolic pressure is more related to the initial metabolic status. Black race is an independent determinant of higher subsequent blood pressure.

▶ As in most studies, the division between normotension and hypertension was 140/90 mm Hg. Those who subsequently developed hypertension, in addition to their larger left ventricular mass, also had initial blood pressures that were higher (although still well below 140/90) than did those who remained normotensive. Obviously, 140/90 is an arbitrary separation, and a person whose pressure goes from 110/70 to 130/85 may be considered to have a significant rise. Moreover, as shown in the Tecumseh population, a tendency toward higher readings even as young as age 8 is typical for those who eventually develop overt hypertension.

In all of these studies, the measurements of blood pressure were by routine sphygmomanometry, although in the Tecumseh study, home measurements were also used. In the future, more such data will be derived from automatic recordings, and we will next consider some of the reasons why.— N. Kaplan, M.D.

Diagnosis and Monitoring

▶ ↓ Before considering issues of blood pressure measurement, findings of a large-scale survey in Norway suggest that, at least in one population with a nationalized health-care system, the detection of hypertension has been much improved over what was found 20 or even 10 years ago.— N. Kaplan, M.D.

Detecting Hypertension: Screening Versus Case Finding in Norway
Holmen J, Forsén L, Hjort PF, Midthjell K, Waaler HT, Bjørndal A (National Institute of Public Health, Community Research Centre, Verdal, National Institute of Public Health, Unit for Health Services Research, Oslo, Norway)
BMJ 302:219–222, 1991   3–5

Background.—The rule of halves, introduced in the 1970s, states that hypertension is diagnosed in only half of the people in a population with it. The detection of hypertension in adults was assessed in the county of Nord-Trøndelag in central Norway to determine whether the situation has changed.

Methods.—The cross-sectional survey included 74,977 persons, representing 88.1% of those aged 20 and over. All 106 general practitioners in the county were involved. Hypertension was assessed according to the blood pressure thresholds used in the Norwegian treatment program. Individuals with elevated readings on screening were examined clinically and placed into treatment groups.

Results.—Overall, 2,399 persons had elevated blood pressure levels on screening. Before screening, 6,210 (8.3%) reported taking antihypertensive drugs, and an additional 3,849 (5.1%) had been having regular blood pressure monitoring. As a result of the screening, drug treatment was begun in 406 persons (.5%) and blood pressure monitoring was begun in another 1,007 (1.3%). Of those taking antihypertensive medicine after screening, 94% had been identified before screening. Of those whose blood pressure was monitored regularly after screening, 79.3% had been identified before screening.

Conclusions.—The best strategy for finding hypertensive patients in need of care has been debated. At the blood pressure screening thresholds used, and when hypertension is defined by an overall clinical diagnosis, general practitioners can find hypertensive patients effectively by the case finding strategy.

▶ In our less organized system of health care, detection of hypertension is certainly not as commonplace as in Norway. Nonetheless, most Americans see a health care provider every year, where a blood pressure can easily be obtained and there is little need for organized screening programs anymore. As an example, almost 25 million high school students in the United States participate each year in organized sports, and they are usually required to have a medical examination, including a blood pressure measurement, before they begin. This examination may provide the first awareness of an elevated blood pressure.—N. Kaplan, M.D.

Tracking of Elevated Blood Pressure Values in Adolescent Athletes at 1-Year Follow-Up
Tanji JL (Univ of California, Davis Med Ctr, Sacramento)
Am J Dis Child 145:665–667, 1991   3–6

Background.—Although borderline hypertension may exist for many years, the diagnosis is often not made until the third or fourth decade. This is partly because young people, particularly adolescents, do not often seek medical attention. Preparticipation physical examinations for high school sports were used to determine whether elevated blood pressures at this examination correlate with elevated blood pressures at 1-year follow-up.

Methods.—Examinations were done on 467 adolescents, 359 boys and 108 girls, with a mean age of 16.2 years. The group was 61.9% white. The criterion for an elevated blood pressure was 142/92 mm Hg or higher. When significant elevations in blood pressure were found, follow-up checks were made within 3 months. Four hundred thirty-six students were reexamined after 1 year.

Results.—Significant elevations of blood pressure were found in 12.2% of patients. Of these, 79.6% had persistently elevated blood pressure at 1-year follow-up. There was a family history of hypertension in 80.7% of students with elevated blood pressure and in 5.6% of normotensive students. Mean body weights were 94.5 kg in the hypertensive group and 75.2 kg in normotensive subjects. The hypertensive patients were also more likely to do heavy resistance training (71.9%) than were normotensive subjects (15.8%).

Conclusions.—Adolescents can be effectively screened for hypertension by routine preparticipation examinations for high school sports. A continued follow-up of this cohort in a prospective, longitudinal study is indicated.

▶ As the authors point out, the relatively high prevalence of elevated pressures in this healthy group of 16–18-year-olds may reflect some special features of high school athletes: excess body weight, involvement in isometric (resistance) training, and perhaps use of anabolic steroids. Because almost 80% of those initially found to have an elevated pressure were still hypertensive 1 year later, it is obvious that they need to be counseled about preventive measures and carefully followed.

Another reason that an elevated pressure was so common was the performance of only one reading in an office setting as part of an examination that likely was associated with considerable stress, because if the adolescent's health status was found to be abnormal, participation in school sports could be prohibited. It does not take much to invoke stress-induced elevations in blood pressure.—N. Kaplan, M.D.

Awareness of High Blood Pressure Increases Arterial Plasma Catecholamines, Platelet Noradrenaline and Adrenergic Responses to Mental Stress
Rostrup M, Mundal HH, Westheim A, Eide I (Univ of Oslo)
J Hypertens 9:159–166, 1991   3–7

Introduction.—Several studies have suggested that prior awareness of hypertension may initiate psychological distress during clinical examination, which by itself could increase sympathetic tone. However, the effects of hypertension awareness on sympathetic tone and responsiveness have not been well studied. The effects of hypertension labeling in individuals with a near-normal blood pressure (BP) were examined.

Study Design.—A group of 19-year-old men undergoing routine medical examination for the military draft during 1987 had their BP taken after sitting for 5 minutes. None of the men were told what the results were. Thirty-six of them belonged to the 95th percentile of mean BP, 110 mm Hg or higher. One year later, 18 men were sent a neutral letter and 18 were sent a letter indicating that their BP was elevated at the initial screening. All were asked to come in 2 weeks later for follow-up examination, at which time their BP and heart rate (HR) were measured. Twenty-six men, 13 in each group, also underwent intra-arterial BP recording and serial arterial catecholamine sampling during cold pressor testing and mental stress tests. The investigators were also blinded as to the blood pressure awareness of the subjects.

Results.—Hypertension awareness significantly increased baseline plasma norepinephrine and epinephrine levels and intraplatelet norepinephrine levels. After sitting for 15 minutes in the testing laboratory, informed men had a significantly higher mean heart rate than noninformed men. The informed men had a significantly higher heart rate and blood pressure in anticipation of a cold pressor test and exaggerated norepinephrine and diastolic BP responses to mental stress compared with the noninformed men.

Conclusion.—Information about high BP may increase both the resting sympathetic tone and the sympathetic and cardiovascular responses to mental stress. Awareness of high BP should be taken into consideration when interpreting studies that investigate the early pathogenesis of essential hypertension.

▶ This study beautifully documents the "labeling" effect: those who are aware of having an elevated blood pressure are more hypertensive and more responsive to pressor stimuli, at least for a short time, simply because of their awareness of the diagnosis. No one can avoid the knowledge that hypertension is the silent killer, and it comes as no surprise that people recently told they are hypertensive are more stressed.

The problem, however, is that we may enter our patients into a vicious cycle: recognize an elevated blood pressure under stressful circumstances, tell the patient about the high reading, further elevate the stress level, and raise the blood pressure further. Two lessons need be learned. First, be gentle and comforting when telling a patient of an elevated pressure, advising that proper management will avert the severe decree. Second, always document an initially high level with many more readings, preferably taken out of the office setting to overcome the "white-coat" effect.

The situation can be complicated by such seemingly minor influences as the gender of the examiner.— N. Kaplan, M.D.

Gender Effects on Blood Pressures Obtained During an On-Campus Screening

McCubbin JA, Wilson JF, Bruehl S, Brady M, Clark K, Kort E (Univ of Kentucky, Lexington)
Psychosom Med 53:90– 100, 1991   3–8

Background.—Blood pressure measurements may be influenced by psychosocial factors. Higher recordings have been observed in some persons when their blood pressure is measured by a physician (i.e., white-coat hypertension), or at a clinic or at work. The impact of psychosocial determinants, including patient personality indices, response styles, and gender, were examined in a carefully controlled blood pressure screening of college students.

Methods.—A screening of 167 volunteers (age range, 18–35 years) was conducted at the University of Kentucky Student Center. After 19 persons were excluded because of their medical histories, 77 men and 71 women were included. Four blood pressure measurements were made at 1-minute intervals using a Dinamap Adult/Pediatric Vital Signs Monitor.

Results.—Average systolic blood pressure correlated significantly with gender, body mass, and reported caffeine intake. Average diastolic blood pressure correlated significantly with age. Multivariate relationships for blood pressures and demographic characteristics demonstrated that males had significantly higher systolic blood pressures than females, as did persons who had recently ingested caffeine. The average difference between the first and the later measures of blood pressure was significantly greater when the measurement was made by a person of the opposite sex of the participant. Males reported significantly higher hostility scores and more pronounced anger scores than females, but no interaction was observed between hostility and blood pressure. Some interaction with the anger expression did affect the participant gender by screener gender interaction.

Somatic anxiety response style significantly moderated the impact of the participant gender by screener gender interaction on the average systolic blood pressure.

Conclusions.—These findings indicate that a potential exists for errors in blood pressure measurements related to the gender of the patient and examiner. Apparently, females experience increases in blood pressure when the measurement is taken by a male, whether by a physician or a nonphysician screener. Males had lower final systolic blood pressure levels when measured by a female. Subtly changing the psychosocial milieu of blood pressure measurement can cause small but important alterations in resting pressures.

▶ The more authoritarian figure of a male examiner may explain the higher prevalence of "white-coat" hypertension in women. Obviously, the blood pressure can be affected by multiple influences, including the outside temperature. In Montreal, where the range of temperature at noon was from −24° C to +27° C, the average office readings in 2,000 patients were 7/3 mm Hg higher on the coldest days than on the warmer days (1).

Because everyone cannot bask in the Florida (or even the Texas) sunshine during the winter, those who live in the north should anticipate somewhat higher readings in their patients when the weather outside is chilly. Climactic differences will not be overcome by out-of-the-office readings, but most of the "white-coat" effect will be. Another study (2) documents that about 15% of patients with persistently elevated office readings will be normotensive by 24-hour ambulatory monitoring. Interestingly, these investigators found that 14% of borderline hypertensives (office blood pressure between 140/90 and 160/95) tended to have lower average ambulatory readings than office readings.

For the near future, conventional sphygmomanometry in the office setting will be most widely used, both for diagnosis and monitoring. In the more distant future, ambulatory monitoring will surely be used more, particularly because less expensive models and criteria for normal and high ranges are now available.—N. Kaplan, M.D.

References

1. Kuneš J, et al: Influence of environmental temperature on the blood pressure of hypertensive patients in Montreal. *Am J Hypertens* 4:422–426, 1991.
2. Enström I, et al: How good are standardized blood pressure recordings for diagnosing hypertension? A comparison between office and ambulatory blood pressure. *J Hypertens* 9:561–566, 1991.

Mean and Range of the Ambulatory Pressure in Normotensive Subjects From a Meta-Analysis of 23 Studies

Staessen JA, Fagard RH, Lijnen PJ, Thijs L, Van Hoof R, Amery AK (Univ of Leuven, Belgium)
Am J Cardiol 67:723–727, 1991
3–9

Background.—Although ambulatory blood pressure (BP) monitoring overcomes many problems in variability of BP measurement, its clinical

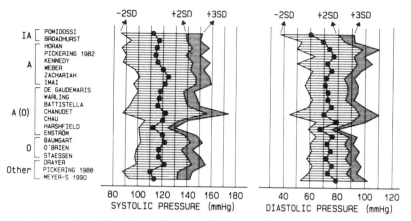

Fig 3–2.—Systolic and diastolic blood pressure (BP) during 24 hours in various studies. The mean and the mean ± 2 and + 3 standard deviations are given. Abbreviations are used to indicate the technique for BP recording: *A*, auscultatory; *A(O)*, auscultatory with oscillometric back-up; *IA*, intra-arterial; *O*, oscillometric. (Courtesy of Staessen JA, Fagard RH, Lijnen PJ, et al: *Am J Cardiol* 67:723–727, 1991.)

relevance is questionable because of the lack of agreement on reference values. A meta-analysis of published reports was therefore done to establish the mean and range of normal ambulatory BP.

Methods.— Twenty-three studies were identified from the English, French, and German literature. The reports included a total of 3,476 normal subjects, with numbers per study ranging from 9 to 815.

Results.—Most studies that reported a mean 24-hour BP were compatible with a range of 115–120/70–75 mm Hg, a mean daytime BP of 120–125/75–80 mm Hg, and a mean nighttime BP of 105–110/60–65 mm Hg (Fig 3–2). Averages were 118/72 mm Hg for 24-hour BP, 123/76 for daytime BP, and 106/64 for nighttime BP after weighting for the number of subjects included in the individual studies. Night/day pressure ratios ranged from .79 to .92 for systolic and from .75 to .90 for diastolic BP, with averages of .87 and .83, respectively. Assuming that the mean standard deviation of 2 in the various studies was normal, the normal ranges were 97–139/57–87 mm Hg for 24-hour BP, 101–146/61–91 mm Hg for daytime BP, and 86–127/48–79 mm Hg for nighttime BP.

Conclusions.—Results of a meta-analysis of 23 studies of normal BP measurements by ambulatory monitoring were evaluated. These values could serve as a temporary reference for clinical practice until the results of prospective studies focusing on the relation between ambulatory BP and the incidence of cardiovascular morbidity and mortality are available.

▶ Based on these 3,476 recordings of normal adult subjects, the authors recommend these lower limits for "probable" or "suspect" hypertension by ambulatory monitoring: average of all 24-hour readings was 139/87; average of daytime, awake readings was 146/91, the average of nighttime or sleep readings was 127/79. Obviously, these daytime values, representing the mean plus 2 standard deviations of over 3,000 recordings, are virtually identical to the 140/90 mm Hg accepted by most everyone for the diagnosis of hypertension based on variable numbers of office recordings by conventional sphygmomanometry.

Nighttime readings have never been included in the ascertainment of hypertension because they cannot be obtained by conventional measurements. Therefore, I strongly believe that they should not be included in the determination of the diagnosis of hypertension by ambulatory monitoring. In most normotensive and hypertensive patients, the nighttime values are considerably lower and, if they are not, the patient likely has left ventricular hypertrophy and dysfunction.

For a complete and balanced presentation of everything you could possibly want to know about ambulatory monitoring, Tom Pickering has just published a terrific book, *Ambulatory Monitoring and Blood Pressure Variability* (Science Press, London, 1991). Among his many pearls, Dr. Pickering comments, "No agreement has been reached about the upper limit of normal ambulatory blood pressure or about how it should be defined. The 95th percentile of the range in 'normotensive' subjects [used by Staessen et al. in the above abstract] gives a value that is probably too high, which is perhaps not surprising since hypertension affects more than 5% of the population."

Elsewhere in his book, Pickering decries the use of such rigid criteria for separating normotension and hypertension using ambulatory monitoring just as his illustrious father, Sir George, did with conventionally obtained measurements.

Nonetheless, clinicians need such criteria to make diagnosis, so it is certain that we will establish them and use them. However, the more important issue is: what blood pressure level should indicate the need for active drug therapy? As many of us have been arguing, much more than the blood pressure should be used to make that critical decision. Along with Tom Pickering, another co-worker of John Laragh's, Michael Alderman, has nicely restated the case for using all of the appropriate risk factors in ascertaining relative risk and the need, thereby, for active drug therapy (1).

One of the determinants of risk included by Dr. Alderman is the level of plasma renin activity, particularly in view of his finding that plasma renin activity did predict the development of heart attacks.—N. Kaplan, M.D.

Reference

1. Alderman MH: Heterogeneity among hypertensive subjects: A tool for clinical decision-making. *Clin Chem* 37:1885–1890, 1991.

Association of the Renin-Sodium Profile With the Risk of Myocardial Infarction in Patients With Hypertension
Alderman MH, Madhavan S, Ooi WL, Cohen H, Sealey JE, Laragh JH (Albert Einstein College of Medicine, Bronx, NY; Cornell Univ Med College, New York)
N Engl J Med 324:1098–1104, 1991   3–10

Background.—A previously published retrospective study suggested that hypertensive patients can be stratified by their pretreatment renin-sodium profiles for treatment outcome. A prospective study to test this hypothesis began in 1981. Data were collected on 1,717 patients with mild or moderate hypertension whose renin-sodium profile was ascertained.

Methods.—Between January 1981 and October 1988, 3,183 employees were screened at a work-site hypertension control program. Of these, 1,717 patients met the following characteristics for inclusion into the study: a 24-hour urinary excretion of sodium between 35 and 240 mmol, a renin profile measured within 6 months of the program, and a follow-up of at least 2 months after the renin determination.

Results.—Overall, 12.3% of the subjects had a high renin-sodium profile, 55.9% had a normal profile, and 31.8% had a low profile. Those with high and low renin profiles differed in age, race, sex, and treatment history. The mean diastolic pressure of subjects with high renin profiles was significantly, but not clinically, higher than in those in the other 2 patient groups, 100 mm Hg versus 97 mm Hg and 96 mm Hg. Drug treatment normalized blood pressure equally in all renin profile groups. A total of 107 fatal or nonfatal events occurred among the 1,717 patients during the 8.3 years of follow-up. The overall rates of myocardial infarction adjusted for age, sex, and race were 14.7 per 1,000 person-years in the high renin profile group, 5.6 in the normal group, and 2.8 in the low profile group. There was no association between strokes and renin profile. The independent association of a high renin profile with myocardial infarction remained after adjustment for other cardiovascular factors and the use of β-blockers.

Implications.—These findings indicate that patients with high renin-sodium profiles have a greater risk of myocardial infarction than those with low or normal renin-sodium profiles despite equal degrees of subsequent control of blood pressure by antihypertensive drug therapy.

▶ It must be heartening for John Laragh and his co-workers to have confirmation by a prospective study of a claim they made in 1972 on the basis of a retrospective analysis, a claim that has been repeatedly attacked and denied by other investigators, including me. However, remember that there were only 27 myocardial infarctions in the entire study and there was no association between plasma renin activity (PRA) and stroke (as had been claimed in 1972). I agree with the authors in their final statement: "The next step will be to confirm and extend the associations observed here between PRA and myocardial infarction and to determine how they can be applied to clinical research and practice."

For me and for now, determination of PRA remains a research tool except in the differential diagnosis of secondary forms of hypertension, as will be covered in the abstracts near the end of the Hypertension section of this YEAR BOOK. However, more evidence for the prognostic value of PRA has come from another of Dr. Laragh's former co-workers.—N. Kaplan, M.D.

Ambulatory Blood Pressure Patterns in Children and Adolescents: Influence of Renin-Sodium Profiles

Harshfield GA, Pulliam DA, Alpert BS, Stapleton FB, Willey ES, Somes GW
(Univ of Tennessee, Memphis; LeBonheur Children's Med Ctr, Memphis)
Pediatrics 87:94–100, 1991   3–11

Introduction.— Renin-sodium profiling may be used to distinguish between different forms of essential hypertension. Studies have shown that casual blood pressure (BP) values do not differ between hypertensives with different renin-sodium profiles, but the relation between ambulatory BP patterns and renin-sodium profiles has never been studied. Because essential hypertension has its origins in childhood, the relationship between ambulatory BP and renin-sodium profiles in normotensive adolescents was studied.

Methods.— Renin-sodium profiles were obtained in 159 black and white healthy, normotensive adolescents. Based on the relationship between plasma renin activity and 24-hour urinary sodium excretion, children were classified as having a high, intermediate, or low renin-sodium profile. Twenty-nine children (18%) had low renin-sodium profiles, 103 (65%) had intermediate renin-sodium profiles, and 27 (17%) had high renin-sodium profiles. Ambulatory BP was monitored for 24 hours. Diaries of activities were kept for each hour the monitor was worn. Casual and awake BP values were then compared with the nomogram constructed from the renin-sodium profiles.

Results.— Casual and awake BP values did not differ significantly among normotensive children with low, intermediate, and high renin-sodium profiles. However, children with high renin-sodium profiles had a smaller decline in systolic BP from awake to asleep (7 vs. 11 mm Hg) and a higher diastolic BP during sleep (65 vs. 62 mm Hg) than children with low or intermediate renin-sodium profiles. Children with high renin-sodium profiles also showed greater BP variance during sleep than children with low or intermediate renin-sodium profiles.

Conclusion.— The blunted nocturnal BP decline and increased nocturnal BP variance among normotensive children with high renin-sodium profiles may be a marker for the future development of essential hypertension.

▶ The observation that normotensive children with higher plasma renin activity (PRA) levels have less of a nocturnal fall in blood pressure may turn out to be as important for the prognostic value of PRA measurements as the finding by Alderman et al. in the previous abstract. This will be true if more of these high PRA subjects develop persistent hypertension or have more left ventricular hypertrophy and cardiovascular dysfunction. If these 2 preliminary observations are confirmed, those of us who have downplayed the value of PRA for prognosis will have to admit that Laragh et al. were right all along. (I write this as the Dallas Cowboys have just won their wild-card game against the Chicago Bears to enter the race for the 1992 Super Bowl. I only wish I had as much faith in their return as John Laragh has had in PRA.)

Before leaving Diagnosis and Monitoring, comment should be directed to the continuing evidence for increased incidences of cardiovascular catastrophes in the early morning, calling further attention to the need for measuring the blood pressure soon after arising from bed when the abrupt rise in pressure occurs (1). In a lovely study, Panza et al. (2) showed that the early morning was a time of higher vascular tone, which was related to increased α-sympathetic vaso-constrictor activity during the morning. They conclude that "This (circadian) variation may contribute to higher blood pressure and the increased incidence of cardiovascular events at this time of day."—N. Kaplan, M.D.

References

1. Khoury AF, et al: The early morning rise in blood pressure (BP) occurs after arising and not before or after awakening [Abstract]. *Am J Hypertens* 4:993, 1991.
2. Panza JA, et al: Circadian variation in vascular tone and its relation to α-sympathetic vasoconstrictor activity. *N Engl J Med* 325:986–990, 1991.

Mechanisms of Hypertension

▶ ↓ The presence of hypertension reflects the interaction between inherited traits and environmental influences. The genetic contribution to systolic and diastolic blood pressure levels has been quantitated in hemodynamic studies of monozygotic and dizygotic twins and found to vary from 22% to as high as 70% under varying conditions of posture and exercise (1). More about the genetic contribution and a great deal more about other possibly predictors of hypertension is provided in the proceedings of a National Institutes of Health workshop published as a supplement to the November 1991 issue of the *American Journal of Hypertension.*

One of the traits that may be inherited is an inability of the kidneys to excrete the large amounts of sodium ingested by most people in industrialized societies. This inability has been explored in 2 studies on normotensive subjects with hypertensive parents, subjects known to be a higher risk for developing hypertension.   N. Kaplan, M.D.

Reference

1. Bielen EC, et al: Inheritance of blood pressure and haemodynamic phenotypes measured at rest and during supine dynamic exercise. *J Hypertens* 9:655–663, 1991.

Blunted Renal Sodium Excretion During Acute Saline Loading in Normotensive Men With Positive Family Histories of Hypertension
Widgren BR, Herlitz H, Hedner T, Berglund G, Wikstrand J, Jonsson O, Andersson OK (Sahlgrenska Hosp, Göteborg, Sweden)
Am J Hypertens 4:570–578, 1991   3–12

Introduction.—There is substantial evidence that individuals with family histories of hypertension are at increased risk for developing elevated blood pressure. To investigate some of the mechanisms involved in this genetic predisposition, the effects of a rapid saline load during usual sodium intake was studied in normotensive healthy young men with or without family histories of hypertension.

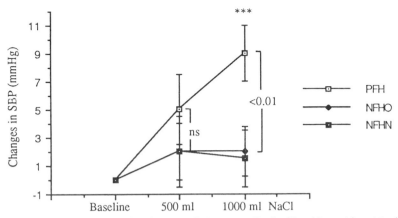

Fig 3–3.—Changes in systolic blood pressure during acute saline load in subjects with positive family histories of hypertension (PFH), controls matched for body mass index (NFHO), and lean controls with negative family histories of hypertension (NFHN). (Courtesy of Widgren BR, Herlitz H, Hedner T, et al: *Am J Hypertens* 4:570–578, 1991.)

Methods.—Eleven of the men recruited for the study had positive family histories of hypertension. They were matched for age with a control group negative for a family history of hypertension. Ten of the controls were matched with the original 11 men for body mass index (BMI) and 11 were lean (normal BMI). For each group, the natriuretic and intra-arterial blood pressure (BP) response to an acute saline load (1,000 mL .9% sodium chloride) was recorded.

Results.—The men with positive family histories of hypertension and the controls matched for BMI had a significantly higher baseline BP than the lean controls. During the saline infusion, individuals with a positive family history disclosed a diminished natriuretic response compared with the 2 control groups. Systolic BP increased significantly in subjects with a positive family history, but not in the 2 control groups (Fig 3–3). Finally, a significant negative correlation was noted between baseline sodium excretion and sodium efflux rate from erythrocytes in the men with positive family histories of hypertension.

Conclusion.—Normotensive young men with positive family histories of hypertension have a blunted natriuretic and an exaggerated blood pressure response to an acute saline load. This blunted renal sodium excretion and increased pressor response to saline may be influenced by neuronal as well as hormonal mechanisms.

Renal Hemodynamics and the Renin-Angiotensin-Aldosterone System in Normotensive Subjects With Hypertensive and Normotensive Parents

van Hooft IMS, Grobbee DE, Derkx FHM, de Leeuw PW, Schalekamp MADH, Hofman A (Erasmus Univ Med School, Rotterdam, The Netherlands; Univ Hosp Dijkzigt, Rotterdam; Zuiderziekenhuis, Rotterdam)
N Engl J Med 324:1305–1311, 1991
3–13

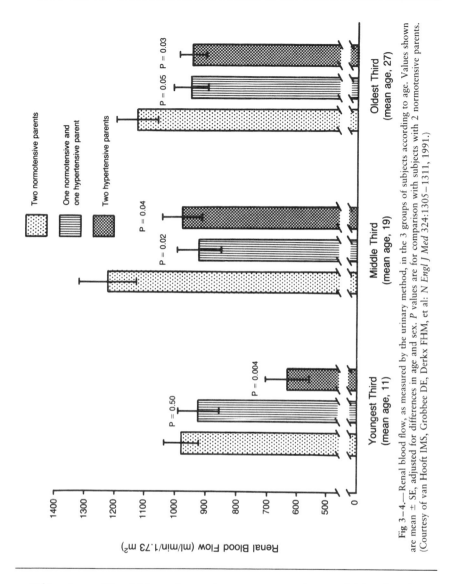

Fig 3–4.—Renal blood flow, as measured by the urinary method, in the 3 groups of subjects according to age. Values shown are mean ± SE, adjusted for differences in age and sex. *P* values are for comparison with subjects with 2 normotensive parents. (Courtesy of van Hooft IMS, Grobbee DE, Derkx FHM, et al: *N Engl J Med* 324:1305–1311, 1991.)

Objective.—The kidney is an important regulator of blood volume and blood pressure, but its influence on the development of essential hypertension is not fully understood. To determine whether young persons at risk for hypertension because of family history have altered renal hemodynamics, 3 groups of normotensive subjects were studied.

Methods.—The 154 participants were taken from a larger group of residents of the town of Zoetermeer, The Netherlands, who were members of a study of blood pressure and other cardiovascular risk factors. Participants ranged in age from 7 to 32. Forty-one had 2 normotensive parents, 52 had 1 normotensive and 1 hypertensive parent, and 61 had 2 hypertensive parents. Renal hemodynamics were measured by the clearance of paraaminohippuric acid and inulin. Characteristics of the renin-angiotensin-aldosterone system were also compared in the 3 groups.

Findings.—Even after adjustments for differences in height, weight, age, and proportion of males, subjects with 2 hypertensive parents had higher systolic and diastolic blood pressure than subjects in the other 2 groups. Hematocrit and the serum level and 24-hour urinary excretion of sodium and potassium were similar in the 3 groups. Renal blood flow was significantly lower in those with 2 hypertensive parents. The most striking differences were noted in the youngest third of the subjects whose mean age was 11 years (Fig 3–4). Members of this group also had a higher filtration fraction and renal vascular resistance. Compared to those with 2 normotensive parents, subjects with 2 hypertensive parents had lower plasma concentrations of renin and aldosterone.

Discussion.—Young persons with a family history of hypertension show an increase in renal vasoconstriction and a decrease in renin and aldosterone secretion. Thus, changes in renal hemodynamics may take place at an early age in the development of familial hypertension.

▶ The delay in renal excretion of an acute sodium load shown by McVeigh et al. could easily reflect the altered renal hemodynamics found by van Hooft et al. in these 2 studies of young normotensive subjects with positive family histories of hypertension (Abstracts 3–12 and 3–13). The larger and more intensive study by van Hooft is perhaps the best analysis of what may very well be the initiating defect in the hemodynamic cascade that eventuates in hypertension. As documented in the young subjects studied by Julius et al. in Tecumseh (see Abstract 3–3), a hyperdynamic circulation may be typical in the earliest stages. This hyperdynamic state could reflect an overfilled vascular volume, resulting from a defect in renal handling of our constantly excessive oral sodium intake.

In the very youngest normotensive subjects with the greatest genetic likelihood of developing hypertension, van Hooft et al. found the most strikingly reduced renal blood flow and increased filtration fraction and renal vascular resistance. Accompanying these changes were lower levels of plasma renin and aldosterone, which certainly could reflect the suppression of renin release by an overfilled vascular bed. It all makes a neat picture for the very beginnings of hypertension.

Before getting carried away by such data, we should realize that there is much more involved in the heterogeneous mosaic of hypertension. For example, transport of sodium across cell membranes is likely altered, perhaps by a circulating inhibitor of the sodium-potassium pump (1). A possible marker of a genetic contribution to sodium transport changes is the sodium-lithium (Na+-Li+) countertransport measured in red blood cells. In the Tecumseh study, subjects with elevated Na+-Li+ countertransport had higher blood pressure and a greater prevalence of hypertension (2).

Another environmental factor is stress, and it too may interact with sodium.—N. Kaplan, M.D.

References

1. Hilton PJ: Na+ transport in hypertension. *Diabetes Care* 14:233–239, 1991.
2. Weder AB, et al: Red blood cell lithium-sodium countertransport in the Tecumseh Blood Pressure Study. *Hypertension* 17:652–660, 1991.

Suppressed Aggression Accelerates Early Development of Essential Hypertension

Perini C, Müller FB, Bühler FR (University Hospitals, Basel, Switzerland)
J Hypertens 9:499–503, 1991   3–14

Background.—Among the factors contributing to elevated blood pressure are casual blood pressure per se, heart rate, cardiovascular hypersensitivity to stress, family history of hypertension, body weight, and rate of urinary sodium excretion. Because psychological factors also appear to play a role, such factors were studied as predictors for subsequent development of essential hypertension.

Methods.—In a prospective study, 98 normotensive and 23 borderline hypertensive men and women aged 16 to 24 were followed up for an average of 2.5 years. Baseline examination included psychological tests and resting and stress-induced cardiovascular and neurohormonal measurements.

Results.—In the normotensive subjects, the best predictor of subsequent borderline hypertension was the height of casual systolic blood pressure at entry. The weakest predictors were stress-induced blood pressure responses, sympathetic nervous system activity, and psychological factors. In the borderline hypertensive group, the single best predictor of sustained borderline or subsequent established hypertension was the peak systolic blood pressure induced by mental stress. In all subjects taken together, the greatest increases in blood pressure were found in those who had suppressed aggression, particularly if they had borderline blood pressure at entry.

Conclusion.—Suppressed aggression and anxiety mediated by elevated sympathetic nervous system activity seems to contribute to the development of hypertension.

▶ This is one of the latest in a number of studies using laboratory-induced acute mental stress to predict the current presence or future development of hypertension. As most of the other studies have shown, laboratory stress is a very poor predictor. However, suppressed aggression or hostility has previously been found to be a common psychological trait in young, borderline hypertensives, and Perini et al. have shown it to be a predictor of short-term rises in blood pressure. Such hostility may be involved in a group who are very prone to hypertension.—N. Kaplan, M.D.

The Association of Skin Color With Blood Pressure in US Blacks With Low Socioeconomic Status

Klag MJ, Whelton PK, Coresh J, Grim CE, Kuller LH (Johns Hopkins Univ, Baltimore; Charles R Drew Univ, Los Angeles; Univ of Pittsburgh)
JAMA 265:599–602, 1991   3–15

Background.—Blacks in the United States have higher age-specific mean blood pressures and a higher prevalence of hypertension than whites. Differences in access to health care, socioeconomic status, diet, and other risk factors for hypertension explain some of this variation. Previous research on the relationship between skin color and blood pressure in blacks has yielded conflicting results. A community-based sample of blacks in the United States was studied to determine whether skin color is associated with blood pressure.

Methods.—Four hundred fifty-seven blacks from 3 cities were studied. Skin color was measured by a reflectometer. The sample excluded anyone taking antihypertensive medications.

Results.—Darker persons had higher average systolic and diastolic blood pressures. Systolic and diastolic pressures increased by 2 mm Hg for every standard deviation in skin darkness. This relationship depended, however, on socioeconomic status, measured by either education or an index consisting of education, occupation, and ethnicity (Green Index). The association was present only in persons at lower socioeconomic levels as measured by either indicator. According to multiple linear regression, the relationship was independent of age, body mass index, and blood glucose, serum uric acid, urinary sodium-to-potassium ratio, and level of education.

Conclusions.—The relationship between skin color and blood pressure in American blacks appears to vary with socioeconomic status. This may be caused by increased susceptibility to psychosocial stress associated with having darker skin. However, it may also result from an interaction between an environmental factor associated with low socioeconomic status and a gene occurring more frequently in darker skinned persons.

▶ Although the authors suggest other explanations for the association of darker skin color and low socioeconomic class with hypertension in blacks in the United States, the most likely one is the greater hostility, often suppressed, that such people must feel.

Beyond sodium and stress, the other major environmental contributor is weight gain and obesity. Recall the findings reported in the first few abstracts in this section relating the development of hypertension to body mass index and weight gain. Obesity anywhere is associated with higher blood pressure and impairment of left ventricular function (1). Obesity in the upper body (abdomen) is associated even more closely, however, not only to hypertension but also to diabetes and dyslipidemias (2).

These associations with upper body obesity, which I called "the deadly quartet," have been expanded to encompass a large proportion of nonobese hypertensive patients as well (3). Gerald Reaven referred to these features as "syndrome X," but they are much better called "the insulin resistance (5) syndrome." I am particularly attracted to the initials, IRS, which clearly connotes a serious and costly condition.

The presence of glucose intolerance as one of the components of IRS has been re-confirmed.— N. Kaplan, M.D.

References

1. Grossman E, et al: Left ventricular filling in the systemic hypertension of obesity. *Am J Cardiol* 68:57–60, 1991.
2. Després J-P: Obesity and lipid metabolism: Relevance of body fat distribution. *Curr Opin Lipidology* 2:5–15, 1991.
3. Ferrannini E: Metabolic abnormalities of hypertension. A lesson in complexity. *Hypertension* 18:636–639, 1991.

Glucose Tolerance and Blood Pressure: Long Term Follow Up in Middle Aged Men
Salomaa VV, Strandberg TE, Vanhanen H, Naukkarinen V, Sarna S, Miettinen TA (National Public Health Institute, Helsinki; University of Helsinki; Jorvi District Hospital, Espoo, Finland)
BMJ 302:493–496, 1991   3–16

Background.—There is a close association between blood glucose concentrations after glucose challenge and blood pressure, but there have been no follow-up studies since this relationship was established. The role of blood glucose concentration after glucose challenge as a predictor of future hypertension and the temporal relations between glucose tolerance and the development of hypertension were assessed in an 18-year follow-up.

Methods.—The retrospective study was based on the results of a general health checkup in middle-aged businessmen in the late 1960s. In 1974, the men were invited to enter a primary prevention trial for cardiovascular disease, at which time they underwent clinical examination for risk factors. The men were examined again in 1979, and follow-up was done in 1986. At all of the first 3 examinations, blood glucose concentrations after glucose challenge test were measured. The study sample included 1,203 men who did not have an intervention in 1974. Of these, 1,120 were examined in 1979 and 945 attended follow-up in 1986. At this time, 131 of the men were taking antihypertensive drugs and 12 were taking drugs for hyperglycemia.

Results.—The 330 men who were hypertensive in 1986 had significantly higher blood pressures after adjustment for body mass and alcohol intake and significantly higher blood glucose concentrations in response to glucose challenge than men who were normotensive in 1986. According to regression analysis, men who had higher blood glucose concentrations in response to glucose challenge in 1968 had higher blood pressure in subsequent years. For men whose blood glucose concentration was between the second and third tertiles in 1968, the risk of having hypertension was significantly higher (odds ratio 1.71) than for those with concentrations below the first tertile.

Conclusions.—Hypertensive men tend to have increased intolerance to glucose as long as 18 years before their hypertension is clinically manifested. Thus, blood glucose concentration in response to glucose challenge test is an important predictor of the development of hypertension. This abnormality, in combination with dyslipidemia, may be important in the development of atherosclerosis and coronary heart disease.

▶ Note that glucose intolerance was associated with the subsequent development of hypertension *after* adjustment for body mass. This fits with the evidence that IRS is present in as many as half of nonobese hypertensive patients, as reviewed in the article by Ferrannini (1).

As tight as this association has been reported to be in multiple groups of white subjects, it may not be present in other racial groups.—N. Kaplan, M.D.

Reference

1. Ferrannini E: Metabolic abnormalities of hypertension. A lesson in complexity. *Hypertension* 18:636−639, 1991.

Racial Differences in the Relation Between Blood Pressure and Insulin Resistance

Saad MF, Lillioja S, Nyomba BL, Castillo C, Ferraro R, De Gregorio M, Ravussin E, Knowler WC, Bennett PH, Howard BV, Bogardus C (Natl Inst of Diabetes and Digestive and Kidney Diseases, Natl Insts of Health, Phoenix; Medlantic Research Found, Washington, DC)
N Engl J Med 324:733–739, 1991   3–17

Background.—Although insulin resistance and compensatory hyperinsulinemia have been implicated in the pathogenesis of hypertension, studies on the relationship between insulin and blood pressure have produced inconsistent results. The possibility that racial differences exist in this relationship was studied.

Methods.—One hundred sixteen Pima Indians, 53 whites, and 42 blacks who were normotensive and did not have diabetes were studied. The mean ages and blood pressures in these groups were comparable. The euglycemic-hyperinsulinemic clamp technique was used to determine insulin resistance during low-dose and high-dose insulin infusions.

Results.—The Pima Indians had higher fasting plasma insulin levels than did whites or blacks. They also had lower rates of whole-body glucose disposal during low-dose and high-dose insulin infusions. However, after adjustment for age, sex, weight, and percentage of body fat, there was a significant correlation between mean blood pressure and fasting plasma insulin levels as well as rate of glucose disposal during low-dose and high-dose infusions in whites only (Fig 3–5).

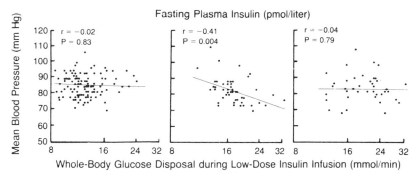

Fig 3–5.—Relation between mean blood pressure and insulin-mediated glucose disposal during low-dose insulin infusions in Pima Indians, whites, and blacks, after adjustment for age, sex, body weight, and percentage of body fat. Differences among the 3 groups in the slopes of the regression lines between mean blood pressure and the fasting plasma insulin concentration and insulin-mediated glucose disposal during low-dose and high-dose insulin infusions were statistically significant (P = .001, .017, and .025, respectively). (Courtesy of Saad MF, Lillioja S, Nyomba BL, et al: *N Engl J Med* 324:733–739, 1991.)

Conclusions.—Plasma insulin levels and insulin resistance are related to blood pressure in whites but not in blacks or Pima Indians. This relationship may be mediated by mechanisms active in whites but not in the other groups. On the other hand, the relationship may not be causal. A common mechanism—genetic or acquired—may be the link between insulin resistance and blood pressure in whites but not in other racial groups.

▶ As seen in Figure 3–5, insulin resistance, measured as decreased whole-body glucose disposal during insulin infusion, was related to blood pressure in whites but not in Pima Indians or in blacks. However, all of these subjects were normotensive, so the data may or may not be pertinent to the situation in hypertensive subjects. Others (1) have found insulin resistance in black hypertensive patients using the same sensitive technique used by Saad et al.

The same pattern of insulin resistance has now been identified in middle-aged nonobese subjects with asymptomatic atherosclerosis (2), further incriminating insulin resistance and/or the resultant hyperinsulinemia as an independent risk factor for atherosclerosis.

The features of IRS include dyslipidemias, mainly hypertriglyceridemia and low high-density lipoprotein cholesterol levels. Gerald Reaven's laboratory has provided an explanation for the low high-density lipoprotein levels.—N. Kaplan, M.D.

References

1. Falkner B, et al: Insulin resistance and blood pressure in young black men. *Hypertension* 16:706–711, 1990.
2. Laakso M, et al: Asymptomatic atherosclerosis and insulin resistance. *Arteriosclerosis Thrombosis* 11:1068–1076, 1991.

High Density Lipoprotein Turnover in Patients With Hypertension

Chen Y-DI, Sheu WH-H, Swislocki ALM, Reaven GM (Stanford Univ; Dept of Veterans Affairs Med Ctr, Palo Alto, Calif)
Hypertension 17:386–393, 1991   3–18

Background.—Hypertensive patients may have hyperinsulinemia and decreased high-density lipoprotein (HDL) cholesterol concentration. However, there are no data regarding the dynamic state of HDL metabolism. To quantify HDL turnover, subjects with and without hypertension were studied.

Methods.—The hypertensive group comprised 12 patients, 10 men and 2 women, mean age 49 years. Their mean blood pressure was 143/96 mm Hg. The normotensive group comprised 8 men and 3 women. The only significant difference between the 2 groups was fasting insulin, which was 21 μU/mL in the hypertensive group compared with 11 μU/mL in controls. Each subject's plasma was measured for insulin, glucose, HDL-cholesterol, and ^{125}I-apolipoprotein AI (apoAI) concentrations. Turnover of HDL was measured using a new pool of purified apoAI every 4 months.

Results.—Concentrations of HDL were lower in the hypertensive group. These patients also had faster fractional catabolic rates of apoAI HDL and total synthetic rates of apoAI. There was a significant correlation between blood pressure and fractional catabolic rate of apoAI/HDL in the experimental population, but there was no such relation when the 2 groups were considered separately. Overall, the subjects had a highly significant positive correlation between apoAI/HDL fractional catabolic rate and insulin concentration.

Conclusions.—Mildly hypertensive and hyperinsulinemic patients appear to have a faster fractional catabolic rate of apoAI/HDL and a lower HDL-cholesterol concentration. These changes appear to result from hyperinsulinemia rather than hypertension itself, as they probably do in patients with noninsulin-dependent diabetes mellitus and hypertriglyceridemia.

▶ Not only are levels of cardioprotective HDL-cholesterol low in hypertensives but these patients tend to have increased levels of LDL and total cholesterol.—N. Kaplan, M.D.

Association Between Blood Pressure and Serum Lipids in a Population: The Tromsø Study

Bønaa KH, Thelle DS (Univ of Tromsø, Norway)
Circulation 83:1305–1314, 1991   3–19

Introduction.—Individuals with both hypertension and hypercholesterolemia are at particularly high risk for coronary heart disease. To better understand the relationship between blood pressure and blood lipids, a large population of young and middle-aged men and women was studied.

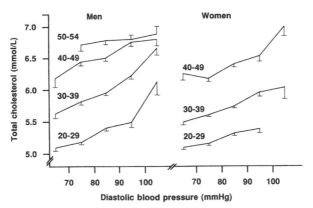

Fig 3–6.—Plot of mean concentrations of serum total cholesterol levels (mmol/L) by diastolic blood pressure in men 20–29, 30–39, 40–49, and 50–54 years old and in women 20–29, 30–39, and 40–49 years old. Cells with less than 20 observations were pooled by adjacent category. *T bars* are SEM. (Courtesy of Bǿnaa KH, Thelle DS: *Circulation* 83:1305–1314, 1991.)

Methods.—All men 20–54 years old and all women 20–49 years old living in one area of Norway were invited to take part in the study; 78%, a total of 8,081 men and 7,663 women, agreed to participate. The subjects were questioned about their medical history, smoking and alcohol habits, physical activity in leisure time, and current use of antihypertensive drugs.

Results.—There was a consistent positive relationship between blood pressure and cholesterol levels, suggesting a biological interrelationship between these 2 major risk factors for coronary heart disease. In both sexes, total and non–high-density lipoprotein (HDL) levels increased significantly with increasing systolic or diastolic blood pressure. The association between blood pressure and total cholesterol level increased with age in women, but decreased with age in men (Fig 3–6). When compared with lean subjects, overweight subjects had greater increases in total cholesterol or triglyceride levels with increases in blood pressure. Smoking, physical activity, and alcohol consumption had little influence on the association between blood pressure and serum lipids.

Conclusion.—Biological interrelationship between hypertension and hypercholesterolemia may influence the mechanisms whereby blood pressure is associated with the risk of coronary heart disease. The 2 risk factors appear to have a synergistic relationship, whereby the increased risk of myocardial infarction is multiplicative rather than additive.

▶ These data confirm what has been previously and consistently noted in smaller populations: dyslipidemias and hypertension coexist more commonly than expected by chance alone. Insulin resistance may be the common denominator.

The combination of glucose intolerance-diabetes, hypertension, and dyslipidemia is bad enough, but the situation may be even worse.—N. Kaplan, M.D.

Hypofibrinolysis in Patients With Hypertension and Elevated Cholesterol

Jansson J-H, Johansson B, Boman K, Nilsson TK (Skellefteå Hospital; Community Health Organisation, Skellefteå; Umeå University, Sweden)
J Intern Med 229:309–316, 1991   3–20

Background.—To examine further the potential way in which hypertension may be involved with atherogenesis, the relationship between hypertension and specific components of the fibrinolytic system was assessed.

Methods.—As part of a program of primary prevention of coronary disease, 84 patients with diastolic blood pressure of 90–109 mm Hg and total serum cholesterol levels of at least 6 mmol L^{-1} were identified as being at high risk. There were 45 men and 39 women, mean age 52 years. This group was matched for age, sex, smoking status, and body mass index to a group of 55 healthy controls. All subjects had measurement of plasminogen activator inhibitor (PAI-1) and tissue plasminogen activator (tPA) antigen and activity before and after venous occlusion; this tested for stimulated release of tPA activity and antigen into the circulation.

Results.—Tissue plasminogen activator activity was significantly lower and PAI-1 levels were significantly higher both before and after venous occlusion in the high-risk patients. Triglyceride levels, diastolic blood pressure, and cholesterol levels were independently associated with PAI-1 levels on multivariate analysis. There was also an independent and inverse association of diastolic blood pressure with resting tPA activity.

Conclusions.—In patients with hypertension and hyperlipidemia, there is reduced activity of the fibrinolytic system. This effect appears unrelated to differences in age, sex, smoking, or body mass index. The association between hypertension and hyperlipidemia and cardiovascular disease is linked to decreased fibrinolytic activity.

▶ These multiple atherogenic relationships may explain why hypertension is associated with increased cardiovascular risk. Another player has been introduced during the last few years: the endothelial lining of the blood vessels wherein vascular damage occurs. Since the discovery of an endothelium-derived relaxing factor (EDRF) in 1980, there has been an ongoing search for both relaxing and constricting factors made by endothelial cells and acting both locally and elsewhere in the circulation. Much of the evidence has been nicely summarized by Tolins et al (1). One of the possible by-products of this research may be the ability to pharmacologically alter these effects and thereby relieve both hypertension and atherosclerosis. A promising lead has been shown in salt-sensitive rats wherein the precursor for EDRF (now known to be nitric oxide) has been found to prevent the development of hypertension (2). In 1992 and beyond, the pharmacological manipulation of EDRF may become common: high levels that likely contribute to the refractory hypotension of septic shock can be reduced by inhibitors of nitric oxide synthesis (3); the impairment of endothelium-dependent dilation of the coronary microcirculation can be restored by infusion of the precursor of nitric oxide, arginine (4).

In the meantime, a more direct role of one of the new endothelium-derived constricting factors, endothelin, has been noted.—N. Kaplan, M.D.

References

1. Tolins JP, et al: Role of endothelium-derived relaxing factor in regulation of vascular tone and remodeling. Update on humoral regulation of vascular tone. *Hypertension* 17:909–916, 1991.
2. Chen PY, Sanders PW: L-Arginine abrogates salt-sensitive hypertension in Dahl/Rapp rats. *J Clin Invest* 88:1559–1567, 1991.
3. Petros A, et al: Effect of nitric oxide synthase inhibitors on hypotension in patients with septic shock. *Lancet* 338:1557–1558, 1991.
4. Drexler H, et al: Correction of endothelial dysfunction in coronary microcirculation of hypercholesterolaemic patients by L-arginine. *Lancet* 338:1546–1550, 1991.

Hypertension Associated With Endothelin-Secreting Malignant Hemangioendothelioma

Yokokawa K, Tahara H, Kohno M, Murakawa K, Yasunari K, Nakagawa K, Hamada T, Otani S, Yanagisawa M, Takeda T (Osaka City University, Japan; University of Tsukuba, Ibaraki, Japan)
Ann Intern Med 114:213–215, 1991   3–21

Background.—Endothelin-1 is known to be an endogenous vasoconstrictor. Plasma levels of endothelin-1 were measured in 2 patients before and after surgical excision of malignant hemangioendothelioma of the scalp.

Case Report 1.—Woman, 80, was seen with a solitary nodule on her scalp and a headache. Her blood pressure was 180/90 mm Hg, and her plasma endothelin-1 level was much higher than the concentration in healthy controls. After surgical excision of the tumor, her blood pressure became normal and the plasma endothelin-1 concentration decreased. On recurrence of the neoplasm, the patient had an increased plasma endothelin-1 concentration and blood pressure of 150/90 mm Hg. After the second excision, blood pressure again returned to normal and plasma endothelin-1 concentration decreased. Endothelin-1 concentration in the tumor tissue was 8 times that of tissue from the normal part of the patient's scalp.

Case Report 2.—Woman, 74, had a solitary pruritic nodule on her scalp and blood pressure of 160/106 mm Hg. After surgical excision of the nodule, her blood pressure fell to 110/70 mm Hg and her plasma endothelin-1 concentration decreased. Her tumor cells exhibited characteristic features of hemangioendothelioma.

Discussion.—These are the first 2 cases of an endothelin-secreting tumor to be reported. Plasma endothelin-1 concentrations and blood pressure levels decreased in both patients after surgical excision of the tumors and increased again with tumor recurrence in 1 patient. Tumor tissue contained much more endothelin-1 than normal tissue, which led to the conclusion that the tumors secreted excessive amounts of endothelin-1. In both patients with malignant hemangioendothelioma, changes in plasma endothelin-1 corresponded with changes in blood pressure, indicating that increased circulating endothelin-1 may contribute to hypertension.

▶ The therapeutic potentials of manipulating both endothelium-derived relaxing and constricting factors are enormous. Next year's YEAR BOOK will likely be full of promising reports to go along with the initial ones of 1991.—N. Kaplan, M.D.

Complications of Hypertension

▶ ↓ With all of the interconnections between hypertension and other cardiovascular risk factors, the progressive increases in the incidence of coronary disease, strokes, and renal failure that accompany every increment in blood pressure are easy to understand. Most of the inconsistencies between levels of blood pressure and the incidence of various cardiovascular morbidities and mortalities can be ascribed to variations of other risk factors.—N. Kaplan, M.D.

Why Do Lean Hypertensives Have Higher Mortality Rates Than Other Hypertensives? Findings of the Hypertension Detection and Follow-Up Program

Stamler R, Ford CE, Stamler J (Northwestern Univ, Chicago)
Hypertension 17:553–564, 1991   3–22

Background.—Excess weight is a risk factor for raised blood pressure, and patients with hypertension are often prescribed a weight reduction program to improve their general health. However, data from the Hypertension Detection and Follow-up Program (HDFP) demonstrated that the patient group with the highest 5-year mortality rate was in the lowest quintile for body mass index (BMI). The present study reports further analysis of the specific causes of death among the 10,908 individuals in the HDFP to explore why those who were lean had a higher mortality rate.

Methods.—The overall study design and methods of the HDFP involved 10,908 hypertensive men and women between the ages of 30 and 67 years who had a baseline BMI measured and were followed for a minimum of 5 years, with the primary endpoint for the study being all cause mortality. The specific underlying cause of death was recorded by nosologist from the death certificate for each decedent.

Findings.—The highest death rate was found in the group with the lowest BMI, with the death rate in the middle BMI quintile being about half that of the lowest 5% of body mass. The mortality rate in the highest BMI decile was similar to that seen in the median BMI level. Whereas mortality rates from cardiovascular diseases were 50% higher among men in the lowest 10% of body mass than in men in the median decile, mortality from noncardiovascular deaths was 2½ times higher in the lean group. The leaner hypertensives had strikingly higher death rates from cirrhosis, malignant neoplasms in men, nonmalignant respiratory disease in men, and violent death. Lean subjects were twice more likely to smoke, and excess deaths particularly from noncardiovascular diseases were mostly seen among smokers. Male smokers in the lowest BMI decile comprised only 3% of the study population but accounted for 8% of all deaths, 11% of noncardiovascular deaths, and 22% of cirrhotic deaths. More deaths occurred early in the follow-up period in lean compared with other patients with hypertension, suggesting that many of the lean patients had occult disease at baseline.

Conclusion.—Excess mortality in lean hypertensive patients may reflect the harmful lifestyles they lead, especially smoking and excess alcohol ingestion. These deleterious practices contribute to both their thinness and a higher risk of death.

▶ Lean hypertensive are at greater risk from noncardiovascular diseases for many reasons that do not directly relate to their hypertension. The obese, on the other hand, suffer from more cardiovascular problems, as described in earlier abstracts. Obese hypertensives also have more left ventricular hypertrophy, and that clearly represents a major risk.—N. Kaplan, M.D.

Relation of Left Ventricular Mass and Geometry to Morbidity and Mortality in Uncomplicated Essential Hypertension

Koren MJ, Devereux RB, Casale PN, Savage DD, Laragh JH (New York Hosp-Cornell Med Ctr, New York)
Ann Intern Med 114:345–352, 1991   3–23

Background.—Echocardiographically detected left ventricular hypertrophy (LVH) has been shown to predict cardiovascular complications within 4 to 5 years in hypertensive men and in healthy persons in the general population. However, the role of LVH in women, its relation to other risk factors, and the impact of left ventricular geometry have not been assessed.

Methods.—Between 1976 and 1981, 280 patients with essential hypertension and no preexisting cardiac disease underwent echocardiography. Two hundred fifty-three of those patients or their family members were contacted for a follow-up interview an average of 10.2 years after the initial echocardiogram.

Results.—Left ventricular mass exceeded 125 g/m^2 in 27% of the patients followed up. A higher proportion of patients with than without left ventricular hypertrophy had cardiovascular events—26% compared with 12%. More patients with increased ventricular mass also suffered cardiovascular death and death from all causes, the proportions being 14% vs. .5% and 16% vs. 2%, respectively. Risk could not be predicted by electrocardiographically detected left ventricular hypertrophy. Patients with normal left ventricular geometry had the fewest adverse outcomes, whereas those with concentric hypertrophy had the most adverse outcomes (Fig 3–7). According to multivariate analysis, age and left ventricular mass were the only independent predictors on all 3 outcome mea-

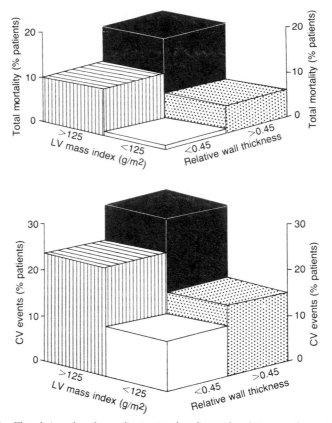

Fig 3–7.—The relation of total mortality (**top**) and cardiovascular *(CV)* events (**bottom**) to patterns of left ventricular *(LV)* geometry in 253 patients with essential hypertension. Mortality and event rates are highest in patients with concentric hypertrophy *(filled squares)*, lowest in patients with normal ventricular geometry *(open squares)*, and intermediate in patients with eccentric hypertrophy *(striped squares)*, and concentric remodeling *(shaded squares)* (*P* < .001 for total mortality and *P* = .03 for CV events by analysis of variance). (Courtesy of Koren MJ, Devereux RB, Casale PN, et al: *Ann Intern Med* 114:345–352, 1991.)

sures. Gender, blood pressure, and serum cholesterol level were not predictors.

Conclusions.—Echocardiographically determined left ventricular mass and geometry identify hypertensive patients at risk independently of and more strongly than blood pressure or other potentially reversible risk factors. Left ventricular mass and geometry may also help to stratify patients as to the need for intensive treatment.

▶ The excess risk associated with echocardiographically measured LVH persisted over a 10+ year follow-up despite the use of conventional antihypertensive therapy in most of the patients over this time. As expected, this therapy consisted primary of diuretics and β-blockers, and the authors question whether a better prognosis might have been shown with "the consistent use of antihypertensive drugs that arc thought to benefit the heart more." This issue will be addressed further in the section on Drug Therapy.

Strokes remain the second most common cause of morbidity and mortality among hypertensives. Although stroke events and deaths have decreased over the past 30 years, the rate of hemorrhagic strokes appears to have increased over the past 10 years (1). Part of this increase may be the result of improved recognition of intracerebral hemorrhages by CT. Use of MRI has also provided evidence for a great deal more cerebrovascular disease than ever suspected.—N. Kaplan, M.D.

Reference

1. Mayo NE, et al: Changing rates of stroke in the province of Quebec, Canada: 1981–1988. *Stroke* 22:590–595, 1991.

Magnetic Resonance Imaging White Matter Lesions and Cognitive Impairment in Hypertensive Individuals
Schmidt R, Fazekas F, Offenbacher H, Lytwyn H, Blematl B, Niederkorn K, Horner S, Payer F, Freidl W (Karl Franzens University, Graz; Steiermärkische Gebietskrankenkasse, Graz, Austria)
Arch Neurol 48:417–420, 1991
3–24

Background.—Asymptomatic hypertensive individuals have been reported to have subtle deficits in performance of neuropsychologic tests. The capability of MRI to test whether functional changes and/or parenchymal damage can cause these changes was tested. Thirty-five asymptomatic hypertensive patients, all under age 50, were studied by MRI and neuropsychologic testing.

Methods.—The patients were 26 men and 9 women, mean age 38.7 years. Patients had essential hypertension for an average of 6 years but had no other known causes for cerebral damage or cognitive impairment. Twenty normotensive controls, mean age 37.9 years, were also studied. Neuropsychologic tests were administered to assess memory and learning ability, attention, vigilance and reaction time, and mood. Signal abnormalities and cerebral atrophy were assessed on MRI scans in blinded fashion.

Results.—The hypertensive group did significantly worse on tests of verbal memory and total learning and memory capacity, regardless of drug treatment. No differences were noted in tests of visual memory, attention, vigilance, and reaction time. On mood subscales, hypertensive patients described themselves as less active but otherwise ranked similarly. Thirty-eight percent of the hypertensive patients had punctate high-signal intensities of the white matter, compared with 20% of the control group. However, test performance was no different between hypertensive patients with and without white-matter lesions.

Conclusions.—Patients with essential hypertension have subtle neuropsychologic deficits and a higher frequency of white-matter signal abnormalities as seen on MRI scan. These findings do not appear to be correlated, however. Thus "functional," as opposed to gross structural, mechanisms appear to be responsible for the deterioration in cognitive performance.

▶ The almost twofold increase in white-matter lesions seen in this presumably asymptomatic group of young patients with uncomplicated hypertension is disturbing, even if their presence is not responsible for their greater degree of cognitive impairment. These data plus the evidence reported by Mayo et al. (1) suggest that the widely held perception that more widespread therapy of hypertension has largely overcome the stroke problem is incorrect. Nonetheless, we shall review new evidence from therapeutic trials that therapy will reduce stroke mortality, and the problem must be a failure to reach many patients at risk.—N. Kaplan, M.D.

Reference

1. Mayo NE, et al: Changing rates of stroke in the province of Quebec, Canada: 1981–1988. *Stroke* 22:590–595, 1991.

Nondrug Therapy

▶ ↓ Along with the need to provide more effective drug therapy to reduce stroke and other cardiovascular morbidity and mortality, there remains an equal need to more effectively use a variety of nondrug therapies. This need covers the larger population who are at risk for developing hypertension or who have relatively mild degrees of elevated pressure. Among them, nondrug therapies may be enough to lower the blood pressure to a safe range while at the same time reducing the extent of other cardiovascular risk factors.

Despite my enthusiasm for their use, nondrug therapies are not as potent as drug therapies, and their use has not been shown to reduce hypertensive complications.—N. Kaplan, M.D.

Cardiovascular Effects of Weight Reduction Versus Antihypertensive Drug Treatment: A Comparative, Randomized, 1-Year Study of Obese Men With Mild Hypertension
Fagerberg B, Berglund A, Andersson OK, Berglund G, Wikstrand J (Sahlgren's Hospital, Gothenburg, Sweden; Lund University, Malmö, Sweden)
J Hypertens 9:431–439, 1991   3–25

Background.—There is controversy regarding the relative benefits of antihypertensive drug treatment and nonpharmacological treatment as the first-line therapy for patients with mild hypertension. The effects of the 2 treatment modalities were compared on left ventricular mass, left ventricular systolic function, and the structure of the peripheral arterial resistance vessels.

Patients.—Men in generally good health, between the ages of 40 and 69 years, and with primary mild hypertension, were recruited for the study. During a run-in period of 6 weeks, any previously prescribed antihypertensive drugs were withdrawn. The men were then randomly allocated to drug treatment (atenolol followed by bendrofluazide and nifedipine) or a nonpharmacologic regimen (reducing body weight and restricting sodium chloride intake). The primary therapeutic goal was a diastolic blood pressure <90 mm Hg.

Results.—At 1-year follow-up, weight decreased by 7.8 kg and salt intake decreased by 42 mmol/day in the diet group. Casual systolic and diastolic blood pressures, as well as heart rate, were significantly reduced in the drug-treated group. The diastolic blood pressure goal was achieved by 73% of the drug and 29% of the diet group. No statistically significant differences in left ventricular morphology or function could be detected between the 2 groups.

Conclusion.—In this group of 61 patients, weight reduction and sodium restriction were inferior to a conventional antihypertensive drug treatment in lowering casual blood pressure. Previous antihypertensive treatment affected the results of intervention on left ventricular mass.

▶ In this study, relatively small degrees of weight loss and sodium restriction were accomplished. Unfortunately, these degrees are similar to what most report in clinical trials, so it is clear that more vigorous pursuit of the goals of nondrug therapies must be attempted. Nonetheless, the diet program came close to showing a significant reduction in left ventricular mass and was associated with a decrease in vascular resistance measured by plethysmography at maximal dilation.

Weight reduction usually lowers the blood pressure and does so in multiple ways.—N. Kaplan, M.D.

Effect of Weight Reduction in Moderately Overweight Patients on Recorded Ambulatory Blood Pressure and Free Cytosolic Platelet Calcium
Scherrer U, Nussberger J, Torriani S, Waeber B, Darioli R, Hofstetter J-R, Brunner HR (Centre Hospitalier Universitaire Vaudois, Lausanne, Switzerland)
Circulation 83:552–558, 1991   3–26

Introduction.—Despite the increasing evidence that weight reduction induced by a hypocaloric diet lowers the blood pressure (BP) in obese hypertensive patients, the mechanism by which weight loss decreases the BP remains unknown. Although studies have shown that platelet cytosolic calcium decreases during drug treatment for hypertension, it is not known whether platelet calcium also decreases during nonpharmacologic BP reduction. This study prospectively examined the relation between platelet cytosolic calcium and ambulatory BP during weight reduction in moderately overweight patients with mild hypertension.

Study design.—Seventeen women and 14 men, aged 21–73 years, with a body mass index (BMI) greater than 25 and mild hypertension were provided with a nutritionally balanced, calorie-restricted diet that would achieve a 5% reduction in BMI within 10 weeks. Body weight, office BP, and pulse rate were monitored at 2-week intervals. Ambulatory BP recordings were obtained at baseline and at the end of weeks 4 and 10 of the diet intervention. Blood samples to measure platelet free cytosolic calcium were obtained at baseline and at the end of the 10-week study period.

Findings.—Patients were classified according to their response to the diet intervention. At the end of the 10-week study period, 19 patients achieved a 5% reduction in their BMI or a mean weight loss of 8.5 kg, a significant decrease in both office and ambulatory BP, and an 11% decrease in free cytosolic platelet calcium. The other 12 patients showed no relevant changes in body weight, BP, or free cytosolic platelet calcium.

Conclusion.—The BP-lowering effects of moderate weight loss correlate with a decrease in platelet calcium. The findings of this study further support a link between intracellular calcium homeostasis and BP regulation.

Obesity-Related Hypertension: Evaluation of the Separate Effects of Energy Restriction and Weight Reduction on Hemodynamic and Neuroendocrine Status

Weinsier RL, James LD, Darnell BE, Dustan HP, Birch R, Hunter GR (Univ of Alabama at Birmingham)
Am J Med 90:460–468, 1991   3–27

Background.—It is unknown whether the fall in blood pressure with weight reduction results from concurrent changes in diet or from the reduction in body mass itself. The independent effects of energy restriction and weight reduction were studied in 24 obese, hypertensive women.

Methods.—The subjects were postmenopausal women, average age 59 years and average of 137% of ideal body weight. All had mild-to-moderate hypertension and normal glucose tolerance. The women followed a tightly controlled diet over 5 months. Throughout the study, the intake of sodium, potassium, and calcium, the polyunsaturated-to-saturated fat ratio, and the proportions of carbohydrate, fat, and protein were held constant. Subjects were hospitalized for 10 days on 4 occasions—twice before weight loss, at energy balance and at an intake of 800 kcal; and twice after weight loss, first at an intake of 800 kcal and then at return to energy balance. Hemodynamic and endocrine status were evaluated at these times.

Results.—During energy restriction, declines were seen in fasting serum insulin, triiodothyronine-to-reverse triiodothyronine ratio, resting metabolic rate, and heart rate, along with negative sodium and potassium balances. No consistent response to changes in energy intake was noted in catecholamines, renin, aldosterone, plasma volume, cardiac output, or blood pressure. However, with weight reduction blood pressure, plasma volume, cardiac output, and plasma renin activity were all independently lowered.

Conclusions.—Weight loss appears to lower blood pressure in a manner that is distinct from energy restriction and appears to be related to changes in blood volume and cardiac output. Increased body mass per se is at least partly responsible for obesity-related hypertension.

▶ These 2 studies (Abstracts 3–26 and 3–27) carefully monitored small groups of moderately obese hypertensive subjects for a few months while on about half of their usual caloric intake. In both studies, those subjects who lost the expected amount of weight achieved significant falls in blood pressure. Scherrer et al. (Abstract 3–26) observed a concomitant fall in cytosolic calcium within platelets, presumably reflecting similar changes within vascular smooth cells. Such falls in intracellular calcium have been shown to lower vascular tone and therefore could be responsible for the fall in blood pressure.

Weinsier et al. (Abstract 3–27) rather ingeniously separated the effects of caloric restriction from weight reduction and found that the blood pressure fell consistently only with weight loss, in turn related to a shrinkage in blood volume and cardiac output. Thus, these studies demonstrate multiple ways by which weight loss causes the blood pressure to fall.

In addition to weight reduction, dietary sodium restriction usually lowers pressure. The effectiveness of moderate sodium restriction was conclusively documented by an analysis of all 78 controlled trials in the literature (1). Two important facts emerge from this analysis: first, it takes at least a month of sodium restriction to demonstrate a significant effect; second, the higher the pressure and the older the patient, the greater the effect. Overall, a 50 mmol/day reduction was shown to lower systolic blood pressure by an average of 5 mm Hg in normotensive people and by 7 mm Hg in those with hypertension. Diastolic pressures fall about half as much. Of greatest significance, Law et al. estimate that a reduction of only 50 mmol/day (an amount less than one third of usual intake, a level of sodium restriction that is easily attainable) by the entire population would lower blood pressure enough to reduce the incidence of stroke by 22% and of coronary heart disease by 16%. Shame on those who would deny such benefit to the population, achieved at no cost and with absolutely no danger.

In addition to the proven benefits of moderate sodium restriction, new evidence supports the effectiveness of increasing dietary potassium intake. Siani et al. (2) showed that 81% of those hypertensives who increased average potassium intake by about 2 grams per day over 1 year were able to reduce their intake of drug therapy by more than half while maintaining control of their blood pressure, and only 29% of those who did not increase potassium intake were able to do so. Of further interest, a 10-day period of dietary potassium restriction that induced a .8 mmol/L fall in plasma potassium caused the blood pressure to rise by 7/6 mm Hg in 12 patients with hypertension (3).

The next nondrug therapy examined intensively in 1991 was physical activity, and most of the findings are positive.—N. Kaplan, M.D.

References

1. Law MR, et al: III-Analysis of data from trials of salt reduction. *BMJ* 302:819–24, 1991.
2. Siani A, et al: Increasing the dietary potassium intake reduces the need for antihypertensive medication. *Ann Intern Med* 115:753–759, 1991.
3. Krishna GG, Kapoor SC: Potassium depletion exacerbates essential hypertension. *Ann Intern Med* 115:77–83, 1991.

Relation Between Leisure-Time Physical Activity and Blood Pressure in Older Women
Reaven PD, Barrett-Connor E, Edelstein S (Univ of California, San Diego)
Circulation 83:559–565, 1991   3–28

Introduction.—There is some evidence that physical activity reduces blood pressure (BP) in young and middle-aged women, but the relation between physical activity and BP in older women has not been well studied. As part of an ongoing population-based study on life-styles and chronic disease in older adults, the effects of self-reported leisure-time activity on BP in older women were examined.

Study Design.—The study sample included 641 white women, aged 50–89 years, who completed a questionnaire assessing their leisure-time activities during the 2-week period before clinical evaluation. Activities were grouped by relative intensity, using activity intensity codes that represent the ratio of metabolic rate during work to basal metabolic rate. Women were rated as light, moderate, or heavy exercisers if they participated in at least 1 activity at that estimated intensity level during the previous 2 weeks, and as sedentary if they had not participated in any leisure-time activity during those 2 weeks. Alcohol consumption, smoking habits, and blood glucose levels were also included in the evaluation.

Results.—Based on the self-reported activity reports, 78 (12%) women were classified as sedentary, 373 (58%) as light exercisers, 154 (24%) as moderate exercisers, and 36 (6%) as heavy exercisers. Women who were physically active were significantly younger and thinner than sedentary women. There were no significant intergroup differences with respect to alcohol consumption, cigarette smoking, or prevalence of coronary heart disease and diabetes. However, prevalence rates of systolic, diastolic, and overall hypertension were significantly lower in active women at all physical activity levels compared with sedentary women. Prevalence rates of diastolic hypertension decreased nearly stepwise with each higher physical activity level. Systolic BP levels in heavy exercisers were approximately 20 mm Hg lower than in sedentary women. These differences remained statistically significant after adjustment for age and body mass index. Physical activity was also associated with lower fasting and 2-hour postchallenge insulin levels. After adjustment for insulin levels, the differences in BP levels among activity groups remained unchanged.

Conclusion.—Routine physical activity performed by older women is associated with lower BP and a lower prevalence of hypertension. Even light or moderately intense physical activity may be sufficient to obtain these benefits.

▶ These relatively crude data are in keeping with others showing lower blood pressure in people who are more physically active and reductions of blood pressure by aerobic exercise, both over the short-term (1) and long-term (2). Although not all studies of regular aerobic exercise have demonstrated significant reductions of blood pressure (3), all-cause mortality has been shown to be progressively lower in normotensive and hypertensive men who are at increasingly higher degrees of physical fitness (4).

Moderation of alcohol intake is another useful nondrug therapy because excessive consumption can raise the blood pressure.—N. Kaplan, M.D.

References

1. Pescatello LS, et al: Short-term effect of dynamic exercise on arterial blood pressure. *Circulation* 83:1557–1561, 1991.
2. Somers VK, et al: Effects of endurance training on baroreflex sensitivity and blood pressure in borderline hypertension. *Lancet* 337:1363–1368, 1991.
3. Seals DR, Reiling MJ: Effect of regular exercise on 24-hour arterial pressure in older hypertensive humans. *Hypertension* 18:583–592, 1991.
4. Blair SN, et al: Physical fitness and all-cause mortality in hypertensive men. *Ann Med* 23:307–312, 1991.

Alcohol Consumption and Blood Pressure in Black Adults: The Pitt County Study

Strogatz DS, James SA, Haines PS, Elmer PJ, Gerber AM, Browning SR, Ammerman AS, Keenan NL (State Univ of New York at Albany; Univ of Michigan, Ann Arbor; Univ of North Carolina, Chapel Hill; Univ of Minnesota, Minneapolis)
Am J Epidemiol 133:442–450, 1991   3–29

Background.—The direct association between alcohol consumption and blood pressure is established, but its form and strength in blacks are uncertain. This relationship was investigated in a random, community-based sample of 1,784 black adults.

Methods.—The subjects, ranging in age from 25 to 50 years, all lived in an eastern North Carolina county. Subjects were interviewed in their homes to gather information about their risk factors for hypertension, including health and health habits, education, occupation, psychosocial resources, psychosocial stressors, and coping styles. Blood pressure and anthropometric measurements and a food frequency questionnaire were included in this session. Alcohol consumption was ranked into 4 categories, ranging from abstention to 7 or more drinks per week.

Results.—Fifty-two percent of the sample were abstinent and 12 percent had 7 or more drinks per week. The systolic blood pressure of the latter group was 6.8 mm Hg higher than that of the nondrinkers for both men and women after adjustment for age and body mass (Fig 3–8). No threshold effect was evident, and diastolic blood pressure showed similar patterns. Subjects in the high consumption group were more likely to have low socioeconomic status, including current unemployment, greater perceived anger and stress, being unmarried, and lacking instrumental and emotional support.

Conclusions.—There appears to be a graded association between alcohol consumption and blood pressure in black adults. Social factors may be important determinants of this association, which cannot be explained

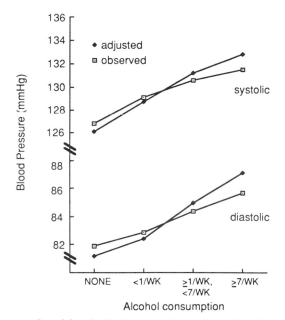

Fig 3–8.—Mean systolic and diastolic blood pressure (observed and adjusted for age, body mass index, and the ratio of waist to hip circumferences) of 25- to 50-year-old black men, by level of alcohol consumption in Pitt County, North Carolina, 1988. (Courtesy of Strogatz DS, James SA, Haines PS, et al: *Am J Epidemiol* 133:442—450, 1991.)

by age, body mass, or body mass distribution. Preliminary analyses also suggest that the difference is unaccounted for by physical activity or dietary factors.

▶ Not all surveys show the progressive rise in pressure with all increments of alcohol intake seen in this group of black adults but virtually every study has shown a significantly higher pressure in those who consume more than 3 drinks per day (1). On the other hand, there is very strong evidence that the consumption of 1 to 2 drinks per day is associated with significantly lower rates of coronary heart disease (2).

In the study by Keil et al., those subjects who smoked tended to have lower blood pressure at all levels of alcohol intake, an association that is usually attributed to the lower body weight of smokers. However, smoking is bad for blood pressure and even worse for cardiovascular complications.—N. Kaplan, M.D.

References

1. Keil U, et al: Alcohol and blood pressure and its interaction with smoking and other behavioural variables: Results from the MONICA Augsburg Survey 1984–1985. *J Hypertens* 9:491–498, 1991.
2. Kaplan NM: Bashing booze: The danger of losing the benefits of moderate alcohol consumption. *Am Heart J* 121:1854–1856, 1991.

Elevation of Ambulatory Systolic Blood Pressure in Hypertensive Smokers: A Case-Control Study

Mann SJ, James GD, Wang RS, Pickering TG (New York Hosp-Cornell Med Ctr, New York)
JAMA 265:2226–2228, 1991   3–30

Background.—When blood pressure is measured in the office, smokers have pressures the same as, or lower than, nonsmokers. This is despite the fact that smoking is known to raise blood pressure acutely, even in chronic smokers. Ambulatory monitoring was used to compare office and 24-hour ambulatory blood pressures of hypertensive smokers and non-smokers. Both groups were mainly white; the smokers tended to be somewhat younger.

Methods.—Fifty-nine cigarette smokers were identified from chart review of patients who had undergone 24-hour blood pressure recordings performed after at least 2 weeks of no blood pressure medications. A group of 118 nonsmokers, matched for age, sex, race, and weight, was then selected for comparison. Blood chemistries, cholesterol levels, renin activity, and blood pressure measurement in the office were obtained within 1 week of the 24-hour blood pressure monitoring.

Results.—When measured in the office, blood pressures were 141/93 for the smokers and 142/93 for the nonsmokers. However, 24-hour monitoring showed that the average awake ambulatory systolic blood pressure in smokers was 145 mm Hg compared with 140 mm Hg for the nonsmokers. Among patients older than age 50 years, this difference was greater—153 mm Hg for smokers compared with 142 mm Hg. In patients younger than age 50 years during the day and in both the younger and older groups during sleep, no difference was seen.

Conclusions.—Daytime ambulatory systolic blood pressure appears to be higher in white hypertensive patients older than age 50 years than in nonsmokers, despite the fact that their blood pressures are similar when measured in the office. The finding that office blood pressure may underestimate ambulatory blood pressure in older smokers may have implications for pharmacotherapy of hypertension in these patients.

Hypertension, Cigarette Smoking, and the Decline in Stroke Incidence in Eastern Finland

Tuomilehto J, Bonita R, Stewart A, Nissinen A, Salonen JT (National Public Health Institute, Helsinki, Finland; University of Auckland, New Zealand; University of Kuopio, Finland)
Stroke 22:7–11, 1991   3–31

Background.—Finland has high rates of both cardiovascular disease and risk factors for cardiovascular disease. Changes in the prevalence of hypertension and cigarette smoking were examined in a sample of the population in 2 rural provinces of Finland, North Karelia and Kuopio, in 1972 and 1977 to study their relation to the development of subsequent stroke over 8 years. The province of North Karelia received an active program of cardiovascular disease risk factor intervention; the province of Kuopio served as a reference area to evaluate the intervention program.

Methods.—In both surveys in both provinces participants had their blood pressure measured and provided data on cigarette use, height and weight, history of stroke, myocardial infarction, diabetes, and other major diseases. They were told their blood pressure values and referred to local primary health facilities if the values were high. Both the 1972 cohort (ages 25–59 years) and the 1977 cohort (ages 30–64 years) were followed up for 8 years through national hospital discharge data and death certificate registers.

Results.—In the 1972 cohort, 146 strokes were recorded in the 8-year follow-up compared with 105 events in the 1977 cohort. In both provinces, the proportion of smokers decreased significantly in men between 1972 and 1977 and increased slightly, although remaining low, in women. The prevalence of hypertension fell for both sexes between 1972 and 1977, with a greater decrease in North Karelia than in Kuopio. Stroke incidence declined 30% in men and 36% in women in both provinces. Overall stroke incidence fell from 15.5 per 1,000 population to 10.4. Data indicated that 28% of all stroke events could be attributed to hypertension, 17% to cigarette smoking, and 43% to the combination of these two. A 29% decline in stroke incidence could be accounted for by the decreases in the prevalence of hypertension and smoking.

Discussion.—Stroke incidence declined significantly during the study period. Results of this study show that blood pressure control had a greater effect than changes in smoking on the decrease in stroke risk. Further efforts to eliminate smoking and control elevated blood pressure are needed to reduce the high incidence of stroke and stroke mortality in Finland.

▶ Smoking is usually considered as a risk mainly for pulmonary and coronary diseases, but it may also raise blood pressure and accelerate the development of stroke. As detailed in the December 14, 1991, issue of *JAMA,* the evil of cigarettes continues to grow among our young people, and physicians are woefully negligent in helping smokers to quit.

Another rather mild addiction, caffeine, does not adversely affect blood pressure. However, drinking unfiltered boiled coffee, Scandinavian style, may cause a slight rise in systolic levels (2). Because drinking unfiltered coffee has also been associated with more coronary disease, let us keep those filters in place.—N. Kaplan, M.D.

References

1. MacDonald TM, et al: Caffeine restriction: Effect on mild hypertension. *BMJ* 303:1235–138, 1991.
2. van Dusseldorp M, et al: Boiled coffee and blood pressure. A 14-week controlled trial. *Hypertension* 18:607–613, 1991.

Drug Therapy

▶ ↓ The most important publications about the therapy of hypertension in 1991 involved the population at highest risk—the elderly. One study documented, for the first time, the benefit of treating isolated systolic hypertension in the elderly; the other conclusively confirmed the benefit of treating combined systolic and diastolic hypertension in the elderly.—N. Kaplan, M.D.

Prevention of Stroke by Antihypertensive Drug Treatment in Older Persons With Isolated Systolic Hypertension: Final Results of the Systolic Hypertension in the Elderly Program (SHEP)
SHEP Cooperative Research Group (Natl Heart, Lung, and Blood Inst, Bethesda, Md)
JAMA 265:3255–3264, 1991   3–32

Purpose.—A multicenter, randomized, double-blind, placebo-controlled trial was designed to determine whether antihypertensive drug treatment reduces the risk of nonfatal and fatal total stroke in otherwise healthy persons aged 60 years and older with isolated systolic hypertension (ISH). Cardiovascular and coronary morbidity and mortality and all-cause mortality were also examined.

Study Design.—Of 4,736 persons with a mean age of 72 years, 2,365 were allocated to active drug treatment and 2,371 to matching placebo. Systolic blood pressure (SBP) ranged from 160–219 mm Hg and diastolic blood pressure (DBP) was under 90 mm Hg. The average BP at entry was 170/77 mm Hg. Chlorthalidone and atenolol were administered in a stepped-care regimen with low-dose chlorthalidone (12.5 mg/day) used initially.

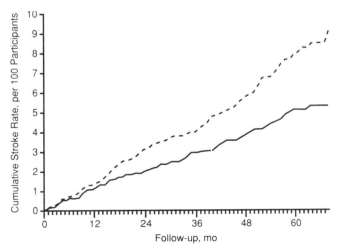

Fig 3–9.—Cumulative fatal plus nonfatal stroke rate per 100 participants in the active treatment *(solid line)* and placebo *(broken line)* groups during the Systolic Hypertension in the Elderly Program. (Courtesy of SHEP Cooperative Research Group: *JAMA* 265:3255–3264, 1991.)

Results.—After a mean follow-up of 4.5 years, 103 persons in the active treatment group and 159 persons in the placebo group had had a stroke. At the end of 5 years, the average BP was 143/68 mm Hg in the active treatment group and 155/72 mm Hg in the placebo group. The 5-year incidence of total stroke was 5.2% with active treatment and 8.2% with placebo (Fig 3–9). Active treatment also lowered the 5-year incidence of nonfatal and fatal major cardiovascular events.

Conclusion.—Antihypertensive stepped-care drug treatment for ISH reduced the incidence of total stroke by 36% in healthy persons aged 60 years and over.

▶ This landmark study settles a long unanswered question: does treating elderly people with isolated systolic hypertension help? The answer is a resounding yes. The treatment in the careful, gentle manner practiced in the SHEP trial, using very low doses of drugs and slowly titrating the systolic pressures down to an average of 145 mm Hg, relatively few patients suffered bothersome side effects.

Before we all rush to apply such therapy to the 10+ million elderly in the United States with isolated systolic hypertension, a few cautions are advised:

- The SHEP subjects were a healthy group of elderly people; 95% had no limitation of daily activity. The elderly with diabetes, coronary disease, or cerebrovascular disease might not be either as responsive to therapy or as resistant to side effects.
- There still may be a danger in lowering systolic or diastolic pressures too much [i.e., a J-curve, as has been seen in multiple trials of younger patients with combined systolic and diastolic hypertension when pressures are lowered below 145/85 mm Hg (1)]. An analysis of the SHEP data regarding the J-curve is in process.
- Whether diuretics and β-blockers, the only drugs available in the early 1980s when SHEP was started, are the best drugs to treat ISH in the elderly is not known. Certainly the low doses of diuretic used in SHEP will cause less metabolic mischief than the higher doses still commonly prescribed. As subsequent abstracts will cover, however, other drugs may be as good as or better than the choices used in SHEP.
- We must be aware of and take precautions to avoid the dangers of postural and postprandial hypotension so commonly seen in elderly patients with systolic hypertension. In the SHEP cohort, postural hypotension (defined as a drop of SBP of 20 mm Hg or more) was found in 17.3% after 1 and 3 minutes of standing from the seated position (2). The frequency would have been even higher if the patients had quickly changed from supine to standing, the better way to look for postural hypotension. Postprandial hypotension is a major problem in the elderly (3): 96% of 113 elderly nursing home patients showed a postprandial fall in SBP that averaged 18 mm Hg, and 36% had a fall of more than 20 mm Hg without standing (4).

With these cautions in mind, we can also take heart in the results of another large trial of elderly patients with combined systolic and diastolic hypertension, the Swedish Trial in Old Patients with Hypertension (STOP-Hypertension) (5). This double-blind study randomly allocated half of 1,627 elderly patients (average age 75.7 years; average BP = 195/102) to placebo or active drug therapy (a diuretic or one of 3 β-blockers). After an average time of 25 months in the trial, those on active therapy (average BP = 166/87) had significantly fewer fatal and nonfatal strokes and total mortality than did those on placebo (average BP = 188/97).

Of additional interest, deaths from coronary disease were not significantly reduced in either SHEP or STOP-Hypertension. This discrepancy—protection against strokes but not against coronary disease—continues to plague diuretic and β-blocker based therapeutic trials. The question remains: can other therapies do better?—N. Kaplan, M.D.

References

1. Farnett L, et al: The J-curve phenomenon and the treatment of hypertension. Is there a point beyond which pressure reduction is dangerous? *JAMA* 265:489–495, 1991.
2. Applegate WB, et al: Prevalence of postural hypotension at baseline in the Systolic Hypertension in the Elderly Program (SHEP) Cohort. *J Am Geriatr Soc* 39:1057–5064, 1991.
3. Mathias CJ: Postprandial hypotension. Pathophysiological mechanisms and clinical implications in different disorders. *Hypertension* 18:694–704, 1991.
4. Vaitkevicius PV, et al: Frequency and importance of postprandial blood pressure reduction in elderly nursing-home patients. *Ann Intern Med* 115:865–870, 1991.
5. Dahlöf B, et al: Morbidity and mortality in the Swedish Trial in Old Patients with Hypertension (STOP-Hypertension). *Lancet* 338:1281–1285, 1991.

A Randomized Controlled Trial of the Effects of Three Antihypertensive Agents on Blood Pressure Control and Quality of Life in Older Women

Applegate WB, Phillips HL, Schnaper H, Shepherd AMM, Schocken D, Luhr JC, Koch GG, Park GD (Univ of Tennessee, Memphis; Columbiana Associates, Ala; Univ of Alabama, Birmingham; Univ of Texas Health Sciences Ctr, San Antonio; Univ of South Florida, Tampa; et al)
Arch Intern Med 151:1817–1823, 1991   3–33

Background.—There have been few randomized studies of antihypertensive agents in older patients. Little is known, in particular, about the efficacy and impact on quality of life of antihypertensive drugs in older women. This question was addressed in a multicenter, randomized, double-blind, parallel group trial of 240 women with stable essential hypertension.

Patients and Methods.—The patients' average age was approximately 70 years. None had other major illnesses that might interfere with the study implementation or results. A placebo run-in phase of 4–6 weeks allowed washout of previously used antihypertensive medications. The patients were randomized to titrated doses of atenolol (50–100 mg once a day), enalapril (5–20 mg once a day), or diltiazem (sustained release 60–80 mg twice a day).

Results.—The effects of the drugs on blood pressure (BP) and quality of life were assessed at 8 and 16 weeks. At both periods, diltiazem demonstrated greater diastolic BP lowering than the other agents. Diastolic BP at week 16 was reduced by −13.7 mm Hg with diltiazem, by −10.8 mm Hg with atenolol, and by −10.5 mm Hg with enalapril. Atenolol was associated with more treatment failures and with a trend for somewhat worse scores on quality-of-life measures.

Conclusion.—All of the study agents effectively lowered BP in these older hypertensive women. The rates of adverse reactions were similar for the 3 medications. Overall, none had a differential clinical impact on quality of life. Atenolol, however, may be less desirable than diltiazem or enalapril as a first-line antihypertensive medication in older women.

▶ In this smaller but still sizable randomized double-blind trial in elderly women, an ACE inhibitor (enalapril) or a calcium blocker (diltiazem) did somewhat better than a β-blocker (atenolol) in lowering blood pressure and preventing side effects. The short duration and small number of subjects precluded any study of morbidity or mortality and, unfortunately, no studies on blood chemistries or lipids were obtained.

Another, even larger, ongoing trial in younger patients with mild hypertension has given some of the latter comparative data.—N. Kaplan, M.D.

The Treatment of Mild Hypertension Study: A Randomized, Placebo-Controlled Trial of a Nutritional-Hygienic Regimen Along With Various Drug Monotherapies
The Treatment of Mild Hypertension Research Group (Univ of Minnesota, Minneapolis)
Arch Intern Med 151:1413–1423, 1991   3–34

Introduction.—Lowering blood pressure (BP) in patients with hypertension results in a reduced incidence of stroke. To determine the effects of BP management on cardiovascular morbidity and mortality, 6 treatments for mild hypertension were compared. Preliminary, 12-month follow-up data were reviewed concerning the effects of the 6 treatments on BP, blood lipid levels, side effects, and quality of life.

Patients.—Study participants ranged in age from 45 to 69 years; their average BP was 140/91 mm Hg. The 902 men and women were randomized to receive nutritional-hygienic intervention in addition to 1 of 6 treatments: placebo, a diuretic (chlorthalidone), a β-blocker (acebutolol), an α_1-antagonist (doxazosin), a calcium antagonist (amlodipine), or an angiotensin-converting enzyme inhibitor (enalapril).

Results.—At the 12-month follow-up, the average weight loss for all 902 patients was 4.7 kg and 21% of the subjects had achieved a 10% reduction in body weight or loss to desirable weight by reducing their energy intake and increasing physical activity. Urinary sodium excretion was reduced for the group as a whole by 23%. Patients receiving antihypertensive medication achieved significantly greater reductions in BP than

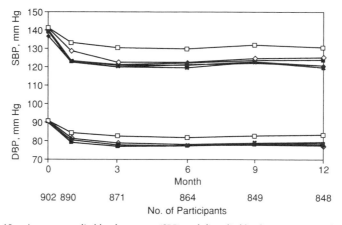

Fig 3–10.—Average systolic blood pressure (SBP) and diastolic blood pressure (DBP) by treatment group. *Open squares* indicate placebo; *solid diamonds*, amlodipine maleate; *Xs*, chlorthalidone; *open diamonds*, doxazosin mesylate; *solid squares*, enalapril maleate; and *open squares with dots* acebutolol. (Courtesy of The Treatment of Mild Hypertension Research Group: *Arch Intern Med* 151:1413–1423, 1991.)

those following a nutritional-hygienic regimen alone and there was no significant difference in the blood pressure reductions by the 5 drugs (Fig 3–10). The average pulse rate decreased in all treatment groups, but the drop was significantly greater in those receiving acebutolol. Improvement in quality of life, as compared with placebo, was greatest for participants given acebutolol and chlorthalidone. All groups had an increased ratio of high-density lipoprotein to total cholesterol level but the effect was greatest in those taking doxazosin. Side effects were reported as often with placebo as with active treatment.

Conclusion.—Nutritional-hygienic treatments for mild hypertension may be effective for many patients. The addition of one of 5 different classes of antihypertensive agents can significantly lower BP with minimal short-term side effects.

▶ This study, referred to as TOMHS, is the very first to compare members of all 5 major classes of antihypertensive agents against one another in sizable numbers of patients who were randomly allocated to receive 1 of the 5 drugs and followed for a long time while carefully assessing a variety of effects including quality-of-life measures, lipid levels, and echocardiography.

As important as these data are, they are intended to serve as only a pilot study to what is sorely needed: a large-scale comparative study that will determine the effects of all available classes on morbidity and mortality. These endpoints are the only ones that count and they can only be determined by a similar study many times larger than the TOMHS pilot study. At this moment, the director of the National Institutes of Health/National Heart, Lung, and Blood Institute is trying to come up with the not inconsiderable amount of money needed to do such a study. Here's hoping it will be done because without such a study, we will continue to have no answer to the most important question in hypertension today: can other therapies than diuretics or β-blockers (the only ones studied) reduce mortality from coronary disease (which has not been shown with diuretic and β-blocker–based therapeutic trials, including the new SHEP and STOP-Hypertension trials).

In the meantime, we must continue to use surrogate endpoints (side effects, biochemical and lipid changes, left ventricular hypertrophy, etc.) to guide us toward the choice of therapy. All of the hypertension gurus (or at least most of us) are advising an individualized approach based on certain patient characteristics and concomitant diseases (e.g., an angiotensin-converting enzyme inhibitor for a hypertensive with congestive heart failure, a calcium blocker for someone with coronary artery disease, an α-blocker for someone with hypercholesterolemia). Such an approach—including substitution of an agent from another class if the initial choice is ineffectual rather than continuing to add one step on top of another—makes sense, but no one knows what, in fact, is really best.

Problems with diuretics and β-blockers, still numbers 1 and 2 in overall usage, continue to arise (despite their successes in the SHEP and STOP-Hypertension trials).—N. Kaplan, M.D.

Excess Mortality Associated With Diuretic Therapy in Diabetes Mellitus
Warram JH, Laffel LMB, Valsania P, Christlieb AR, Krolewski AS (Joslin Diabetes Ctr, Boston; Harvard School of Public Health, Boston; Hospital San Raffaele, Milan, Italy)
Arch Intern Med 151:1350–1356, 1991   3–35

Background.—Diabetic patients receiving treatment for hypertension have been found to have a high mortality rate. Since a large number of diabetic hypertensives were treated at the Joslin Clinic between 1972 and 1979 as part of a clinical trial on retinopathy, their records were reviewed to determine whether the high mortality rate could be attributed to associated risk factors or to a deleterious effect of antihypertensive therapy.

Methods.—The series included 759 diabetics, 94% of whom were followed for a median period of 4.5 years. They were white, aged 35–69, and had normal serum creatinine levels. Most were taking insulin, and the average duration of diabetes was 18 years. The population was subdivided according to proteinuria status. Among the 496 patients without initial proteinuria, 47% were hypertensive; among the 263 with proteinuria, 66% were hypertensive. Within each group of hypertensive diabetics, about one third were not treated, about 20% were treated with diuretics alone, another 20% with other antihypertensives only, and another 20% with diuretics plus other agents.

Results.—Cardiovascular mortality over the median follow-up of 4.5 years was higher in those hypertensives treated for hypertension than in those left untreated. This higher mortality rate was not explained by a clustering of other cardiovascular risk factors or by the severity of nephropathy or diabetes. The excess mortality was found primarily in those hypertensives treated with diuretics alone, even though these patients had the lowest blood pressure while on therapy. After adjustment for differences in other risk factors, cardiovascular mortality was 3.8 times higher in those hypertensive diabetics treated with diuretic alone than in those hypertensive patients left untreated.

Conclusion.— In view of the excess mortality found with diuretic therapy of diabetic hypertensives, the use of diuretics in such patients must be reconsidered.

▶ As I noted in an editorial that accompanied this paper (1), these findings could reflect the use of overly large doses of diuretics, as were commonly prescribed in the late 1970s when this study was going on. Moreover, diabetic hypertensives may be particularly susceptible to diuretic-induced metabolic mischiefs such as hypokalemia and hypercholesterolemia. A further worsening of diabetic control might also contribute to this susceptibility, particularly since hydrochlorothiazide has been shown to further worsen insulin sensitivity (2). Regardless, these striking findings must be taken as a real concern about the use of diuretics.

Concerns about the use of β-blockers, the second most popular group of antihypertensive drugs, also continue to surface. In addition to their tendency to aggravate insulin resistance as reviewed by Lithell, they tend to lower cardioprotective HDL-cholesterol levels, an effect that rather surprisingly has been shown to be ameliorated by concomitant use of chromium (3).

Another commonly perceived side effect of β-blockers—depression—was not noted in a large prospective study (4). Moreover, no worsening of the rate of depression was seen among the 111 patients in this trial who took reserpine, leading the authors to encourage the use of this drug as a "low-cost alternative" for the considerable number of hypertensive patients who are poor.

With increasing pressure to cut down on the costs of medical care, we may very well end up with 2 large categories of antihypertensive therapy: inexpensive generic diuretics, β-blockers and a bit of reserpine for the poor and uninsured; and the newer and more expensive ACE inhibitors, calcium blockers and α-blockers for those who can afford them. I include α-blockers because of some of their attractive features even though their use has been limited in the past.—N. Kaplan, M.D.

References

1. Kaplan NM: Two dilemmas of diabetes. *Arch Intern Med* 151:1270–1272, 1991.
2. Lithell HOL: Effect of antihypertensive drugs on insulin, glucose, and lipid metabolism. *Diabetes Care* 14:203–209, 1991.
3. Roeback JR Jr, et al: Effects of chromium supplementation on serum high-density lipoprotein cholesterol levels in men taking beta-blockers. A randomized, controlled trial. *Ann Intern Med* 115:917–924, 1991.
4. Prisant LM, et al: Depression associated with antihypertensive drugs. *J Fam Pract* 33:481–485, 1991.

Effects of Doxazosin on Serum Lipids: A Review of the Clinical Data and Molecular Basis for Altered Lipid Metabolism

Pool JL (Baylor College of Medicine, Houston)
Am Heart J 121:251–260, 1991
3–36

Background.—In addition to the reduction of high blood pressure, antihypertensive therapy must aim to effectively manage increased cholesterol levels and other risk factors of coronary heart disease. A new, long-acting, postsynaptic α_1-adrenoreceptor inhibitor, doxazosin, is a prime candidate for the comprehensive therapies now needed. It has positive effects on both high blood pressure and adverse lipid levels.

Discussion.—Controlled clinical trials have shown that doxazosin has antihypertensive effectiveness similar to other antihypertensive agents. In these trials, doxazosin lowered the levels of total cholesterol, low-density lipoprotein (LDL) cholesterol, and triglycerides and raised the levels of high-density lipoprotein (HDL) cholesterol (Fig 3–11). Doxazosin may inhibit the development of CHD in 2 ways: it binds to the α_1-adrenoreceptor and inhibits receptor-mediated responses to epinephrine and norepinephrine. In addition it has direct and indirect effects on lipid metabolism. It increases LDL receptor activity, reduces intracellular LDL synthesis, decreases the synthesis and secretion of very low density lipoprotein (VLDL) cholesterol, stimulates lipoprotein lipase activity, and decreases the rate of cholesterol absorption. Doxazosin may inhibit platelet aggregation. First-year results from the Treatment of Mild Hypertension Study showed the expected drops in blood pressure for all 5 antihypertensive drugs studied. Lipid changes have varied with the type of antihypertensive therapy but have been favorable with doxazosin.

Conclusions.—Doxazosin can lower both blood pressure and serum lipid levels. It appears to reduce circulating lipid levels by enhancing LDL catabolism and depressing intracellular LDL and VLDL synthesis. Long-

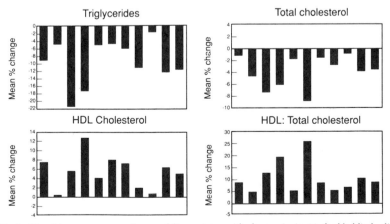

Fig 3–11.—Mean percentage change of lipoproteins with doxazosin in 11 double-blind, clinical comparison studies. (From Pool JL: *Am Heart J* 121:251–260, 1991. (Courtesy of Pool JL, Taylor AA, Nelson EB: *Am J Med* 87[suppl 2A]:57S–61S, 1989.)

term studies are needed to better define the implications of these findings, and to determine whether doxazosin therapy can lower death rates associated with CHD.

Effects of Doxazosin and Atenolol on the Fibrinolytic System in Patients With Hypertension and Elevated Serum Cholesterol
Jansson J-H, Johansson B, Boman K, Nilsson TK (Skellefteå Hospital, Skellefteå, Sweden; Ulmeå Hospital, Ulmeå, Sweden)
Eur J Clin Pharmacol 40:321–326, 1991   3–37

Introduction.—Antihypertensive drug therapy may adversely affect the fibrinolytic system and thus increase cardiovascular morbidity and mortality. Tissue plasminogen activator (t-PA) and plasminogen activator inhibitor (PAI-1) are considered to be the key components of the fibrinolytic system. Atenolol is a selective β_1-adrenoceptor blocker and doxazosin is an α_1-adrenoceptor inhibitor. The effects of atenolol and doxazosin on t-PA and PAI-1 plasma levels were assessed in 84 patients with previously untreated mild-to-moderate hypertension and elevated serum cholesterol levels.

Methods.—Forty-two patients were randomly allocated to therapy with atenolol and 42 were treated with doxazosin. Both groups were well matched for clinical and metabolic variables. The t-PA and PAI-1 levels in citrated plasma were measured before and after venous occlusion at baseline and at the end of the 6-month study period.

Results.—Doxazosin and atenolol both significantly decreased the systolic and diastolic blood pressures. After 6 months of doxazosin therapy, t-PA activity after venous occlusion and t-PA capacity were significantly increased compared with baseline values. There was no significant change in any of the fibrinolytic variables in patients treated for 6 months with atenolol. Thus, doxazosin but not atenolol improved the activity of the fibrinolytic system.

Conclusion.—Because the level of fibrinolytic activity in hypertensive patients with elevated cholesterol levels is considered a predictor of cardiovascular events, the significant improvement in the activity of the fibrinolytic system seen with doxazosin therapy may represent an additional therapeutic benefit.

▶ I have long been an advocate of α-blocker therapy for hypertension and the favorable effects on lipids, and the fibrinolytic system noted in these 2 abstracts, along with their ability to improve insulin sensitivity as noted in the prior reference by Lithell, will (I believe) encourage more use of the 2 longer-acting α-blockers now available, terazosin and doxazosin. Meanwhile, calcium-blockers and ACE inhibitors are the 2 classes of drugs whose use is growing most rapidly. There are a lot of good reasons for this growth.—N. Kaplan, M.D.

Normalization of Left Ventricular Mass and Associated Changes in Neurohormones and Atrial Natriuretic Peptide After 1 Year of Sustained Nifedipine Therapy for Severe Hypertension

Phillips RA, Ardeljan M, Shimabukuro S, Goldman ME, Garbowit DL, Eison HB, Krakoff LR (Mount Sinai Med Ctr, New York)
J Am Coll Cardiol 17:1595–1602, 1991   3–38

Background.—Because left ventricular hypertrophy is a powerful predictor of cardiovascular morbidity and mortality, the effects of therapy with the extended-release formulation of nifedipine alone or in combination with a thiazide diuretic on left ventricular function and structure were studied, and the associated neuroendocrine response was characterized.

Methods.—Sixteen patients with severe hypertension (diastolic pressure of 120 mm Hg or more) were identified on the basis of emergency department screening. Eleven were women, 9 were black, and mean age was 56 years. Mean supine blood pressure was 196/122 mm Hg. The initial 30-mg nifedipine dose was titrated to a maximum of 150 mg to achieve a diastolic blood pressure of 95 mm Hg or less. Chlorthalidone, 50 mg/day, was added if blood pressure remained above 95 mm Hg or if the patient could not tolerate the higher nifedipine dose. Over the 1-year treatment period, serial changes in left ventricular mass index and associated alterations were evaluated.

Results.—Mean seated blood pressure declined from 200/122 to 144/89 mm Hg at 1 year. Left ventricular mass reduced from 121 to 96 g/m² at 6 months, and this 19% reduction was sustained at 1 year (Fig 3–12). Significant reductions in the septal and posterior wall thicknesses were seen. Prevalence of left ventricular hypertrophy decreased from 63% to 25%, and left ventricular fractional shortening increased from 34% to 41%. No change was seen in the relation between fractional shortening and end-systolic stress. Over 1 year, peak velocity of early fill-

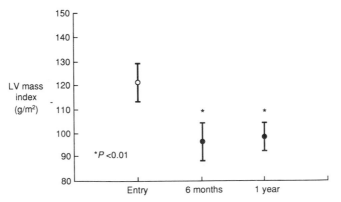

Fig 3–12.—Effect of treatment on left ventricular *(LV)* mass index in 16 patients. The prevalence of left ventricular hypertrophy was reduced from 63% to 25% after 6 months of treatment. (Courtesy of Phillips RA, Ardeljan M, Shimabukuro S, et al: *J Am Coll Cardiol* 17:1595–1602, 1991.)

ing increased from 57 to 63 cm/sec. There was no change in the peak velocity of late filling and a significant decrease in the ratio of late to early peak left ventricular filling velocity. Plasma atrial natriuretic peptides decreased from 70 to 41 pg/mL, and there were no changes in plasma renin activity and catecholamine levels. Although a trace of peripheral edema was noted in almost half of the subjects, none withdrew from therapy because of side effects.

Conclusions.—In patients with severe hypertension, 1 year of treatment with extended-release nifedipine resulted in regression of left ventricular mass and maintenance of left ventricular systolic function. Atrial natriuretic peptide was reduced, and there was no detectable activation of the sympathetic or renin system. Side effects were easily tolerated.

▶ Regression of left ventricular hypertrophy has been frequently observed with calcium blockers, ACE inhibitors, α-blockers and centrally acting α-agonists such as methyldopa. Whether this regression will provide better clinical cardioprotection remains to be seen but, like God and motherhood, it should be helpful.

Despite some lingering confusion, calcium blockers are equally effective in younger as well as in older patients.— N. Kaplan, M.D.

Analysis of Advancing Age on the Response to Nicardipine Among 467 Adult Hypertensive Patients

Kuramoto K, Ikeda M, Kaneko Y, Omae T, Yoshinaga K, Yamada K (Tokyo Metropolitan Geriatric Hospital; Jichi Medical School, Oomiya, Japan; Yokohama Hypertension Research Center, Japan; Natl Cardiovascular Center, Suita, Japan; Tohoku University, Sendai, et al)
J Hypertens 9:59–63, 1991   3–39

Background.—Reports regarding possible increased effectiveness of calcium entry-blockers in treatment of hypertension in elderly patients are contradictory and are based on small patient populations. The antihypertensive responses to nicardipine in 467 hypertensive patients (age, 30–74 years) were analyzed.

Methods.—Patients were grouped according to age and started on 10 mg or 20 mg of nicardipine 3 times a day, with dosages adjusted according to symptoms. Nicardipine was administered for 12 weeks, with blood pressure, heart rate, and subjective symptoms monitored every 2 weeks. Antihypertensive response was defined as a reduction of blood pressure of 20/10 mm Hg for reduction of blood pressure to below 149/89 mm Hg.

Results.—Between 64.5% and 77.1% of patients responded to nicardipine, with a difference in response rates between youngest and oldest groups of less than 5%. Response rate in patients younger than 39 years of age was 64.5%; in those aged 40–49 years, 67.1%; in those aged 50–59 years, 76.9%; in those aged 60–69 years, 77.1%; and in those older than 70 years, 68.8%. Similar blood pressure reduction was achieved in each age group after nicardipine treatment, with an average reduction in systolic blood pressure of 25 mm Hg and in diastolic blood pressure of 14 mm Hg. Mean heart rate before treatment was 74.4 beats/min; after treatment it was 73.9 beats/min.

Conclusions.—These findings indicate that pretreatment blood pressure is a better indicator than relative age of the patient in considering calcium entry-blockers for treatment of hypertension. Although greater blood pressure reduction occurs in older hypertensive patients, this seems to be a result of the higher baseline blood pressure among older patients. No age-related trend was noted in the percentage of blood pressure decrease.

▶ This large scale study should pretty well put to rest the issue about a major difference in responsiveness of the elderly to calcium blockers. The elderly and blacks obviously do respond well to them (1), and these drugs are attractive vasodilatory agents for elderly hypertensives, particularly if the patient also has occlusive vascular disease in his or her coronary, cerebral, renal, or peripheral vessels. Another of their attractive features is their mild natriuretic effect (2), which translates into a lesser need for diuretics and, perhaps, a somewhat lesser additive effect when diuretics are combined with calcium blockers.

When calcium blockers are used, there are few interactions that interfere with their effectiveness, but patients should be warned about which liquid they use to help swallow the tablets.—N. Kaplan, M.D.

References

1. Zing W, et al: Calcium antagonists in elderly and black hypertensive patients. Therapeutic controversies. *Arch Intern Med* 151:2154–2162, 1991.
2. Krishna GG, et al: Natriuretic effect of calcium-channel blockers in hypertensives. *Am J Kidney Dis* 18:566–572, 1991.

Interaction of Citrus Juices With Felodipine and Nifedipine
Bailey DG, Spence JD, Munoz C, Arnold JMO (Victoria Hospital, Univ of Western Ontario, London, Ont)
Lancet 337:268–269, 1991   3–40

Background.—In a study on ethanol-drug interactions, it was found by chance that citrus fruit juices may greatly augment the bioavailability of some drugs. This possible food-drug interaction was further explored.

Methods.—Six white men aged 48 to 62 years with borderline hypertension and 6 normotensive white men aged 18 to 45 years were studied. The hypertensive men took felodipine, 5 mg, with water, grapefruit juice, or orange juice. The 6 healthy men took nifedipine, 10 mg, with water or grapefruit juice.

Results.—The mean felodipine bioavailability with grapefruit juice was 284% of that with water (range 164% to 469%) and diastolic blood pressure fell more with grapefruit juice than with water (−20 vs −11 mm

Hg). Heart rate was higher with grapefruit juice than with water and vasodilation-related side effects occurred more often. These effects did not happen with orange juice. In the normotensive group, bioavailability of nifedipine with grapefruit juice was 134% of that with water, with a range of 108% to 169%.

Conclusions.—This is the first demonstration of a pharmacokinetic interaction between citrus juice and a drug in keeping with the observation that 200 mL of grapefruit juice tripled the bioavailability of felodipine tablets. Orange juice, which contains similar amounts of basic nutrients, did not produce these effects.

▶ Grapefruit juice contains bioflavonoids, which may inhibit the breakdown of felodipine (and other drugs) involving oxidation by cytochrome P450. The lesson is simple: patients should take whatever medications they use over long periods under similar circumstances of time of day, food ingestion, etc., to avoid unexpected variations in drug effects. Who would ever have thought that grapefruit juice could make such a difference?

Along with calcium blockers, ACE inhibitors are being used in more and more hypertensives, particularly if the patients have congestive heart failure. Another group being targeted for therapy with ACE inhibitors is the diabetic hypertensive population. That group may soon be expanded to include the normotensive diabetic population as well.— N. Kaplan, M.D.

Efficacy of Captopril in Postponing Nephropathy in Normotensive Insulin Dependent Diabetic Patients With Microalbuminuria
Mathiesen ER, Hommel E, Giese J, Parving H-H (Hvidøre Hospital, Klampenborg, Denmark; Glostrup Hospital, Copenhagen, Denmark)
BMJ 303:81–87, 1991   3–41

Introduction.—Animal studies have suggested that angiotensin-converting enzyme (ACE) inhibition might reduce glomerular hypertension, restrict increases in urinary albumin excretion, and slow the development of structural glomerular lesions. A 4-year randomized study was done to assess the efficacy of ACE inhibition in preventing nephropathy in diabetic patients.

Study Design.—The subjects were 44 patients with insulin-dependent diabetes. All were normotensive, mean blood pressure was 127/78 mm Hg, and all had persistent microalbuminuria of 30–300 mg/24 hours. Patients were paired according to urinary albumin excretion, blood pressure, hemoglobin A_{1c} concentration, and glomerular filtration rate. One patient in each pair received captopril, starting at a dose of 25 mg/day and increasing to 100 mg/day in the first 16 months. After 30 months, thiazide was added. The other patients were given no antihypertensive drugs.

Observations.—In the captopril group, urinary albumin excretion decreased gradually from 82 to 57 mg/24 hours, whereas this measure increased from 105 to 166 mg/24 hours in the control group (Fig 3–13).

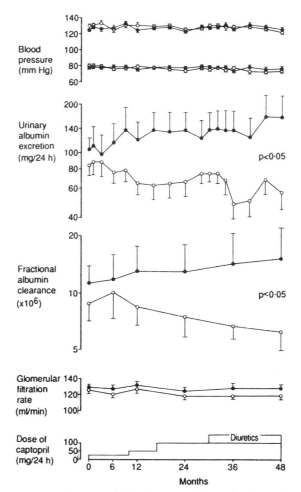

Fig 3–13.—Time course of mean arterial blood pressure, urinary albumin excretion, fractional albumin clearance, and glomerular filtration rate in normotensive insulin-dependent patients with diabetes and microalbuminuria. Twenty-one patients received captopril *(open circle)* and 23 served as untreated controls *(filled circle)*. Ordinates of urinary albumin excretion and fractional albumin clearance are log scales. *Bars* are SEM. (Courtesy of Mathiesen ER, Hommel E, Giese J, et al: *BMJ* 303:81–87, 1991.)

Urinary albumin was consistently lower in the captopril group after 16 months of treatment. Diabetic nephropathy occurred in 7 patients in the control group compared with none of the captopril-treated patients. In both groups, there were no significant changes in blood pressure, glomerular filtration rate, hemoglobin A_{1c} concentration, and urinary sodium and urea excretion.

Conclusion.— In normotensive, insulin-dependent patients with diabetes and persistent microalbuminuria, ACE inhibition may delay the appearance of overt diabetic nephropathy. Captopril treatment reduces urinary excretion of albumin with no significant change in blood pressure or glomerular filtration rate. Longer follow-up is needed before this treatment can be recommended in normotensive diabetics.

▶ This beautifully conducted clinical trial confirms what these investigators (1) and other have shown in hypertensive and, to a lesser degree, normotensive diabetics with early nephropathy: ACE inhibitors will retard the progression of renal damage. Despite some experimental data suggesting that ACE inhibitors may be better in doing this than other drugs, the clinical evidence is less convincing.— N. Kaplan, M.D.

Reference

1. Parving H-H: Impact of blood pressure and antihypertensive treatment on incipient and overt nephropathy, retinopathy, and endothelial permeability in diabetes mellitus. *Diabetes Care* 14:260–269, 1991.

Comparison Between Perindopril and Nifedipine in Hypertensive and Normotensive Diabetic Patients With Microalbuminuria

Melbourne Diabetic Nephropathy Study Group (St Vincent's Hosp, Fitzroy, Australia)
BMJ 302:210–216, 1991   3–42

Background.—To determine the relative efficacy of 2 different classes of antihypertensive drugs on retarding the progression of diabetic nephropathy, an angiotensin converting enzyme (ACE) inhibitor was compared with a calcium antagonist in diabetic patients with microalbuminuria.

Methods.—Fifty diabetic patients were randomly assigned to treatment with perindopril or nifedipine for 12 months and monitored for 1 or 3 months after treatment, depending on whether they were hyperten-

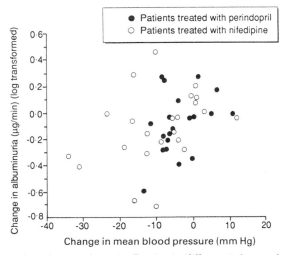

Fig 3–14.—Correlation between change in albuminuria (difference in log transformed albumin excretion rate) and change in mean blood pressure during drug treatment (*r* = .37, *P* = .016). (Courtesy of Melbourne Diabetic Nephropathy Study Group: *BMJ* 302:210–216, 1991.)

sive or normotensive. Of the 43 patients who finished the study, 30 were normotensive and 13 were hypertensive. Nineteen patients had type I diabetes and 24 had type II. The main outcome measures were albumin excretion rate, blood pressure, and glomerular filtration rate.

Results.—Both drugs significantly decreased mean blood pressure. During treatment, there were no significant between-group differences in albuminuria or mean blood pressure. Changes in mean blood pressure and albuminuria were significantly correlated (Fig 3–14). Both perindopril and nifedipine significantly reduced mean blood pressure and albuminuria in hypertensive patients. Normotensive patients had no significant decreases in albuminuria with either drug.

Conclusions.—Blood pressure appears to be an important determinant of urinary albumin excretion in diabetic patients with microalbuminuria. Perindopril and nifedipine had similar effects on urinary albumin excretion. Both prevented increases in albuminuria in normotensive patients and reduced albuminuria in hypertensive patients.

▶ These results suggest that, to retard the progression of diabetic nephropathy, it matters little how the blood pressure is lowered as long as it is lowered. The final answer is not yet available and additional, larger comparative studies are now in process. In the meantime, ACE inhibitor usage will continue to expand. These drugs have well-documented efficacy in relieving congestive heart failure, and preliminary evidence suggests that these drugs will relieve angina (1).

Meanwhile, about 1 in 6 patients given chronic ACE inhibitor therapy will develop a dry, hacking cough that may be accompanied by voice change and sore throat (2). It is not dangerous, but it sure can be a bother.

More serious but much less common is acute, usually reversible, renal failure when an ACE inhibitor is given to patients with unrecognized bilateral renovascular hypertension or polycystic kidney disease (3). Even less common is acute renal artery thrombosis in patients with unilateral renovascular disease (4). These circumstances all involve the abrupt removal of high levels of angiotensin II needed to maintain renal perfusion.

In view of these real and potential problems with ACE inhibitors, another possible way to treat diabetic hypertensives may be particularly attractive.—N. Kaplan, M.D.

References

1. Akhras F, Jackson G: The role of captopril as single therapy in hypertension and angina pectoris. *Int J Cardiol* 33:259–266, 1991.
2. Yeo WW, et al: Prevalence of persistent cough during long-term enalapril treatment: Controlled study versus nifedipine. *Q J Med* 81:763–770, 1991.
3. Chapman AB, et al: Reversible renal failure associated with angiotensin-converting enzyme inhibitors in polycystic kidney disease. *Ann Intern Med* 115:769–773, 1991.
4. Hannedouche T, et al: Acute renal thrombosis induced by angiotensin-converting enzyme inhibitors in patients with renovascular hypertension. *Nephron* 57:230–231, 1991.

Treating Insulin Resistance in Hypertension With Metformin Reduces Both Blood Pressure and Metabolic Risk Factors

Landin K, Tengborn L, Smith U (Sahlgrenska Hospital, University of Göteborg, Sweden)

J Intern Med 229:181–187, 1991   3–43

Background.—Insulin resistance and hyperinsulinemia may have an important part in the development of hypertension and its accompanying metabolic aberrations.

Patients.—To further investigate this possibility, 9 middle-aged men with untreated hypertension were treated with metformin. The men were nonsmokers who were not obese and did not have diabetes. Metformin was given orally at a dose of 850 mg twice a day for 6 weeks.

Outcomes.—Metformin reduced total and low-density-lipoprotein cholesterol, triglyceride, fasting plasma insulin, and C-peptide levels. The treatment increased glucose disposal, an indicator of insulin action measured by the euglycemic clamp method. Tissue plasminogen activator (t-PA) activity also rose, whereas t-PA antigen dropped. Plasminogen activator inhibitor and fibrinogen were not affected. Body weight also did not change. On metformin withdrawal, both blood pressure and metabolism returned toward initial levels (Fig 3–15).

Conclusions.—In mildly hypertensive men, metformin therapy increased insulin action, lowered blood pressure, improved metabolic risk

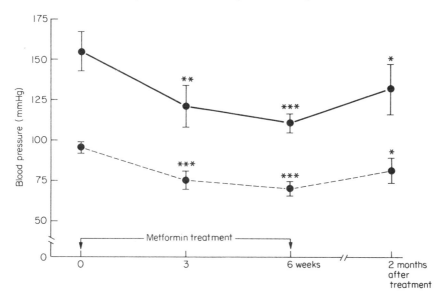

Fibrinolysis

Fig 3–15.—Effect of metformin on systolic *(solid line)* and diastolic *(broken line)* blood pressure in hypertensive men (N = 9). Mean values ± 1 SD are shown. Significances of differences are calculated for changes compared with initial results. $*P < .05$, $**P < .01$, $***P < .001$. (Courtesy of Landin K, Tengborn L, Smith U: *J Intern Med* 229:181–187, 1991.)

factor profile, and tended to raise fibrinolytic activity. These findings support the notion that insulin resistance has an important role in hypertension, which may open new possibilities for alleviating the abnormalities associated with cardiovascular disease.

▶ This preliminary study was done in nondiabetic hypertensive patients, so it obviously needs confirmation in larger groups of diabetic subjects. Metformin is being used widely in Europe and will likely soon become available in the United States for treatment of diabetes. If it does all of the good things in diabetic hypertensives that it did in these few nondiabetic hypertensives, it may be an important addition to the therapy.

The improvements in insulin sensitivity, lipids, and fibrinolysis support the possible use of metformin in nondiabetic hypertensives as well, but that will take a lot more study.

In addition to diabetics, another group of patients who are at high risk for hypertensive complications are those who are resistant to therapy.—N. Kaplan, M.D.

Resistant Hypertension in a Tertiary Care Clinic
Yakovlevitch M, Black HR (Yale Univ)
Arch Intern Med 151:1786–1792, 1991   3–44

Introduction.—Estimates of the frequency of resistant hypertension (HTN) differ considerably, but the condition is thought to be more common (up to 13%) in referral centers. To determine the prevalence and causes of resistant HTN among patients at a tertiary care clinic, a total of 436 charts were reviewed.

Patients and Methods.—During a 3-year period (1986–1988), 91 patients who met criteria for resistant HTN were seen more than once. These patients had been treated with at least 3 antihypertensive drugs simultaneously, but their blood pressure (BP) remained elevated. Follow-up continued until their BP was controlled or until March 1990.

Results.—A cause of resistant HTN was found in 83 of the 91 patients (table). Most (53) had drug-related reasons for resistance, such as a suboptimal regimen. Nine patients had not complied with treatment and 2 had high alcohol consumption. A secondary cause was found in 10 patients, 6 with renovascular HTN and 4 with primary aldosteronism. Seven patients had psychological causes and 6 had elevated pressures only in the physician's office. In the 53 patients without secondary HTN, control of BP was achieved in 42 and improved in 9, most commonly by the addition of a diuretic. Control or improvement was also achieved in 7 of the 10 patients with secondary HTN.

Conclusion.—Resistant HTN is common in a tertiary care clinic setting, but BP can be controlled or significantly improved in the majority of these patients. Better tolerated newer agents and the proper use of diuretics to control volume expansion are recommended treatment strategies.

Primary Cause of Resistant Hypertension

Primary Cause of Resistance*	No. of Patients	No. Ultimately Controlled	No. Significantly Improved
Group 1: noncompliance (without medication intolerance)	9	3	1
Group 2: drug related Suboptimal medical reigmen	39	29	6
Drug interaction	1	0	1
Objective medication intolerance	13	4	1
With noncompliance	7	1	0
Without noncompliance	6	3	1
Group 3: interfering substances Alcohol abuse	2	2	0
Group 4: secondary hypertension Renal artery stenosis	6	2	1
Primary aldosteronism	4	4	0
Group 5: psychological causes Subjective medication intolerance	7	2	0
Group 6: office resistance	2	2	0
Cause undetermined	8	0	0

*In addition to the primary problems listed, 7 patients had a suboptimal medical regimen, 6 patients had a drug interaction, 5 patients were noncompliant, and 2 had office resistance as a contributory but not major cause of resistance.
(Courtesy of Yakovlevitch M, Black HR: *Arch Intern Med* 151:1786–1792, 1991.)

▶ These data confirm previous reports of the prevalence and causes of resistant hypertension. One fact shines through: most patients who are resistant to therapy are resistant because they have not been given appropriate therapy by their physicians, usually not enough of a diuretic. As the authors state: "Physicians and patients have become way of using these drugs, and this undoubtedly reflects their concerns about the adverse effects of diuretics." In fact, failure to use a diuretic or a large enough dose of one has been repeatedly noted to be the most common cause for resistance to therapy even before we were aware of the metabolic mischief induced by diuretics.

For most uncomplicated hypertensives, only a little bit (i.e., 12.5 mg of hydrochlorothiazide) is needed, and some can get away with no diuretic, particularly if given drugs that are natriuretic themselves (calcium blockers) or that block the renin-aldosterone mechanism (ACE inhibitors). However, once hypertension becomes more severe, and particularly when multiple drugs are needed, the tendency for volume retention increases and patients often end up with a dilated vascular bed that is still overfilled with an expanded fluid volume.

Many of those who are resistant are also severely hypertensive, and an immediate reduction in blood pressure may be needed. There are many drugs that can accomplish that.—N. Kaplan, M.D.

Comparison of Sublingual Captopril and Nifedipine in Immediate Treatment of Hypertensive Emergencies: A Randomized, Single-Blind Clinical Trial
Angeli P, Chiesa M, Caregaro L, Merkel C, Sacerdoti D, Rondana M, Gatta A
(University of Padua; Hospital of Padua, Italy)
Arch Intern Med 151:678–682, 1991   3–45

Background.—There is controversy about the best immediate treatment of hypertensive emergencies. Several drugs are available, but controlled randomized studies are lacking because of the rarity with which such conditions are encountered. A randomized, single-blind study was done to compare the safety and effectiveness of sublingual captopril tablets and sublingual nifedipine capsules for initial treatment of hypertensive emergencies.

Methods.—Twenty-two patients were studied during a 2-year period. All patients received sublingual placebo and were monitored for 20 minutes; in 2 cases, the diastolic blood pressure dropped more than 10 mm Hg, and these patients were excluded. The remaining patients were randomized to receive either 25 mg of sublingual captopril or 10 mg of sublingual nifedipine. If diastolic blood pressure dropped less than 10 mm Hg 20 minutes after drug administration, patients were classified as nonresponders and received intravenous therapy.

Results.—Nine of 10 patients responded to sublingual captopril. At 50 minutes, their mean blood pressure dropped from 245/144 to 190/115 mm Hg. This effect lasted a mean of 4 hours. In 6 of these 9 patients, the lowered blood pressure was associated with improvement of end-organ function within 60 minutes. No side effects were seen in this group. Eight of 10 patients responded to sublingual nifedipine. Its hypotensive effect was seen in 10 minutes for diastolic blood pressure and 20 minutes for systolic blood pressure compared with 20 and 30 minutes for captopril. However, there was no difference in time or magnitude of the peak hypotensive effects of these drugs, or in the duration of the effect. Of these 8 patients, 6 had improvement of end-organ function within 60 minutes. Minor side effects were seen in 3 patients.

Conclusions.—Sublingual captopril appears to be a safe and effective means of lowering arterial blood pressure in hypertensive emergencies. It may even be suited for use as a drug of first choice, although further studies in larger populations are needed.

▶ The effectiveness of both drugs used sublingually was equal. In other studies, the sublingual route has actively been shown to slow the onset of action of liquid nifedipine, which is more rapidly absorbed through the gastric mucosa. However, the sublingual route is preferable because the blood pressure should not be brought down too quickly and too much to avoid hypoperfusion of vital organs (brain and heart).

Actually, the number of true hypertensive "urgencies" that require such rapid reduction of pressure is much smaller than the number of times these drugs are used. Most patients with severe hypertension but who are in no immediate danger are better treated with usual oral therapy and given a few hours to more slowly and safely bring their pressures down.

Recall that in the study by Yakovlevitch and Black, a secondary cause for hypertension was the second most common mechanism for resistance, leading us into the last section of our coverage.—N. Kaplan, M.D.

Secondary Causes

▶ ↓ In most series, the most common type of secondary hypertension is renal parenchymal disease, followed by renovascular disease. The former is easily recognized, the latter may be tough to identify. The need is particularly great among those with resistant hypertension, and this includes blacks who have usually been said to suffer from renovascular hypertension (RVHT) only infrequently. Among 67 blacks with severe or resistant hypertension, 9% turned out to have RVHT, whereas RVHT was the diagnosis in 18% of 97 whites, with similar clinical features (1).

In this series, the diagnosis of RVHT was based on captopril-stimulated peripheral blood renin measurements and renal arteriography. In the study by Svetkey et al. the post-captopril renin levels were distinctly elevated in 48% of the whites with proven RVHT but in only 17% of the blacks. Others have also found the captopril test to have poor sensitivity and accuracy even when renography is also performed along with the measurement of plasma renin levels.—N. Kaplan, M.D.

Reference

1. Svetkey LP, et al: Similar prevalence of renovascular hypertension in selected blacks and whites. *Hypertension* 17:678–683, 1991.

The Value of Tests Predicting Renovascular Hypertension in Patients With Renal Artery Stenosis Treated by Angioplasty
Postma CT, van Oijen AHAM, Barentsz JO, de Boo T, Hoefnagels WHL, Corstens FHM, Thien T (University Hospital, Nijmegen, The Netherlands)
Arch Intern Med 151:1531–1535, 1991   3–46

Introduction.—Renal artery stenosis can be diagnosed with certainty only retrospectively, after the stenosis has been relieved. To evaluate tests predicting renovascular hypertension, these procedures were compared: selective renal vein renin sampling, captopril-stimulated plasma renin activity, and renal scintigraphy after capropril. A secondary aim of the study was to identify clinical characteristics that show a relationship to blood pressure outcome after percutaneous transluminal renal angioplasty (PTRA).

Patients.—Study participants included 30 hypertensive patients with a documented stenosis of at least 50% of the luminal diameter of 1 of the renal arteries and 1 patient with bilateral stenoses. After PTRA, patients were initially seen every 4 weeks, then every 3 months after stabilization of blood pressure.

Results.—At the 12-month follow-up, PTRA resulted in a cure in 8 patients, improvement in 12, and failure in 11, yielding a benefit rate of 65%. Two mathematical models used to analyze the renal vein renin assays gave accuracies of 44% and 60%. The captopril test had a sensitivity of 36% and an accuracy of 43%, whereas the sensitivity of renal captopril ^{99m}Tc-labeled pentetic acid scintigraphy was 60% (Fig 3–16). Age appeared to be the only significant factor differentiating the groups with

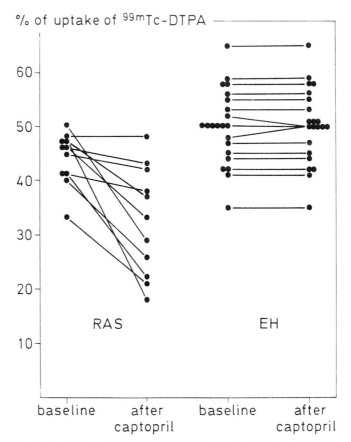

Fig 3–16.—Renal technetium Tc 99m (99mTc)-labeled pentetic acid scintigraphy in 11 patients with renal artery stenosis (RAS) and in 11 patients with essential hypertension (EH). Of the patients with RAS, the uptake in the kidney behind the stenosis is depicted. In the patients with EH, the uptake in both kidneys is shown. (Courtesy of Potsma CT, van Oijen AHAM, Barentsz JO, et al: *Arch Intern Med* 151:1531–1535, 1991.)

benefit and failure. The mean age of patients was 40.6 years for those whose blood pressure improved and 54 years for those without blood pressure response.

Conclusion.—Because patients without true renovascular hypertension will not be helped by PTRA, it is important to identify those who will benefit from the procedure. The tests currently available are not of great predictive value, but age may have an important influence on outcome.

Captopril Renography in the Diagnosis of Renal Artery Stenosis: Accuracy and Limitations
Mann SJ, Pickering TG, Sos TA, Uzzo RG, Sarkar S, Friend K, Rackson ME, Laragh JH (Cornell Univ, New York)
Am J Med 90:30–40, 1991   3–47

Introduction.—Captopril has been shown to improve the diagnostic accuracy of renal scintigraphy in patients with renal artery stenosis because it exaggerates the asymmetry of function between an ischemic and a normal contralateral kidney. However, the usefulness of captopril renography in the detection of bilateral stenosis and its ability to distinguish between parenchymal and renovascular disease have not been clearly established.

Patients.—Renography was performed before diagnostic renal angiography in 55 patients with a high clinical index of suspicion for renovascular hypertension. Hemodynamically significant renal artery stenosis was defined as stenosis exceeding 70%. Renography was performed on 2 consecutive days, with 25 mg of captopril administered orally 1 hour before the second study. Post-captopril radionuclide studies were compared with pre-captopril studies to assess the magnitude of the captopril-induced changes. Renography was performed with technetium-99m-diethylenetriamine pentaacetic acid (DTPA) as a measure of glomerular filtration rate and iodine-131-orthoiodohippurate as a measure of renal blood flow.

Results.—Thirty-five patients had significant renal artery stenosis on arteriography; 21 had unilateral and 14 had bilateral stenosis. Twenty patients did not have significant renal stenosis and were diagnosed as having essential hypertension. The 3 criteria for diagnosing renal artery stenosis by the DPTA scan were asymmetry of uptake, time to peak uptake, and retention seen at 15 minutes. In patients with bilateral disease, the finding of asymmetry identified the more severely affected kidney, but the presence or absence of stenosis in the contralateral kidney could not be determined reliably. A comparison of pre-captopril and post-captopril studies revealed that captopril-induced DPTA scintigraphic changes were highly specific for renal artery stenosis, but they occurred in only 51% of the cases. Thus, the sensitivity of this technique is low. Iodine-131-orthoiodohippurate scintigraphy gave similar results although with slightly lower sensitivity and specificity.

Conclusion.—Asymmetric DTPA uptake, time to peak uptake, or DTPA retention on a single post-captopril renogram is a highly sensitive and specific finding for renal artery stenosis, but it does not distinguish unilateral from bilateral disease. The presence of captopril-induced change is highly specific for renal artery stenosis, but the sensitivity of this finding is low.

▶ In both of these series, captopril renography provided only about a 50% sensitivity for the diagnosis of RVHT. Whereas it was highly specific, giving few false positives, its ability to correctly diagnose only half of patients with the disease means that it cannot serve as an appropriate screening test.

Better results with captopril renography have been reported by others. Setaro et al. (1) performed both the pre- and post-captopril DPTA studies on the same day in 94 patients who were strongly suspected by clinical criteria of having RVHT, of whom 47% had renal artery stenosis. Captopril renography was 91% sensitive and 94% specific in identifying or excluding RVHT. Erbslöh-Möller et al. (2) also reported similarly excellent results with ^{131}I-hippuran renography followed by intravenous furosemide, measuring residual cortical activity of the isotope at 20 minutes.

Because of the multiple variations used by different investigators and the widely divergent results reported, a 2-day meeting on captopril renography was held on November 28–29, 1990, with 12 groups presenting their data. These papers and more are published as a supplement to the *American Journal of Hypertension* (volume 4, number 12, part 2, December 1991). The final 3 papers provide about as good a consensus on the indications, performance, and interpretation of the procedure as is now feasible. My interpretation of all this is that the procedure should serve as an adequate screening study to rule out RVHT in populations with fairly low prevalence of the disease, but it is not sensitive enough to firmly exclude the process in those patients with a high clinical suspicion. For them, renal arteriography remains the preferable initial study.

Beyond RVHT, mention will be given to important papers about other secondary causes:

- Chronic renal failure: Hypertension remains a major contributor to mortality in patients with end-stage renal disease (3). Those on chronic dialysis who are hypertensive usually have volume overload (4).
- Pheochromocytoma: MIBG-I^{131} scintigraphy may be useful in establishing the diagnosis in patients with borderline biochemical studies (5).
- Primary aldosteronism: Severe hypertension and a high prevalence of vascular complications was observed in 32 patients seen at one hospital in Yokohama (6).
- Coarctation of the aorta: Long-time survival after surgical correction is common, but deaths from coarctation or its repair continue to occur, mostly more than 20 years after the operation (7).—N. Kaplan, M.D.

References

1. Setaro JF, et al: Simplified captopril renography in diagnosis and treatment of renal artery stenosis. *Hypertension* 18:289–298, 1991.
2. Erbslöh-Möller B, et al: Furosemide-^{131}I-hippuran renography after angiotensin-converting enzyme inhibition for the diagnosis of renovascular hypertension. *Am J Med* 90:23–29, 1991.

3. Rostand SG, et al: Cardiovascular complications in renal failure. *J Am Soc Nephrol* 2:1053–1062, 1991.
4. Thylén P, et al: Hypertension profiling by total body water (TBW) determinations in patients on chronic hemodialysis. *Int J Artif Organs* 14:18–22, 1991.
5. Hanson MW, et al: Iodine 131-labeled metaiodobenzylguanidine scintigraphy and biochemical analyses in suspected pheochromocytoma. *Arch Intern Med* 151:1397–1402, 1991.
6. Young S-C, et al: Hypertension complications in patients with primary aldosteronism. A retrospective study. *Curr Ther Res* 50:317–325, 1991.
7. Bobby JJ, et al: Operative survival and 40 year follow up of surgical repair of aortic coarctation. *Br Heart J* 65:271–276, 1991.

Sleep Apnea and Systemic Hypertension: A Causal Association Review
Hoffstein V, Chan CK, Slutsky AS (Univ of Toronto, Ont)
Am J Med 91:190–196, 1991   3–48

Introduction.—A number of prospective studies have demonstrated that hemodynamic changes that could lead to significant cardiovascular end-organ damage occur during apneic episodes. Hypertension is prevalent in patients with sleep apnea syndrome (SAS), but it is not clear whether hypertensive persons should be routinely screened for SAS.

Literature Review.—A search of the literature revealed 5 epidemiologic studies done between 1978 and 1989 that dealt with the causal association between SAS and systemic hypertension. A case-control approach was used in 4 of these investigations. The strength of the association was quite variable even when a conservative cutoff value for the apnea index was chosen. There is some evidence suggesting a dose-response relationship between SAS and hypertension, but the risk association was unstable, with the relative risk estimate for SAS and hypertension varying from 1.3 to 40.

Conclusions.—The data available indicate a positive association between sleep apnea and hypertension but do not justify performing polysomnography as part of the routine work-up of hypertensive patients. Prospective longitudinal studies are needed to define changes in blood pressure from the time SAS is diagnosed through treatment and follow-up. Polysomnography should be done in suspect cases.

▶ When hypertension is found in association with sleep apnea, nasal continuous positive airway pressure (nCPAP) may markedly reduce the blood pressure. In 12 such patients, nocturnal intra-arterial blood pressure fell from 140/82 to 126/69 and indirectly measured daytime blood pressure fell from 169/104 to 138/87 after 6 months of nCPAP (1).—N. Kaplan, M.D.

Reference

1. Mayer J, et al: Blood pressure and sleep apnea: Results of long-term nasal continuous positive airway pressure therapy. *Cardiology* 79:84–92, 1991.

▶ ↓ A good deal of important information has been published about pregnancy-induced hypertension or preeclampsia.—N. Kaplan, M.D.

Calcium Excretion in Preeclampsia

Sanchez-Ramos L, Sandroni S, Andres FJ, Kaunitz AM (Univ of Florida, Jacksonville)
Obstet Gynecol 77:510–513, 1991   3–49

Background.—Some studies have found that preeclampsia is associated with hypocalciuria, but others have found no relationship. One hundred forty-three pregnant women were studied to determine whether patients with preeclampsia have decreased urinary calcium excretion and evaluate the usefulness of urinary calcium level in screening for preeclampsia.

Methods.—Preeclampsia was diagnosed on the basis of a blood pressure of 140/90 mm Hg or a rise of 30 mm Hg in systolic or 15 mm Hg in diastolic pressure, along with significant proteinuria. Fifty-eight patients were normotensive; 52 had gestational hypertension, and 33 had preeclampsia. The 3 groups showed no significant differences in mean maternal age, race, or parity.

Results.—Excretion of total calcium was 130 mg/24 hours in patients with preeclampsia, significantly lower than the 284 mg/24 hour value in normotensive patients and the 233 mg/24 hour value in patients with gestational hypertension. The preeclampsia group also had significant increases in mean arterial pressure and excretion of total protein. A urine calcium threshold of 12 mg/dL was chosen as predictive of preeclampsia according to the receiver operator curve. This threshold had a sensitivity of 85%, specificity of 91%, positive predictive value of 85%, and negative predictive value of 91%.

Conclusions.—Preeclampsia may be distinguished from other hypertensive disorders of pregnancy on the basis of urinary calcium levels. A level less than 12 mg/dL is suggestive of preeclampsia. However, further studies must be done before this test can be recommended for screening purposes.

▶ These data and those in another group of 41 patients (1) confirm the observation noted by Taufield et al. (2) in 1987 that women with preeclampsia have low levels of urinary calcium excretion. Of even more clinical importance, Belizan et al. (3) have reconfirmed their original evidence that calcium supplementation after the 20th week of pregnancy will reduce the risk of developing hypertension by some 37%.

Even more impressive reductions (by 65%) in the risk of developing preeclampsia have been noted in 6 controlled trials of the use of low-dose aspirin in women considered at high risk for developing the syndrome (4).

Rather than routinely giving supplemental calcium or low-dose aspirin, it will probably be more cost-effective to treat those women at increased risk for developing preeclampsia. In a case-control study of 139 preeclamptic women and 132 control women (5), preeclamptic women were more likely to be multiparous or to have had preeclampsia in a previous pregnancy. They were more likely to have higher body mass, to work during pregnancy, to have a family history of hypertension and, among nulliparous women, to be black.—N. Kaplan, M.D.

References

1. Huikeshoven FJM, Zuijderhoudt FMJ: Hypocalciuria in hypertensive disorder in pregnancy and how to measure it. *Eur J Obstet Gynecol Reprod Biol* 36:81–85, 1990.
2. Taufield PA, et al: Hypocalciuria in preeclampsia. *N Engl J Med* 316:715–718, 1987.
3. Belizán JM, et al: Calcium supplementation to prevent hypertensive disorders of pregnancy. *N Engl J Med* 325:1399–1405, 1991.
4. Imperiale TF, Petrulis AS: A metanalysis of low-dose aspirin for the prevention of pregnancy-induced hypertensive disease. *JAMA* 266:260–264, 1991.
5. Eskenazi B, Fenster L, Sidney S: A multivariate analysis of risk factors for preeclampsia. *JAMA* 266:237–241, 1991.

▶ ↓ Lastly, there is continued good news about the protective effects of postmenopausal estrogen therapy.—N. Kaplan, M.D.

Short-Term Effects of Estrogen and Progestin on Blood Pressure of Normotensive Postmenopausal Women
Regensteiner JG, Hiatt WR, Byyny RL, Pickett CK, Woodard WD, Moore LG
(Univ of Colorado, Denver)
J Clin Pharmacol 31:543–548, 1991   3–50

Introduction.—Blood pressure starts to rise progressively at the time of menopause, but it is not clear whether aging itself or lowered production of estrogen and progestin is chiefly responsible.

Study Design.—Twelve healthy normotensive women with a mean age of 51 years who had complete ovariectomy and hysterectomy an average of 5 years before the study received estrogen and progestin, separately and together, in a placebo-controlled study. Conjugated equine estrogens were given in a dose of 2.5 mg daily, and medroxyprogesterone acetate was given in a dose of 60 mg daily. Treatments were given for 1 week with another week of no treatment between each new treatment.

Results.—Neither progestin nor estrogen alone affected blood pressure. Combined treatment reduced systolic pressure by 7 mm Hg and diastolic pressure by 5 mm Hg. The order of treatment did not influence the results. Body weight did not change during the study.

Summary.—Combined estrogen and progestin treatment lowered mean arterial pressure by 6% in these healthy postmenopausal women. Doses were higher than those generally administered so the results may not be applicable to women given typical hormonal replacement doses.

▶ Women will certainly not be given postmenopausal estrogen replacement therapy (ERT), particularly in the large doses used in this study, in an attempt to lower their blood pressure. But the multiple benefits of ERT are being increasingly recognized, and I believe that most postmenopausal women should receive these benefits (1). Despite the known propensity of oral contraceptives to raise blood pressure, ERT will not, so concerns about hypertension should not interfere with the use of ERT.

All in all, it has been an interesting year, with significant advances in our understanding of the mechanisms and management of hypertension. We may be on the threshold of even more exciting preventative moves, including aspirin for preeclampsia, ACE inhibitors for nephropathy, and EDRF-enhancing agents for hypertension. Meanwhile, we certainly can be more optimistic about the treatment of elderly hypertensive patients.—N. Kaplan, M.D.

Reference

1. Kaplan NM: A plea for two actions that need to be taken. *Am J Cardiol* 67:641–642, 1991.

4 Pediatric Cardiovascular Disease

Introduction

Every year provides many learning experiences and this one is no exception. We learn about some new treatments and some that disappoint us by imperfect results. We find some new insights into pathogenesis of congenital heart disease and of the psychological implications of being born with a defect or of undergoing new and inventive surgical measures to repair the problem. We find once again that much is exciting in the field of pediatric cardiovascular disease and that much more remains to be investigated. Here are some highlights of the articles that follow.

Arrhythmias continue to be a problem in some patients in long-term follow-up of the surgical procedures used to help them, especially after repair of tetralogy of Fallot, physiologic repair of transposed great arteries, and the Fontan procedure.

Wolff-Parkinson-White syndrome sometimes requires more than medical management when patients fail to get relief of recurrent tachycardia. Results of surgery and of the newer radiofrequency ablation of bypass tracts are reported.

The conduction disturbance selected is fetal complete heart block, with a note about long-term (5 years) use of pacemakers in children.

The section on congenital heart disease offers insights into one truly complex anomaly and then a group of articles on conceptually simpler malformations that are nonetheless challenging. These involve various levels of obstruction to left ventricular outflow. Rare but nonetheless interesting are 2 articles on familial clustering of congenital heart disease.

Echocardiography and especially transesophageal echocardiography in the laboratory and in the operating room provide increasingly sophisticated information about anatomy and function.

Extracorporeal membrane oxygenation (ECMO) is a dramatic "last-ditch effort" to save infants with critically severe respiratory distress. The article reports a salvage of ⅔ of the infants so treated.

Adult concerns about risk factors for coronary artery disease are tested in children for race (black or Hispanic) and for type A behavior.

In addition to some comments in other sections about exercise testing for arrhythmias or for postoperative function, 3 articles merit singling out in the section on Exercise. These relate to application of exercise ECG in detection of arrhythmias and the role of chronotropic impair-

193

ment on exercise. In addition, the role of lung function and pulmonary valve regurgitation are addressed.

Kawasaki disease continues to occur in young children, for reasons unknown. We learn that it is not caused by a retrovirus, that there are some epidemiologic relations to recent rug handling, and that there may be a possible confirmatory test of diagnosis. Most importantly comes the new multicenter report that a single dose of 2 gm/kg of intravenous gamma globulin is more effective than the 4-day treatment of 400 mg/kg daily.

Patients with myocarditis were treated with immunosuppressive medications and improved in a preliminary report.

We learn more about the pharmacokinetics of captopril, an agent used in adults in cardiac failure for more than a decade, which is now increasingly used in children.

To treat the patient as a whole has long been an injunction to medical students and practitioners. The 25-year follow-up study from the Mayo Clinic addresses the psychological implications of congenital heart disease. There follows a preliminary report of early effects on cognitive development of infants undergoing the Jatene procedure of arterial switch for transposed great arteries.

As usual, the surgical section is the largest. It is broken down into 4 malformations, with surgical results: coarctation of the aorta, the Fontan circulation, transposition of the great arteries, and that always challenging malformation for which the late and great Dr. Helen Taussig coined the term "pseudotruncus arteriosus." Most pediatric cardiologists and surgeons now refer to it as tetralogy of Fallot with pulmonary atresia.

The final section enhances our knowledge of the rapidly expanding field of interventional/therapeutic cardiac catheterization in 5 selected situations.

What a year! Let's keep reading and learning together.

Mary Allen Engle, M.D.

Arrhythmias and Conduction Disturbances

POSTOPERATIVE

Ventricular Late Potentials and Induced Ventricular Arrhythmias After Surgical Repair of Tetralogy of Fallot

Zimmermann M, Friedli B, Adamec R, Oberhänsli I (University Hospital, Geneva, Switzerland)
Am J Cardiol 67:873–878, 1991   4–1

Background.—Rarely, a patient will die suddenly late after repair of tetralogy of Fallot. Although programmed ventricular stimulation has proved helpful in identifying patients with coronary artery disease who are at risk of sustained ventricular tachycardia (VT) or sudden death, this has not been confirmed in those with surgically treated tetralogy.

Study Plan.—Thirty-one patients having tetralogy of Fallot repaired a mean of 5 months previously were prospectively studied by right heart

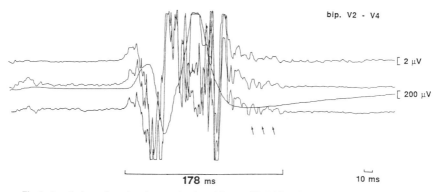

Fig 4–1.—Body surface signal-averaging in a 15-year old child with postoperative tetralogy of Fallot. Three successive high-gain (2 μV/cm) signal-averaged recordings are displayed together with a reference ECG (200 μV/cm). Bipolar (*bip*.) chest lead between V_2 and V_4; recording speed 1,000 mm/sec; filters 100 and 300 Hz. Ventricular late potentials are present (*arrows*) in this patient. Total filtered QRS duration is 178 msec and I-40 is 90 ms. (Courtesy of Zimmermann M, Friedli B, Adamec R, et al: *Am J Cardiol* 67:873–878, 1991.)

catheterization, 24-hour Holter monitoring, body-surface and intracavitary signal-averaging recordings, and programmed ventricular stimulation. All the patients were free of symptoms.

Findings.—Ventricular late potentials were found in one third of patients (Fig 4–1), and spontaneous ventricular arrhythmia in 12 patients (39%). In no patient did programmed stimulation produce sustained VT, but 3 patients exhibited nonsustained VT. The presence of ventricular premature complexes (VPCs) during Holter monitoring correlated with inducible VT. Both VPCs and late potentials were 100% sensitive in predicting VT inducibility, but late potentials were somewhat more specific (75% vs. 68%).

Conclusions.—The finding of spontaneous VPCs or ventricular late potentials shortly after repair of tetralogy raises the risk of inducible VT being present. The absence of such findings may predict a low risk of later ventricular arrhythmia.

▶ Fortunately rare, but nonetheless frightening, is the possibility of sudden death after intracardiac repair of tetralogy of Fallot. This prospective study added the determination of ventricular late potentials and induction of ventricular arrhythmias to the more standard studies of Holter monitoring and cardiac catheterization. They found that early abnormalities in these 2 parameters could identify those at greater and at less risk of subsequent ventricular arrhythmias.—M.A. Engle, M.D.

Cardiac Rhythm After Mustard Repair and After Arterial Switch Operation for Complete Transposition

Kramer H-H, Rammos S, Krogmann O, Nessler L, Böker S, Krian A, Bircks W (Heinrich-Heine-Universität, Düsseldorf, Germany)
Int J Cardiol 32:5–12, 1991   4–2

Background.—Arrhythmias are a common problem after Mustard's repair of complete transposition (concordant atrioventricular and discordant ventriculo-arterial connections). Recently, the arterial switch operation has been performed for primary repair of complete transposition. The arterial swtich procedure (anatomical repair) is more likely to avoid systemic ventricular dysfunction than the venous switch procedure (physiologic repair) because the left ventricle is re-established as the systemic ventricle. With the arterial switch, major surgery within the atria is avoided so the risk of arrhythmias caused by dysfunction in the sinus node or within the atria is lessened. The prevalence of arrhythmias was compared in 45 patients after arterial switch operation, in the most recent 47 patients who underwent Mustard repair in infancy, between 1981 and and in a second group of 49 patients undergoing the Mustard repair procedure about 4 years before 1981.

Methods.—Both groups were monitored with Holter ECG at similar periods of follow-up. The second group of 49 patients who had earlier undergone the Mustard repair at an older age were included to determine the frequency of disturbances of rhythm during later postoperative years (Fig 4–2).

Results.—Symptomatic brady-/tachyarrhythmia syndrome occurred in 1 patient who had recently undergone the Mustard procedure and in 5 patients who had the Mustard repair at an older age, but no patients in the arterial switch group had symptomatic brady-/tachyarrhythmia syndrome. Bradyarrhythmias indicating sinus node dysfunction did not occur in the arterial switch group but did occur in both of the Mustard repair groups (14 and 18, respectively). Three patients who underwent Mustard repair in the earlier years had complete atrioventricular block.

Conclusions.—In the arterial switch group, there were normal findings

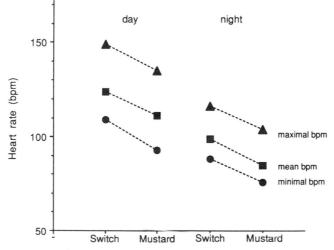

Fig 4–2.—Heart rate of patients with complete transposition after arterial switch operation and after Mustard repair (recent group) during 3 hours of day and night time. (Courtesy of Kramer H-H, Rammos S, Krogmann O, et al: *Int J Cardiol* 32:5–12, 1991.)

in 93% of the cases. Only 51% of the Mustard repair group and 29% of the group repaired at a later age had normal findings. In both of the Mustard repair groups almost a third had bradyarrhythmias indicating sinus node dysfunction. The arterial switch operation was superior to the Mustard repair in terms of rhythm disturbances.

▶ This report from Düsseldorf compared recent results of the arterial switch operation with almost as recent results of the Mustard operation and of long-term results of the venous switch operation. They found a similar freedom from arrhythmias after the arterial switch, and a similar increase in arrhythmias over time after the venous switch, as has been reported previously. They appropriately cautioned that it is still too soon to know whether arrhythmias will develop over time after the arterial switch.—M.A. Engle, M.D.

Electrophysiologic Findings After Fontan Repair of Functional Single Ventricle

Kürer CC, Tanner CS, Vetter VL (Univ of Pennsylvania, Philadelphia)
J Am Coll Cardiol 17:174–181, 1991   4–3

Background.—Life-threatening arrhythmias are a well-known postoperative complication after Fontan repair for complex congenital anomalies. However, the optimal surgical approach for avoiding postoperative arrhythmias has not yet been determined. The electrophysiologic findings in 30 patients who were tested after undergoing a modified Fontan repair are described.

Patients.—Twenty boys and 10 girls, median age 6.4 years, underwent cardiac catheterization with electrophysiologic study a mean of 1.9 years after undergoing modified Fontan repair. Indications for operation included tricuspid atresia in 11 children, single left ventricle in 6, heterotaxy syndrome in 5, mitral atresia in 3, single right ventricle in 2, and other complex lesions in 3. Three patients had preoperative arrhythmias.

Findings.—None of the patients had significant residual intracardiac shunting, but 6 patients had small residual interatrial baffle leaks. Fifteen patients (50%) had sinus node dysfunction or ectopic pacemaker automaticity as demonstrated by a prolonged corrected sinus node or a prolonged pacemaker recovery time. Fifteen patients with normal sinus rhythm had a prolonged total sinoatrial conduction time. Only 13 (43%) patients had entirely normal sinus node or ectopic atrial pacemaker function. The predominant atrial rhythm was normal sinus in 21 (70%) patients and ectopic atrial or junctional in 9 (30%). Atrial effective periods (ERPs) and functional refractory periods (FRPs) were determined in 28 patients. None of the patients had an abnormal ERP during basal rhythm (BR) or at a paced cycle length (CL) of 600 ms, but 10 (36%) had a prolonged ERP at a paced CL of 400 ms. The FRP was prolonged in 5 (21%) of 24 patients during BR, in 1 (4.5%) of 22 patients at a paced CL of 600 ms, and in 12 (43%) of 28 patients at a paced CL of 400 ms (Fig 4–3). Abnormalities of atrial ERPs and FRPs were most pronounced

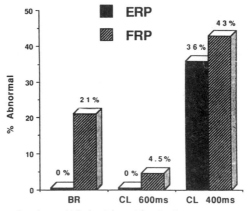

Fig 4–3.—Analogue data from which the right atrial activation map was constructed. Electrocardiograpic leads I, aVF, V_1, and V_6 are shown with intracardiac electrograms from the low medial right atrium (LMRA), residual atrial (At) septum, low lateral right atrium (LLRA), high right atrium (HRA), midlateral right atrium (MLRA), proximal right ventricular apex (RVA 3,4), distal right ventricular apex (RVA 1,2), and 10 ms time lines (TL). The site of orgin of the rhythm (*dashed vertical line*) is the LMRA. (Courtesy of Kürer CC, Tanner CS, Vetter VL: *J Am Coll Cardiol* 17:174–181, 1991.)

at faster paced CLs. Atrial endocardial catheter mapping showed intraatrial conduction delays between adjacent sites in 76% of patients tested and in 8 of 9 patients with inducible intraatrial reentry. Programmed atrial stimulation induced nonsustained supraventricular arrhythmias in 3 patients (10%) and sustained arrhythmias in 8 (27%). None of the patients had inducible ventricular arrhythmias with programmed ventricular stimulation.

Conclusion.—Because the predictive value of electrophysiologic testing after Fontan repair is unknown, continued surveillance is necessary to determine which patients will develop clinically significant arrhythmias.

▶ The group from Philadelphia Children's Hospital, already noted for the excellence of their electrophysiologic studies after surgery for several forms of congenital heart disease, presents the first systematic analysis in post-Fontan patients. The 30 patients had been operated on 1.9 ± 1.3 years before the study. Their ages at surgery ranged from 1.7 to 17.7 years (median 6.4). Three patients had preoperative arrhythmias, 5 had early postoperative arrhythmias, and 8 had late postoperative arrhythmias. Twenty were taking cardiac medications.

The authors found electrophysiologic abnormalities that included sinus mode dysfunction, atrioventricular block, prolongation of atrial refractoriness, delayed intraatrial conduction, and inducible atrial and supraventricular arrhythmias. Figure 4–3 illustrates some of the abnormalities.

These findings were compared with those after extensive intraatrial surgery of the Mustard operation for transposition of the great arteries. Findings were similar. The similar combination of delayed intraatrial conduction and abnormalities of atrial refractoriness with unidirectional block may provide the substrate for reentrant atrial arrhythmias, noted for both procedures.

We should be alert to the possible increasing frequency of arrhythmias as we maintain long-term surveillance of these patients and as surgeons seek modifications of the Fontan procedure in an effort to prevent these electrophysiologic abnormalities.—M.A. Engle, M.D.

Cardiac Arrhythmias After Surgical Correction of Total Anomalous Pulmonary Venous Connection: Late Follow-Up
Saxena A, Fong LV, Lamb RK, Monro JL, Shore DF, Keeton BR (Southampton General Hospital, Southampton, England)
Pediatr Cardiol 12:89–91, 1991   4–4

Background.—Postoperative arrhythmias in cardiac surgery patients may be related to the surgical procedure but may also be caused by a preexisting cardiac abnormality. Total anomalous pulmonary venous connection (TAPVC) requires surgery to the atrial septum and atria to repair the anomaly that causes right atrial and right ventricular dilatation. The results of 24-hour ECG monitoring after total repair of TAPVC performed in infancy were evaluated.

Methods.—Sixteen patients, aged 7 months to 20 years, who had undergone TAPVC in the first year of life were monitored by ECG for assessment of cardiac rhythm. Nine patients also had maximal exercise treadmill tests. None of the patients had any symptoms of an arrhythmia, and the resting ECG was normal in all but 1 patient.

Results.—Despite being asymptomatic, 6 of 16 patients showed significant arrhythmias on 24-hour ECG monitoring. Five of the 6 patients with significant arrhythmias were monitored more than 6 years after surgery. Three of the patients with arrhythmias and 1 other patient showed an inappropriate chronotropic response on maximal exercise treadmill testing.

Conclusions.—In 16 patients who had undergone surgery for TAPVC in infancy, none had any symptoms of an arrhythmia. However, 24-hour ECG monitoring showed significant arrhythmias in 6 of the 16 patients as long as 6 years after surgery. Long-term follow-up after TAPVC is recommended, even if patients are asymptomatic.

▶ We have learned that some patients who underwent successful surgery to close an atrial septal defect may later develop supraventricular arrhythmias, much as happened in the natural history of unoperated atrial septal defect, although we hope, less frequently. This follow-up report 7 months to 20 years after surgery in the first year of life teaches us that, in this situation as well, cardiac arrhythmias can be detected on Holter monitoring or on exercise stress testing.

The same mechanical factors exist as for patients with an atrial septal defect (namely a distended right atrium and atrial incision and suture line). Their young age at surgery (first year of life) informs us that it is not the older age of the patient at atrial surgery that is the primary factor in late postoperative arrhythmias.—M.A. Engle, M.D.

THERAPY

Percutaneous Radiofrequency Catheter Ablation for Supraventricular Arrhythmias in Children

Van Hare GF, Lesh MD, Scheinman M, Langberg JJ (Univ of California San Francisco School of Medicine)
J Am Coll Cardiol 17:1613–1620, 1991   4–5

Background.—Although there is a large body of experience with direct current catheter ablation in adults, such experience in children is limited. Transcatheter application of radiofrequency energy, which has also been used successfully in adults, may be useful in children because of the absence of barotrauma. Initial experience with the use of this technique in children with sustained symptomatic supraventricular tachyarrhythmias was evaluated.

Patients.—Seventeen patients, ranging in age from 10 months to 17 years, underwent catheter radiofrequency procedures for management of malignant or drug-resistant supraventricular tachyarrhythmias. Twelve of the patients had accessory pathway-mediated tachycardia, 4 had atrioventricular (AV) node reentrant tachycardia, and 1 had junctional ectopic tachycardia.

Results.—For the ablation of accessory pathways, 20 W to 40 W of energy were used. The procedure was successful in 11 accessory pathways and failed in 2. There were no recurrences of accessory pathway-mediated tachycardia. In AV node modification for AV node reentrant tachycardia, 15 W of energy were applied until first-degree AV block occurred. After ablation, there was a prolonged AH interval and tachycardia could not be induced. One patient had recurrent tachycardia. In the patient who had junctional ectopic tachycardia, 15 W to 18 W of energy were delivered at the site of the maximal His bundle electrogram until sinus rhythm and normal AV conduction were noted. Although the condition recurred in this patient, a second procedure abolished both tachycardia and AV conduction. Overall, the radiofrequency catheter ablation was initially successful in 17 of 19 procedures, the ultimate rate of cure was 82%, and there were no serious complications.

Conclusions.—For children with supraventricular tachyarrhythmias, radiofrequency catheter ablation appears to be a safe and effective method of treatment. The technique may also obviate the need for surgical management or lifelong drug therapy, and it avoids the barotrauma complications of direct current shock ablation.

▶ The group from San Francisco report with enthusiasm on the outcome of treatment by radiofrequency ablation for children with recurrent tachyarrhythmias unresponsive to pharmacotherapy. In a group of 12 patients with accessory pathways, radiofrequency ablation succeeded in 11 and failed in 2 pathways. In 4 patients with AV nodal reentrant tachycardia, tachycardia was no longer inducible in 3. One patient with junctional ectopic tachycardia needed 2 sessions before the tachycardia was abolished. The therapeutic successes were accomplished with no major complications. The authors compared these results with those obtained by ablation using direct countershock, with its possible complications from barotrauma, and concluded that the technique using radiofrequency energy was safe and effective for those children in whom pharmacotherapy is ineffective.—M.A. Engle, M.D.

Deceptive Surgical Results in Three Siblings With Familial Wolff-Parkinson-White Syndrome
Patruno N, Coltorti F, Pulignano G, Urbani P, Critelli G (Univ of Rome 'La Sapienza,' Rome)
Eur Heart J 11:1116–1119, 1990   4–6

Introduction.—Surgical ablation of the accessory pathways in the treatment of life-threatening or disabling tachyarrhythmias has a high success rate. The case reports of 3 siblings with the Wolff-Parkinson-White syndrome in whom surgical ablation of the accessory pathways proved to be deceptive are presented.

Case Reports.—Two brothers aged 18 and 20 years, and a sister aged 23 years, with a family history of pre-excitation syndrome and 2 instances of sudden death, underwent electrophysiologic study, which documented multiple accessory pathways in all 3 siblings. They had never experienced episodes of tachycardia and had no organic heart disease. All 3 patients underwent surgical ablation of the bypass tracts. Abolition of the accessory pathway conduction was confirmed postoperatively. However, follow-up electrophysiologic studies performed 2 to 8 years later showed resumption of conduction over the anomalous connections with life-threatening arrhythmias during induced fast atrial rhythms. Thus, ablation surgery had been ineffective in all 3 siblings. One patient underwent a second operation that resulted in the disappearance of accessory pathway conduction. However, a rapid ventricular response during atrial pacing, probably because of enhanced atrioventricular node conduction, was still present. The other 2 siblings showed persisting rapid ventricular responses with wide QRS during either incremental atrial pacing or induced atrial fibrillation.

Conclusion.—The apparent success of ablation surgery for the pre-excitation syndrome as demonstrated during postoperative electrophysiologic studies may be illusory in some patients, because accessory pathway conduction can return later.

▶ Electrophysiologic (EP) studies and surgical or nonsurgical ablation of accessory pathways in patients with Wolff-Parkinson-White syndrome and refractory tachyarrhythmias have contributed much to the management of these patients. We have grown accustomed to expecting a satisfactory outcome that is lasting.

This is not always so, as shown by this report of 3 siblings in a family with 2 instances of sudden death. They underwent 4 operative ablations because of their life-threatening arrhythmias caused by multiple accessory pathways with short antegrade refractory period and rapid ventricular responses during atrial fibrillation. Although postoperative EP studies demonstrated abolition of the accessory pathways, nonetheless, later follow-up studies showed resumption of conduction over anomalous connections. The above experience is fortunately quite different from the excellent results in a large number of patients treated in Michigan (see Addendum).—M.A. Engle, M.D.

Addendum

Bolling SF, Moraday F, Calkins H, et al: Current treatment for Wolff-Parkinson-White syndrome: Results and surgical implications. *Ann Thorac Surg* 52:461–468, 1991.

▶ From Ann Arbor, Michigan, comes a report of 123 patients with surgery of aberrant conduction pathways and often of associated congenital anomalies as well, compared with a more recent series of 124 patients with radiofrequency ablation. They had no operative mortality, a 7% initial failure rate that was 3% after reoperation. After catheter ablation, there was a 10% failure rate.

Overall, both of these procedures offered excellent results. Long-term follow-up, however, is essential.—M.A. Engle, M.D.

Perinatal Outcome of Fetal Complete Atrioventricular Block: A Multicenter Experience
Schmidt KG, Ulmer HE, Silverman NH, Kleinman CS, Copel JA (University of Heidelberg, Germany; Univ of California, San Francisco; Yale Univ)
J Am Coll Cardiol 91:1360–1366, 1991   4–7

Introduction.—With the advent of 2-dimensional and M-mode echocardiographic and Doppler ultrasound techniques, more uses of complete atrioventricular (AV) block are being diagnosed before delivery. Data from 3 centers that perform prenatal cardiac diagnosis and treatment were used in studying the clinical course and outcome of 55 fetuses with complete AV block.

Findings.—These fetuses were identified by echocardiography performed in 7,200 pregnant women. Median gestational age of the fetuses was 26 weeks. Twenty-nine fetuses had associated structural cardiac defects. Nineteen of the remaining 26 were carried by mothers with connective tissue disease or who had tested positive for antinuclear antibodies. Hydrops was revealed at ultrasound in 22 fetuses.

Outcome.—Five of the pregnancies were terminated and 24 fetuses or neonates died. Associated structural heart defects, hydrops, an atrial rate no more than 120 beats/min, and a ventricular rate of no more than 55 beats/min were all significantly related to fetal or neonatal death. No fetus with hydrops survived, and only 4 fetuses with an associated structural cardiac defect survived the neonatal period. All the fetuses with left atrial isomerism died. Positive or negative maternal serologic findings did not significantly influence neonatal outcome.

Discussion.—Although fetuses with complete AV block can be identified before delivery, effective forms of therapy have not been established. Nine of 13 infants who received a permanent pacemaker survived the neonatal period. However, only 1 of 4 fetuses treated by transplacental sympathomimetic drugs survived.

▶ This interesting multicenter fetal echocardiographic study extends our knowledge of congenital complete heart block (CCHB) back into the prenatal condition. Remarkable was the progression in 5 fetuses from normal conduction or second degree block to complete heart block. Such progression is rare in postnatal heart block.

Sobering is the outcome, which was worse in those with other structural heart defects (only 4 of 29 surviving) than in those with otherwise normal hearts. Just as in postnatal CCHB, atrial tachycardia and ventricular bradycardia below 55 beats/min were indicators of a poor prognosis. At the end of the neonatal period, a little over half (26 of 50) of unterminated pregnancies survived. Despite permanent pacemaker therapy in 13, only 9 survived.—M.A. Engle, M.D.

Addendum

Kerstjens-Frederikse MWS, Bink-Boelkens MTE, de Jongste MJL, et al: Permanent cardiac pacing in children: Morbidity and efficacy of follow-up. *Int J Cardiol* 33:207–214, 1991.

▶ This long-term follow-up (for around 5 years) provides important information about success and complications. Patients' survival at 5 years (78%) was greater than that of the pacemakers (48%). Epicardial leads are often placed at the time of surgery if it is anticipated that a pacemaker will be needed postoperatively. The authors observed that these produce more problems than do endocardial leads, which the authors therefore recommend. Transtelephonic transmittal is especially important for the first 3 months after implantation because that is the time when exit block is most apt to occur.—M.A. Engle, M.D.

Congenital Heart Disease

Diagnosis and Management

▶ ↓ The first selection relates to an unusually complex combination of defects. A series of 4 papers follows relating to diagnosis and management of 4 kinds of obstruction to left ventricular outflow. The last section pertains to familial congenital heart disease.—M.A. Engle, M.D.

Straddling Mitral Valve With Hypoplastic Right Ventricle, Crisscross Atrioventricular Relations, Double Outlet Right Ventricle and Dextrocardia: Morphologic, Diagnostic and Surgical Considerations
Geva T, Van Praagh S, Sanders SP, Mayer JE Jr, Van Praagh R (Harvard Med School, Boston)
J Am Coll Cardiol 17:1603–1612, 1991   4–8

Background.—A straddling mitral valve is an uncommon congenital cardiac malformation that almost always occurs in association with a conotruncal anomaly. Straddling mitral valve is most often associated with left ventricular hypoplasia and right ventricular (RV) hypoplasia is rarely found. The clinical, surgical, and pathologic findings in 5 patients with straddling mitral valve and RV hypoplasia are examined.

Patients.—Three children, aged 7.2–10.7 years, were studied by 2-dimensional and Doppler echocardiography, cardiac catheterization, and angiocardiography. The hearts of 2 patients who died at ages 19 and 23.8 years were studied at autopsy. Straddling mitral valve was diagnosed when chordal attachments were found on both sides of the ventricular septum.

Findings.—All 5 patients had a similar, distinctive, and consistent combination of anatomical findings, which included dextrocardia, tricuspid stenosis or hypoplasia, hypoplastic RV sinus inflow with large RV infundibulum outflow, severe subpulmonary stenosis, conoventricular septal defect, superoinferior ventricles with well-developed pulmonary arteries, crisscross atrioventricular relations with a double outlet right ventricle, with the combination of visceroatrial situs solitus, a concordant ventricular D-loop, and malposition of the aorta. The 3 surviving patients underwent a modified Fontan procedure. Follow-up cardiac catheterization showed a competent mitral valve, low pulmonary vascular resistance, and low left ventricular end-diastolic pressure. All 3 patients were doing well at reexamination 2.2–5.8 years after operation.

Conclusion.—Major malposition of the highly mobile infundibuloventricular part of the heart relative to the fixed atria appears to have a major role in the morphogenesis of straddling mitral valve. Two-dimensional echocardiography is the optimal diagnostic technique for imaging a straddling mitral valve.

▶ Straddling of the mitral valve sprang into clinical relevance when 2-dimensional echocardiography developed and color Doppler studies added function and flow to form. The Van Praagh group has for a long time been working with cardiologists and cardiac surgeons for the mutual edification of us all in these 3 disciplines. This description of clinical, surgical, and pathologic findings in 5 cases of this particular variation on the straddling mitral valve moves us another step up the ladder of learning and helping.—M.A. Engle, M.D.

Addenda

Bartelings MM, Gittenberger-de Groot AC: Morphogenetic considerations on congenital malformations of the outflow tract: Part 2. Complete transposition of the great arteries and double outlet right ventricle. *Int J Cardiol* 33:5–26, 1991.

▶ The excellent anatomical and embryologic studies from these authors in Leiden nicely complement the complex anatomy described above from Boston. From the embryologists' standpoint, double outlet right ventricle is not an embryologic entity but a feature that may occur with concordant or discordant ventricular-arterial connection.—M.A. Engle, M.D.

Vuillemin M, Pexieder T, Winking H: Pathogenesis of various forms of double outlet right ventricle in mouse fetal trisomy 13. *Int J Cardiol* 33:281–304, 1991.

▶ From the Institute of Embryology in Lausanne comes an interesting approach to the pathogenesis of this malformation. The authors analyzed karyotyped trisomic embryos and traced the development of double outlet right ventricle with or without pulmonary infundibular atresia. They concluded that the pathogenesis of these malformations differs from most known hypotheses based on deductions from human malformed hearts.—M.A. Engle, M.D.

Critical Aortic Stenosis in Early Infancy: Anatomic and Echocardiographic Substrates of Successful Open Valvotomy
Leung MP, McKay R, Smith A, Anderson RH, Arnold R (Royal Liverpool Children's Hospital, Liverpool; University of Liverpool, England)
J Thorac Cardiovasc Surg 101:526–535, 1991   4–9

Introduction.—The operative mortality of open valvotomy in infants with critical aortic stenosis caused by left ventricular (LV) outflow obstruction is high. Recent studies found LV cavity size to be a determinant of survival. This study tried to identify morphologic features predictive of valvotomy outcome by reviewing the clinical course and real-time echocardiograms of infants operated on for critical aortic stenosis.

Methods.—Twenty heart specimens with the diagnosis of critical aortic stenosis from infants under 3 months of age who died after undergoing open valvotomy were examined. The clinical course and preoperative real-time echocardiograms of 20 infants in the same age group who underwent open valvotomy were also studied. Echocardiographic and postmortem measurements were available for 5 hearts.

Findings.—The heart specimens showed a spectrum of valvular, ventricular, and vascular abnormalities that could be accurately identified by echocardiography. A small LV cavity was usually associated with a narrow ventriculoaortic junction, a small ascending aorta, and a narrow subaortic region (Fig 4–4). The mitral valve usually had a single or grossly hypoplastic papillary muscle with short or arcuate tendinous cords. Inflow and outflow orifices were wider in a dilated LV cavity, and the tension apparatus of the mitral valve was either normal or supported by hypertrophic papillary muscles (Fig 4–5). There were significant differences between survivors and nonsurvivors in the echocardiographic dimensions of the LV, subaortic region, ventriculoaortic junction, ascending aorta, and mitral valve orifice. In addition, early nonsurvivors invariably had single or hypoplastic mitral valve papillary muscles with short, tendinous cords. Infants with unfavorable cardiac anatomy tended to be seen earlier and to have a lower systemic blood pressure. These infants

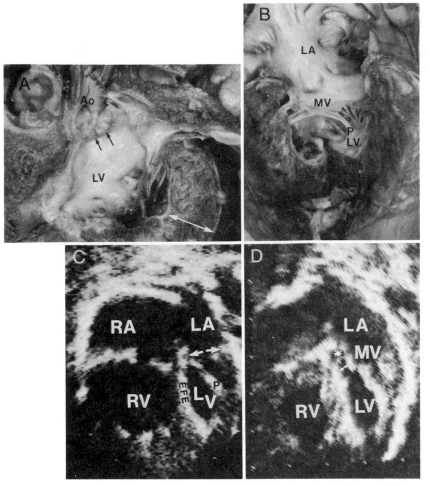

Fig 4–4.—Echocardiographic-morphologic correlate of critical aortic stenosis with a small left ventricular cavity. **A,** heart specimen with dysplastic knobby aortic valve leaflets and cauliflower formation, a narrow ventriculoaortic junction, and small ascending aorta (*Ao*) associated with a diminutive left ventricle (*LV*). **B,** another heart specimen with a diminutive left ventricle and small mitral valve (*MV*) orifice. Note the hypoplastic papillary muscles (*P*), short tendinous cords, and arcuate malformation of the tension apparatus of the mitral valve. There is also endocardial fibroelastosis and a thick posteroapical wall of the left ventricle. *LA*=left atrium. **C,** echocardiogram of a small left ventricle (*LV*) in 4-chambered view. The mitral valve orifice (*arrows*) is small and associated with a hypoplastic papillary muscle (*P*) and short tendinous cords. Endocardial fibroelastosis (*EFE*) and thick posteroapical walls of the left ventricle can be seen. **D,** echocardiogram of the same patient in long-axis view. Note the associated narrow ventriculoaortic junction (*asterisk*) and subaortic region (*arrows*). *LA*=left atrium; *LV*=left ventricle; *RV*=right ventricle; *MV*=mitral valve. (Courtesy of Leung MP, McKay R, Smith A, et al: *J Thorac Cardiovasc Surg* 101:526–535, 1991.)

always required prostaglandin E_2 to maintain right ventricular support of the circulation through a persistent arterial duct.

Conclusion.—Infants with a small LV, a narrow ventriculoaortic junction, and a small mitral valve orifice will not survive aortic valvotomy

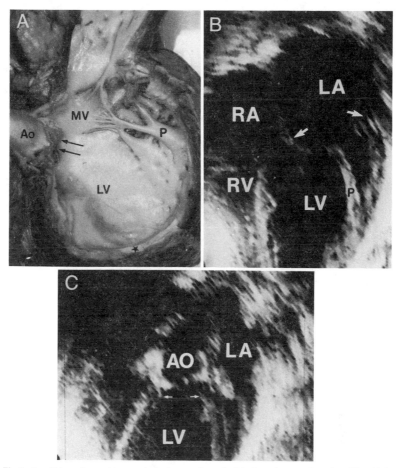

Fig 4–5.—Echocrdiographic-morphologic correlate of critical aortic stenosis with a dilated left ventricle. **A,** heart specimen with a dilated left ventricle and thick endocardial fibroelastosis (*asterisk*). The aortic valve is dysplastic but the ventriculoaortic junction and ascending aorta (*Ao*) are of good size. The mitral valve (*MV*) and its tension apparatus are essentially normal. *LV*=left ventricle; *P*=papillary muscle. **B,** echocardiogram of a dilated left ventricular cavity. Note the large mitral valve orifice (*arrows*) and the rather prominent (reflective) papillary muscle (*P*). **C,** echocardiogram of the same patient in long-axis view. Note the thickened aortic valve with a wide ventriculoaortic junction, subaortic region, and ascending aorta. (Courtesy of Leung MP, McKay R, Smith A, et al: *J Thorac Cardiovasc Surg* 101:526–535, 1991.)

and should be considered for cardiac transplantation or the Norwood-type palliation for hypoplastic left heart syndrome.

▶ This paper from Liverpool addresses the questions of anatomical variations, echocardiographic identification, and outcome. Although the focus is surgical, the same features should be applicable if balloon valvuloplasty is being considered.

The authors reviewed 20 specimens from infants under 3 months and the clinical course and echocardiographic features of 20 other infants of similar age and the same diagnosis. Two patterns emerged, one less favorable to repair than the other.

Unfavorable anatomy is a small LV cavity, which is often associated with a narrow ventriculoaortic junction, small ascending aorta, and narrow subaortic region, often together with a mitral valve that has a single papillary muscle with "arcuate" tendinous cords. More favorable is a dilated LV cavity with wider inflow and outflow and more nearly normal support for the mitral valve. These features are identifiable by real-time echocardiography and are well illustrated in the paper (Figs 4–4 and 4–5).

Although variations in coronary arteries are not discussed, the spectrum of valvular, ventricular, and vascular abnormalities forms an important focus for diagnosis and treatment of babies with a difficult problem.—M.A. Engle, M.D.

Addendum

Parsons MK, Moreau GA, Graham TP, Johns JA, Boucek RJ: Echocardiographic estimation of critical left ventricular size in infants with isolated aortic valve stenosis. *J Am Coll Cardiol* 18:1049–1055, 1991.

▶ The pediatric cardiologists at Vanderbilt studied data from cardiac catheterization and echocardiography in 25 infants less than 3 months of age undergoing aortic valvotomy to develop echocardiographic criteria for LV size. They found that echocardiographically measured LV cross-sectional area, 2 cm² and LV end-diastolic dimension <13 mm were risk factors for early mortality. They found good correlation between these measurements and angiographically determined LV end-diastolic volume.—M.A. Engle, M.D.

Morphologic Features of the Hypoplastic Left Heart Syndrome—A Reappraisal
Aiello VD, Ho SY, Anderson RH, Thiene G (Heart Institute of Sao Paulo, Brazil; National Heart & Lung Institute, London; University of Padova, Italy)
Pediatr Pathol 10:931–943, 1990   4–10

Introduction.—The anatomical features of hypoplastic left heart syndrome have been well studied, but some anatomical features warrant further investigation. One hundred two heart specimens with hypoplastic left heart syndrome were examined and the morphologic findings related to survival and operative palliation.

Materials.—All 102 hearts showed severe aortic stenosis or atresia. Only hearts with either a concordant atrioventricular (AV) connection or absence of the left AV connection were included. Hearts with hypoplastic left ventricle but with double-outlet right ventricle were excluded.

Results.—All 102 specimens had hypoplastic left heart chambers.

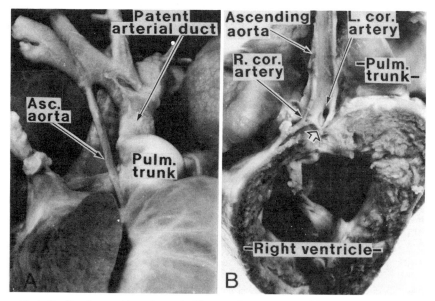

Fig 4–6.—Two hearts with aortic atresia. The ascending aorta is strandlike in (A). In (B) the ascending aorta is wider but blind ending (*open arrow*). In this heart the pulmonary trunk originates from the right ventricle, but there is muscular separation between the aorta and the right ventricle. (Courtesy of Aiello VD, Ho SY, Anderson RH, et al: *Pediatr Pathol* 10:931–943, 1990.)

Sixty-six hearts had a concordant AV connection. The mitral valve was patent but miniaturized in 54 of those, imperforate in 4, and dysplastic in 7. Six dysplastic valves were stenotic, and 1 was insufficient. The left AV connection was absent in 36 hearts. In 23 of these, the aorta was connected to the left ventricle and the aortic valve was patent. The other 79 hearts had aortic atresia (Fig 4–6). In 5 hearts, aortic atresia was the result of an imperforate valve, but the ventriculoarterial connection was otherwise concordant. The aortic trunk ended blindly in the other 74 specimens. Eighty-eight hearts had an intact ventricular septum and 14 had a ventricular septal defect. Forty-four hearts had aortic coarctation, with the site of the coarctation lesion being preductal in 42. There was a statistically significant correlation between the presence of coarctation and the diameter of the ascending aorta in that coarctation was significantly more common in hearts with an ascending aorta of <3 mm in diameter.

Conclusion.—The morphologic features of hypoplastic left heart syndrome are of practical importance because of the options for palliative surgery that are now available.

▶ This common developmental anomaly was observed by means of fetal echocardiography, to develop as growth of the fetus and specifically the right side of the heart proceeds. When a baby is born with this usually rapidly lethal condition, the physician and the family have difficult choices to consider: to let the natural history of the anomaly run its course and the parents try again for a healthy baby, or to undertake a Norwood procedure as initial palliation in the centers that do such an operation, or to consider a heart transplant in the few centers that do this.

This report describes in detail the morphologic features of 102 specimens with hypoplastic left heart syndrome, a survey that may help in understanding the variations in the malformation and the options for management.—M.A. Engle, M.D.

Addendum

Anderson NG, Brown J: Normal size left ventricle on antenatal scan in lethal hypoplastic left heart syndrome. *Pediatr Radiol* 21:436–437, 1991.

▶ These authors showed the echocardiographic images from fetal echocardiogram at routine 20-week antenatal ultrasound screening and the apical view on the fourth day of life shortly before death in severe cardiac failure. The first study showed normal and equal size of the 2 ventricles. Postnatally the left ventricle was small, as were the mitral valve and ascending aorta. The cause of cessation of growth of these important left heart structures was not known. The authors made the important point that on fetal screening by a single view one cannot exclude the development of hypoplastic left heart syndrome by birth.—M.A. Engle, M.D.

Fixed Subaortic Stenosis: Anatomical Spectrum and Nature of Progression
Choi JY, Sullivan ID (Hospital for Sick Children, London)
Br Heart J 65:280–286, 1991   4–11

Background.—Fixed subaortic stenosis can occur in isolation or associated with other structural heart defects, but it is rarely diagnosed in infancy. Fixed subaortic stenosis progresses in severity over time and may appear as an acquired condition. The mechanism of stenosis progression is as yet unknown.

Patients.—The preoperative echocardiograms of 58 infants and children with fixed subaortic stenosis were reviewed retrospectively. The mean age at diagnosis was 4.8 years. In 8 of the 58 patients the diagnosis was made in infancy. Forty-one patients (71%) had associated cardiac abnormalities and 17 (29%) had fixed subaortic stenosis as an isolated lesion.

Results.—Four types of subaortic stenosis were identified. Forty-seven patients (81%) had short segment stenosis, 7 (12%) had long segment narrowing, 3 (5%) had a posteriorly displaced infundibular septum complicated by an additional discrete subaortic lesion, and 1 (2%) had unusual redundant tissue obstructing the left ventricular (LV) outflow tract. Echocardiographic studies performed in 9 patients before the diagnosis of fixed subaortic stenosis showed a normal LV outflow tract in 6 and posterior deviation of the infundibular septum in 3. Serial echocardiographic studies performed in 16 patients after the diagnosis of fixed subaortic stenosis but before surgical repair of the LV outflow tract showed rapid evolution of short segment to long segment narrowing in 1 patient and the development of tethering of the aortic or mitral valve in another 4 patients. Aortic or mitral valve involvement was not seen before age 3 years, but was present thereafter in 25% of patients.

Conclusion.—Fixed subaortic stenosis may appear as an "acquired" lesion that may cause progressively more severe obstruction of the LV outflow tract. Short segment narrowing is by far the most common form of fixed subaortic stenosis.

▶ This condition, sometimes termed discrete subaortic stenosis, is fascinating from several aspects. One is that it is uncommon as an isolated lesion. Another is that it appears to be acquired in some patients under follow-up by echocardiography for other congenital anomalies. A third is that it may progress to severe obstruction. A fourth is that the aortic valve becomes damaged over time, and a fifth is that surgery does not always effect a cure.

The article by Choi and Sullivan from London's Hospital for Sick Children analyzes these features in 58 consecutive infants and children with the diagnosis of fixed subaortic stenosis and shows the value of echocardiography in describing the natural history, the development and the progression of conditions such as this.—M.A. Engle, M.D.

Spectrum of Cardiovascular Anomalies in Williams-Beuren Syndrome
Zalzstein E, Moes CAF, Musewe NN, Freedom RM (Hospital for Sick Children, Toronto)
Pediatr Cardiol 12:219–223, 1991   4–12

Introduction.—Williams et al. and later Beuren et al. described an association of supravalvular aortic stenosis with mental retardation and a typical facial appearance. Beuren et al. subsequently described peripheral pulmonary stenosis in children with this syndrome. An attempt was made to delineate the spectrum of cardiovascular anomalies in 49 patients with the Williams-Beuren syndrome seen in 1966–1988.

Findings.—The patients had a mean age of 39 months at diagnosis, and they were followed for a mean of 10 years. Twenty-eight children had isolated supravalvular aortic stenosis, but 4 of them had additional anomalies (Fig 4–7). Seven of these patients had increased supravalvular obstruction during follow-up and were operated on, most often undergoing resection and pericardial patching. Eight patients had isolated pulmonary artery branch stenosis. Eleven patients had combined right and left outflow obstruction. In 6 of them, supravalvular aortic narrowing in-

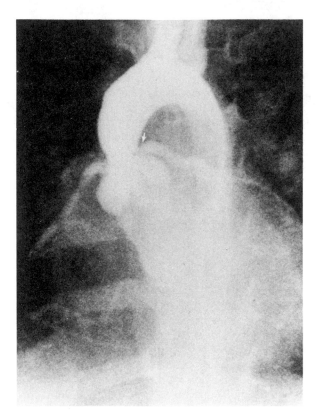

Fig 4–7.—Aortogram of a boy, aged 7 years 5 months. Supravalvular aortic stenosis is seen. The origin of the left coronary artery is stenotic (*arrow*), and there is mild poststenotic dilatation. (Courtesy of Zalzstein E, Moes CAF, Musewe NN, et al: *Pediatr Cardiol* 12:219–223, 1991.)

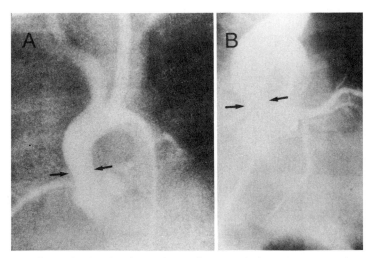

Fig 4–8.—Aortogram. **A,** male infant aged 7 months. Supravalvular aortic stenosis is demonstrated (*arrows*) just distal to the origin of the coronary arteries. **B,** same patient at age 5 years. The supravalvular aortic stenosis persists and appears slightly more severe because of dilatation of the aortic sinuses and poststenotic dilatation of the ascending aorta. (Courtesy of Zalzstein E, Moes CAF, Musewe NN, et al: *Pediatr Cardiol* 12:219–223, 1991.)

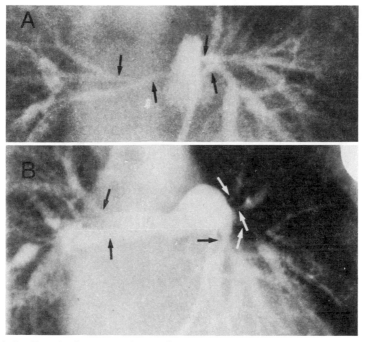

Fig 4–9.—Frontal pulmonary arteriogram. **A,** same patient as in Figure 4–8 at age 7 months. Both pulmonary arteries are diffusely small, the right being more severely affected. There are multiple areas of stenosis (*arrows*) with areas of poststenotic dilatation. **B,** patient at age 5 years. The right pulmonary artery has increased markedly in size, although areas of stenosis persist peripherally (*arrows*). The left pulmonary artery shows little change. (Courtesy of Zalzstein E, Moes CAF, Musewe NN, et al: *Pediatr Cardiol* 12:219–223, 1991.)

creased (Fig 4–8), whereas the pulmonary branch stenosis improved (Fig 4–9). Five of these patients had surgical relief of supravalvular obstruction. Eight patients in this group had associated anomalies (Fig 4–10). Two other patients had isolated lesions—mitral valve prolapse in 1 patient and aortic coarctation in the other.

Discussion.—One third of the patients in this study had progression of supraventricular aortic narrowing and required operative relief. Patients with pulmonary branch stenosis tended to remain stable or improve spontaneously, and they required surgery only infrequently.

▶ This long-term study reviews an interesting syndrome over a 22-year period at a large pediatric cardiologic center (Hospital for Sick Children in Toronto). Forty-nine children were diagnosed and followed. The largest group (28 patients) had pure supravalvular aortic stenosis. Six worsened and were operated on, and 17 with mild stenosis stayed mild. A second group of 8 patients had pure pulmonic stenosis that stayed mild. The third group of 11 who had combined aortic and pulmonic supravalvar stenoses split 5 and 5 for needing surgery or showing improvement. A fourth group had only coarctation (1) or mitral prolapse (1).—M.A. Engle, M.D.

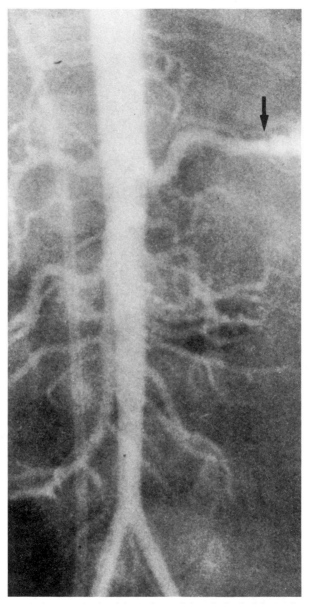

Fig 4–10.—Boy aged 1.5 years. The abdominal aorta below the level of the renal arteries becomes progressively more narrow. There is stenosis of the splenic artery distally (*arrow*). (Courtesy of Zalzstein E, Moes CAF, Musewe NN, et al: *Pediatr Cardiol* 12:219–223, 1991.)

Pathogenesis of Persistent Left Superior Vena Cava With a Coronary Sinus Connection
Nsah EN, Moore GW, Hutchins GM (Johns Hopkins Med Institutions, Baltimore)
Pediatr Pathol 11:261–269, 1991   4–13

Introduction.—The lumen of the left superior vena cava (LSVC) is usually obliterated late in the embryonic period. Patency of the LSVC is commonly associated with cardiovascular malformations. Factors responsible for obliteration of the LSVC or that favor its persistence have not been identified. Previous studies have suggested that mechanical factors are involved in many cardiovascular malformations. The possibility that mechanical factors are involved in LSVC patency was examined.

Methods.—The study material comprised 351 staged, serially sectioned normal human embryos and 1,208 specimens from hearts with congenital malformations. The presence or absence of 66 anatomical features was recorded for each of the 351 normal embryos. Each of the 1,208 specimens of hearts with malformations was assigned to 1 of 22 groups according to its major diagnosis.

Results.—In the normal embryo, obliteration of the LSVC does not begin until stage 21, when all other major structures in the heart have formed. The LSVC undergoes luminal obliteration by compression between the left atrium and the hilum of the left lung. Among the 1,208 specimens of malformations, there were 104 hearts (9%) with persistent LSVC and coronary sinus connection. Persistent LSVC was significantly more frequently associated with atrioventricular canal defects, cor triatriatum, and mitral valve atresia. It was significantly less frequently associated with atrial septal defect or primary patent foramen ovale. The normally late embryonic obliteration of the LSVC suggests that its persistence results from reduced left atrial compression or earlier redistribution of blood flow. The malformations associated with persistent LSVC support that view.

Conclusion.—Identification of a persistent LSVC with coronary sinus connection should suggest an associated malformation, especially atrioventricular canal, cor triatriatum, or mitral atresia.

▶ This extensive review of 1,208 specimens of congenital cardiovascular anomalies in the Johns Hopkins Pathology Collection and systematic study of 351 staged and serially sectioned human embryos in the Carnegie Embryological Collection give us the opportunity to review the development of the systemic venous system. The article offers an explanation for the abnormal and persistent connection of the left superior vena cava with the coronary sinus, a finding in 9% of the pathologic specimens. Normally that connection obliterates late in embryonic development by compression. Its persistence and its association with lesions such as atrioventricular septal defect, cor triatriatum, and mitral atresia suggest reduced left atrial compression or redistribution of blood flow.—M.A. Engle, M.D.

FAMILIAL CONGENITAL HEART DISEASE

Familial Ebstein's Anomaly: A Report of Six Cases in Two Generations Associated With Mild Skeletal Abnormalities
Balaji S, Dennis NR, Keeton BR (Southampton General Hospital, Southampton, England)
Br Heart J 66:26–28, 1991   4–14

Background.—Ebstein's anomaly is a poorly understood cardiac problem with a wide spectrum of clinical presentation. Familial Ebstein's anomaly is rare. A family in which 8 of 11 persons in 3 generations had either Ebstein's anomaly or a characteristic pattern of mild skeletal anomalies or both was described.

Discussion.—Five of the 6 family members with Ebstein's anomaly had mild skeletal anomalies of restricted finger extension, with or without limitation of larger joints, and externally rotated little toes. Two other family members had the skeletal features without Ebstein's anomaly. The 4 female patients were only mildly affected, but 3 of the 4 male patients were severely affected. The findings suggest autosomal dominance for the inheritance of Ebstein's anomaly and skeletal abnormalities.

Conclusion.—This group of 8 members in 3 generations of a family with Ebstein's anomaly, skeletal anomalies, or both, is the largest group reported. Symptoms ranged from mild to severe, with the males more severely affected. The mechanism of inheritance in this family appears to be autosomal dominance.

▶ To me, Ebstein's anomaly has long been a fascinating rarity. This report of a remarkable family with the rare familial occurrence of the rare cardiac abnormality together with (but not necessarily in association with) skeletal abnormalities is interesting. The Ebstein's anomaly varied from so severe as to cause death in 1 neonate and cardiac failure in another, through moderate in a woman who had several pregnancies without a cardiac problem, to very mild.—M.A. Engle, M.D.

Addendum

Donnelly JE, Brown JM, Radford DJ: Pregnancy outcome and Ebstein's anomaly. *Br Heart J* 66:368–371, 1991.

▶ Because Ebstein's anomaly itself is rare, and so is familial Ebstein's anomaly, this report from Queensland, Australia, is all the more remarkable. They studied 12 women with 42 pregnancies and reported good news. Unless the mother was cyanotic or had arrhythmias, the pregnancy was well tolerated. As is usual when the mother is cyanotic, there was an increased risk of prematurity and dysmaturity, but there was only 1 neonatal death among the 36 live-born infants and none with congenital cardiac or other anomalies.—M.A. Engle, M.D.

The Inheritance of Conotruncal Malformations: A Review and Report of Two Siblings With Tetralogy of Fallot With Pulmonary Atresia

Wulfsberg EA, Zintz EJ, Moore JW (Uniformed Services Univ of the Health Sciences, Bethesda, Md; Walter Reed Army Med Ctr, Washington, DC)
Clin Genet 40:12–16, 1991   4–15

Discussion.—Congenital heart defects (CHD) in humans have a combined incidence of about 1%. Congenital heart defects associated with chromosome abnormalities account for approximately 4% to 5% of CHD, single gene syndromes account for 1% to 2%, known teratogens cause 1% to 2%, and the rest are presumably determined multifactorially. During development, conotruncal septation divides the single heart tube into 2 distinct outflow tracts. This report of a brother and sister with tetralogy of Fallot with pulmonary atresia examines the inheritance of familial conotruncal anomalies. The difficulty in genetic counseling for these defects is deciding if a family cluster represents single gene inheritance or is multifactorially determined. The small number of family clusters of conotruncal anomalies and the rare instances of consanguinity in nonsyndromal conotruncal defects are consistent with multifactorial determination. It may still be prudent to raise the possibility of single gene inheritance when counseling families with 2 or more individuals with conotruncal CHD.

▶ In reporting on a brother and sister with the severe form of tetralogy in which there is pulmonary atresia, the authors reviewed the 4 previously reported cases and judged that there was multifactorial determination of the anomaly. Documentation of such cases, together with this review of the literature, should help physicians who counsel parents with an affected child.—M.A. Engle, M.D.

Echocardiography

The Agreement Between Pulmonary and Systemic Blood Flow Measurements in Babies by Dual Beam Doppler Echocardiography

Kapusta L, Hopman JCW, Daniëls O (St Radboud University Hospital, Nijmegen, The Netherlands)
Eur Heart J 12:112–116, 1991   4–16

Background.—Dual-beam Doppler is a new development in echocardiography that measures cardiac output independently of the aortic root diameter and beam-vessel angle. Previous studies found a significant correlation between dual-beam Doppler-derived and thermodilution-derived cardiac output in critically ill adults. The accuracy of dual-beam Doppler was assessed in healthy prematurely born babies and infants.

Technique.—Dual-beam Doppler measures the systolic cross-sectional area directly at the same site and at the same time that the aortic velocity is measured. Because the wide beam completely encircles the aortic cross-sectional area, which is already determined by flow, noncircular cross-sectional areas are measured accurately without the need to assume a specific velocity profile.

Patients.—Cardiac output within the great arteries was measured in 27 infants. Twelve were premature, 5–57 days old, weighing between 1.09 kg and 2.82 kg. The other 15 were between 2 and 323 days old and weighed from 2.5 kg to 8.3 kg. None of the children had any cardiac or other physical abnormalities. Cross-sectional echocardiographic imaging of the ascending aorta and the main pulmonary artery was performed first. Thereafter, dual-beam, pulsed-wave Doppler was used to estimate blood flow rates in the same vessels. The difference between pulmonary and systemic blood flow was used as a measure of accuracy.

Results.—Adequate dual-beam Doppler signals from both arteries were obtained in all 27 babies. The mean difference between pulmonary and systemic blood flow measurements was .02 L/min^{-1}.

Conclusion.—Dual-beam Doppler echocardiography is a promising noninvasive method for estimating cardiac output within the great arteries of healthy infants. Further studies to evaluate the accuracy of this method for assessing infants with intracardial shunts should be undertaken.

▶ Determination, simply and noninvasively, of cardiac output has clinical relevance. The investigators from the Netherlands reported on determining cardiac output using dual-beam echocardiography. The authors investigated the feasibility of using this technique in 27 infants, 12 of whom were premature. They reported that the study could be done and that correlation was good for pulmonary and systemic blood flows (cardiac output). I agree that this methodology looks promising and merits confirmation by other studies.—M.A. Engle, M.D.

Usefulness of Color-Flow Doppler in Diagnosing and in Differentiating Supracristal Ventricular Septal Defect From Right Ventricular Outflow Tract Obstruction

Ludomirsky A, Tani L, Murphy DJ, Huhta JC (Baylor College of Medicine, Houston)

Am J Cardiol 67:194–198, 1991   4–17

Background.—Two-dimensional and Doppler echocardiography provide complementary procedures for noninvasive anatomical and hemodynamic assessment of ventricular septal defect (VSD). Two-dimensional echocardiography can detect the location and size of the VSD, whereas pulsed and continuous-wave Doppler echocardiography measure hemodynamic factors. The use of color Doppler echocardiography in the noninvasive diagnosis of supracristal VSD and the ability of color Doppler to differentiate between supracristal VSD and right ventricular (RV) outflow tract blockage were evaluated.

Methods.—Twenty-eight consecutive patients (age, 3 days to 23 years) who had catheter-diagnosed supracristal VSD or RV outflow tract obstruction were examined. Electrocardiographic gating was used to clarify systolic from diastolic events and to time the flows through the heart cycle.

Results.—All 28 patients had cardiac catheterization. Fourteen had a supracristal VSD, and 14 experienced various kinds of RV outflow tract blockage as seen on angiography and hemodynamic measurements, including 10 with isolated pulmonary valve stenosis and 4 with RV infundibular stenosis. The location of the VSD was accurately identified in all 14 patients with this defect. Six patients with aortic regurgitation had a prolapse of the right coronary cusp toward the RV outflow tract. All patients with pulmonary valve stenosis had thickened and domed pulmonary valve cusps. The pulsed-wave Doppler study identified the area of blockage in all patients with RV outflow tract stenotic defects. All patients with supracristal VSD had a continuous-wave Doppler that showed a high velocity jet across the ventricular septum. In patients with an RV outflow tract obstruction, the continuous-wave Doppler measured the pressure gradient across the stenotic region. Color-flow Doppler demonstrated a turbulent flow across the VSD that was directed toward the RV outflow tract in those with a supracristal VSD. The VSD jet in all patients exhibited a turbulent character lasting through systole. Color-flow Doppler mapping identified the location of the RV outflow tract blockage in all patients.

Conclusions.—These findings indicate that a differential diagnosis can be made when supracristal VSD occurs because the jet from the left to the right ventricle is directed toward the pulmonary valve early in systole. The use of color-flow Doppler mapping is required for localization, measurement, and differentiation of transeptal jet from the RV outflow tract flow in neonates and infants who have a supracristal VSD.

▶ When someone with congenital heart disease has a systolic murmur in the second left interspace (the pulmonary area), differential diagnosis favors real or relative pulmonary stenosis (PS) because that is far more frequent than supracristal ventricular septal defect (VSD), except in Asian people. The group at Texas Children's Hospital set out to determine whether echocardiographic techniques could distinguish the 2 in patients whose diagnosis was known from cardiac catheterization.

Not surprisingly they found that pulsed and continuous-wave Doppler correctly identified 14 of 14 patients with pulmonary stenosis. The VSD was identified in this manner in 10 of 14. The other 4 required color flow with ECG gating for diagnosis. The differential diagnosis is based on the fact that when supracristal VSD is present, the jet from left to right ventricle is directed toward the pulmonic valve. It occurs early in systole before outflow tract flow.

Of incidental interest is the presence of aortic regurgitation or fistula in 6 of those with the VSD, a common complication of this particular location of the septal defect.—M.A. Engle, M.D.

The Value of Transesophageal Echocardiography in Children With Congenital Heart Disease
Stümper O, Kaulitz R, Elzenga NJ, Bom N, Roelandt JRTC, Hess J, Sutherland GR (Academic Hospital Rotterdam Dijkzigt; Interuniversity Cardiology Institute, Rotterdam, the Netherlands)
J Am Soc Echocardiogr 4:164–176, 1991   4–18

Introduction.—The use of transesophageal echocardiography (TEE) in adult patients is well established, but there are few reports of its use in congenital heart disease, particularly in the pediatric age group. Transesophageal echocardiography using dedicated pediatric single-plane probes was evaluated prospectively in children with congenital heart disease. The TEE findings were correlated with those from established imaging techniques or surgical findings.

Patients.—During a 10-month period, 102 children with congenital heart disease aged 2.5 months to 14.9 years, with a mean age of 5.2 years, underwent TEE. Of 102 children, 40 were studied before surgical correction, 24 in the perioperative period, 9 during interventional cardiac catheterization, and 29 during follow-up.

Results.—In 101 children, TEE could be completed. Additional information was provided by TEE for 49 children (48.4%); the information was relevant to patient management in 21 (20.6%). Relevant new findings for medical or surgical management in the 21 patients included 1 juxtaposition of the atrial appendages, 4 anomalous systemic and pulmonary venous connections, 2 sinus venosus atrial septal defects, 1 atrioventricular septal defect, 1 mitral valve endocarditis, 2 left ventricular (LV) outflow obstructions, 1 doubly committed ventricular septal defect, 1 residual shunt post-Fontan, 2 LV function and filling, 3 Mustard baffle obstructions, 1 Mustard baffle leakage, and 2 Fontan obstructions. The TEE was considered nondiagnostic in 2 children and failed to detect lesions in 8. There were 3 complications. Inherent limitations were the semi-invasive nature of the procedure, the need for heavy sedation or general anesthesia, and the limited imaging planes provided.

Conclusion.—Important additional diagnostic information on a wide spectrum of congenital cardiac lesions in children can be provided by TEE.

▶ Transesophageal echocardiography (TEE) is already much appreciated in adult cardiology and its role is beginning to be established in pediatric cardiology. Postoperative Fontan patients need follow-up over their lifetime, and noninvasive methods have a distinct advantage in this regard. This paper from the Netherlands demonstrates the merits of this technique in such monitoring.— M.A. Engle, M.D.

Intraoperative Echocardiography in Infants and Children With Congenital Cardiac Shunt Lesions: Transesophageal Versus Epicardial Echocardiography

Muhiudeen IA, Roberson DA, Silverman NH, Haas G, Turley K, Cahalan MK
(Univ of California, San Francisco)

J Am Coll Cardiol 16:1687–1695, 1990   4–19

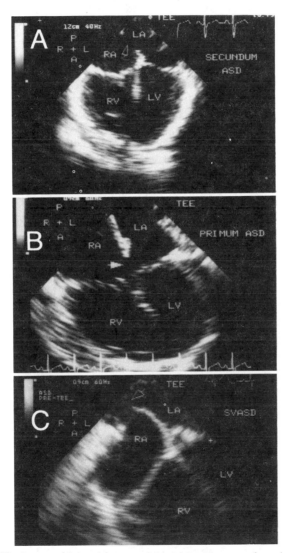

Fig 4–11.—The 3 types of interatrial communication (*arrows*) as seen from the transesophageal 4-chamber view. **A,** ostium secundum atrial septal defect; **B,** ostium primum atrial septal defect; **C,** Sinus venosus atrial septal defect. *Abbreviations: A,* anterior; *ASD* atrial septal defect; *L,* left; *LA,* left atrium; *LV,* left ventricle; *P,* posterior; *R,* right; *RA,* right atrium; *RV,* right ventricle; *SVASD,* sinus venosus arial septal defect; *TEE,* transesophageal echocardiogram. (Courtesy of Muhiudeen IA, Roberson DA, Silverman NH, et al: *J Am Coll Cardiol* 16:1687–1695, 1990.)

Introduction.—Before the recent development of a miniaturized transesophageal echocardiographic probe, intraoperative echocardiography of infants and small children was limited to epicardial imaging. The diagnostic accuracy and limitations of intraoperative transesophageal and epicardial echocardiography were determined for intracardiac shunt lesions in infants and children undergoing surgical treatment.

Patients.—The 50 patients studied were aged 4 days to 16 years and weighed 3 to 45 kg. All 50 patients underwent intraoperative transesophageal echocardiography (Fig 4–11), and 46 also underwent epicardial echocardiography, before and after cardiopulmonary bypass. The miniaturized probe was used in 36 patients weighing 20 kg or less. Epicardial imaging was performed with a 5-MHz pediatric transducer.

Results.—Epicardial imaging could be completed only in 46 of 49 patients in whom it was attempted because of induction arrhythmias in 2 and hypotension in 1 caused by epicardial probe contact. Of the 50 patients, 39 had corrective and 11 had palliative procedures. Overall, transesophageal echocardiography did not provide an adequate intraoperative examination in 3 patients (6%), and epicardial echocardiography failed to provide an adequate study in 4 (8%). The difference was not statistically significant. The complication rates were 6% for epicardial echocardiography and none for transesophageal echocardiography.

Conclusion.—Transesophageal echocardiography in infants and children provides an accurate and immediate assessment of the adequacy of surgical repair.

Transesophageal Echocardiography in Evaluation and Management After a Fontan Procedure

Stümper O, Sutherland GR, Geuskens R, Roelandt JRTC, Bos E, Hess J (Academic Hospital, Rotterdam, The Netherlands; Erasmus University, Rotterdam, The Netherlands)

J Am Coll Cardiol 17:1152–1160, 1991   4–20

Introduction.—Patients who undergo a Fontan procedure for the palliation of congenital cardiac lesions require close postoperative monitoring. Precordial ultrasound is commonly used to assess the functional status in these patients but often yields limited information. Transesophageal echocardiography (TEE) is widely used in adults with acquired cardiac lesions. The availability of pediatric probes now enables the use of this technique in children.

Patients.—Eleven children and 7 adults aged 1.6–34 years underwent a total of 24 TEE studies after undergoing a Fontan procedure. Five adults and 1 child were studied twice. Five patients were studied in the immediate postoperative period and 12 during the follow-up period. The mean interval between operation and TEE study was 3.4 years. Each patient had a complete precordial study before undergoing TEE. Eleven patients also had cardiac catheterization.

Findings.—Transesophageal echocardiography was uneventful in 17 patients. One child had a self-limiting arrhythmia that did not require treatment. Residual atrial shunting was documented during TEE in 3 patients and subsequently confirmed in 2 patients during cardiac catheterization. The third patient underwent early reoperation based on the TEE findings alone. Pulmonary artery obstruction was documented by TEE study and confirmed by cardiac catheterization in 3 patients. Transesophageal echocardiography documented the function of a Glenn anastomosis in 8 of 9 patients. In 1 patient, interposition of the right main bronchus precluded the evaluation. Earlier precordial studies allowed assessment of a Glenn shunt in only 3 patients. Atrioventricular valvular regurgitation was documented by TEE in 11 patients, but by precordial studies in only 5 patients. Thrombus formation was documented by TEE in 3 patients. Assessment of the anterior Fontan connections was successful in 5 of 8 patients and of the posterior Fontan connections in all 10 patients. A coronary artery fistula was identified by TEE in 2 patients, whereas precordial studies did not document this finding in either patient.

Conclusion.—Transesophageal echocardiography is an important diagnostic and monitoring technique after the Fontan procedure. The TEE examination is far superior to precordial ultrasound studies and provides supplementary information to cardiac catheterization.

▶ Pediatric cardiologists and cardiac surgeons are committed to providing the best, most accurate diagnoses to achieve success in surgical repair of congenital cardiovascular lesions. We used to say that "The operating room is no place to make the diagnosis. We need to make the precise diagnosis before the child is accepted for surgery so that time under anesthesia and in the operating room will be as short as possible and the surgeon's time will be devoted to working effectively on the identified problem." Although the goals remain the same, the premise has changed and there is a place in the operating room for improving the accuracy of diagnosis and the outcome of repair. Transesophageal and epicardial echocardiography is proving valuable, as this review of the indications and results (including shortcomings) of the methodology in 50 patients shows: 94% accuracy for the former and 92% for the latter.—M.A. Engle, M.D.

Addendum

Stümper O, Sutherland GR, Sreeram N, Van Daele MERM, Hess J, Bos E, Quagebeur JM. Role of Intraoperative Ultrasound Examination in Patients Undergoing a Fontan-type Procedure. *Br Heart J* 65:204–210, 1991.

▶ A specific application of intraoperative ultrasound is its use in patients undergoing a Fontan-type operation. This report from Rotterdam with 16 patients states that the technique not only refined diagnoses but also monitored ventricular function and excluded residual lesions.—M.A. Engle, M.D.

▶ Transesophageal echocardiography (TEE) is already much appreciated in cardiology in adults and is beginning to establish its role in pediatric cardiology.

Postoperative Fontan patients need follow-up over their lifetime, and noninvasive methods have a distinct advantage in this regard. This paper from the Netherlands demonstrates the merits of this technique in such monitoring.— M.A. Engle, M.D.

Tricuspid Valve Disease With Significant Tricuspid Insufficiency in the Fetus: Diagnosis and Outcome

Hornberger LK, Sahn DJ, Kleinman CS, Copel JA, Reed KL (Univ of California-San Diego Med Ctr, San Diego; Yale-New Haven Hosp, New Haven, Conn; Univ of Arizona Med Ctr, Tucson)
J Am Coll Cardiol 17:167–173, 1991   4–21

Introduction.—Preliminary studies suggest a poor prognosis for fetuses with tricuspid valve disease, particularly when associated with significant tricuspid insufficiency. Follow-up data on infants with prenatally detected tricuspid valve disease are not available. The echocardiographic studies and clinical courses of 27 fetuses at a mean gestational age of 26.9 weeks with tricuspid valve disease and significant tricuspid regurgitation were retrospectively reviewed. One fetus was excluded from analysis because a more complex heart lesion was found at autopsy.

Findings.—Of 26 fetuses, 17 had Ebstein's malformation of the tricuspid valve, 7 had tricuspid valve dysplasia, and 2 had an unguarded tricuspid valve orifice with little or no leaflet tissue. All 26 fetuses had massive right atrial dilation, and several who were studied serially had progressive right-sided cardiomegaly. Six fetuses had hydrops fetalis and 5 of these had atrial flutter. Additional cardiac lesions included pulmonary stenosis in 4 fetuses and pulmonary atresia in 2.

Outcome.—Three fetuses with Ebstein's malformation were electively aborted. Eleven (48%) of the remaining 23 fetuses died in utero at a gestational age ranging from 21 to 38 weeks. Of the 12 fetuses who survived to delivery, 8 died within the first 2 weeks of life. Only 4 infants survived beyond the neonatal period. One of the 4 survivors, who had undergone shunt placement at age 10 hours, died suddenly at 4 months of age despite an apparently functioning shunt. The 3 other survivors had moderate Ebstein's anomaly at postnatal echocardiographic study, but all 3 progressively improved and none required prolonged ventilation or supplemental oxygen.

Conclusion.—The prognosis for fetuses with tricuspid valve disease and significant tricuspid regurgitation diagnosed in utero by echocardiography is extremely poor.

▶ What happens when significant tricuspid insufficiency is diagnosed by fetal echocardiography? The answer from the 3-center study of 27 such fetuses is, unfortunately, "nothing very good." The study documented the presence or the acquisition of pulmonic stenosis or atresia or massive right-sided cardiomegaly. In 6 instances, hydrops occurred; in 5 others, atrial flutter developed; in 48% (23) death occurred in utero. Lung hypoplasia was noted in 10 of 19 autopsies. Only 4 infants survived, and 3 lucky ones had a benign neonatal course.—M.A. Engle, M.D.

Extracorporeal Membrane Oxygenation (ECMO)

Follow-Up of Infants Treated With Extracorporeal Membrane Oxygenation for Newborn Respiratory Failure
Schumacher RE, Palmer TW, Roloff DW, LaClaire PA, Bartlett RH (Univ of Michigan, Ann Arbor)
Pediatrics 87:451–457, 1991   4–22

Introduction.—Extracorporeal membrane oxygenation (ECMO) provides a period of complete lung rest without the damaging effects of mechanical ventilation in severely ill term newborns with respiratory failure. An adverse outcome has been reported in 10% to 25% of ECMO survivors. The follow-up findings in 92 infants treated with ECMO at 1 institution were evaluated.

Patients.—During an 8-year period, 118 newborns of greater than 34 weeks' gestation received ECMO for severe respiratory failure, 103 of whom (87%) survived and were available for follow-up at 1–7 years of age. Newborns treated with ECMO were at an estimated mortality risk of 80% or greater. Data were collected from 265 follow-up clinic visits by 92 children, of whom 81 were seen when between 4 and 12 months of age.

Results.—During the first year of life, 25 infants (31%) had to be rehospitalized, most of them for lower respiratory tract illness. An additional 25 infants (31%) were treated as outpatients for lower respiratory tract illness. Five children (6%) were seen for new or nonstatic neurologic problems. Twenty-one infants (26%) had some evidence of growth failure. No new medical problems were identified after the first year of life. At their latest clinic visit, 16% of children exhibited moderate-to-severe neurologic abnormalities and 8% had moderate-to-severe cognitive delay. Four percent had sensorineural hearing loss, 9% were receiving speech and language therapy, and an additional 6% had speech and language delay. Overall, 16 children (20%) had some type of handicap. Assuming a pre-ECMO mortality risk of 80%, there are now 65 infants alive who would have died with conventional therapy. The use of ECMO has resulted in 49 more children being alive without handicap and 13 children now being alive with handicap.

Conclusion.—Outcome after ECMO appears comparable with that seen in less ill cohorts of infants treated with more conventional therapy. However, long-term follow-up of all ECMO-treated infants remains essential.

▶ This report presents important follow-up data 1 to 7 years after ECMO was used as a life-saving last resort in 92 infants. Those under follow-up were among 103 survivors (87%) out of 118 treated with ECMO. This large series is but a small part of the more than 3,000 newborns treated in ECMO centers through 1989.

Not surprisingly, when infants are so desperately ill in respiratory distress, some residua or sequelae were found. These related to recurrent respiratory tract infections in the first year of life in 62% and in neurologic impairment (16%) or sensorineural hearing loss in 4%.

The authors summarized their experience with the statement that 65 infants were alive who would likely have died without ECMO, and 49 of these had no handicap detected. They emphasized the importance of long-term continuing follow-up.—M.A. Engle, M.D.

Epidemiology

Cardiovascular Risk Factors in Hispanic, White, and Black Children: The Brooks County and Bogalusa Heart Studies
Webber LS, Harsha DW, Phillips GT, Srinivasan SR, Simpson JW, Berenson GS (Louisiana State Univ Med Ctr, New Orleans; Children's Heart Inst of Texas, Corpus Christi)
Am J Epidemiol 133:704–714, 1991   4–23

Purpose.—Previous studies demonstrated that Hispanic Americans have greater frequencies of cardiovascular disease risk factors than white Americans. However, these studies were carried out in adults. Cardiovascular risk factor studies in children can contribute to the understanding of the development of heart disease in adulthood.

Methods.—Risk factors for cardiovascular disease were compared in 401 Hispanic, 2,072 white, and 1,207 black children. The Hispanic children represented a 25% random sample of all school children in a rural county in south Texas, where 95% of the population is Hispanic. The white and black children were enrolled in the Bogalusa Heart Study, a long-term epidemiologic investigation of cardiovascular risk factors in a semirural community in Louisiana, where 65% of the population is white and 35% is black. Both sites used standardized protocols for assessing anthropometrics, blood pressure, and health habits. Serum samples were analyzed for lipid and lipoprotein content.

Results.—Beginning at ages 7–8 years, Hispanic children were about 4 cm shorter than white and black children. For boys, there were no differences in body weight among the 3 groups. However, beginning at age 11 years, black girls were 3–4 kg heavier than white girls and 5–6 kg heavier than Hispanic girls. Triceps skinfolds were similar in Hispanic and white children and were 2–3 mm greater than in black children. Blood pressure levels for the 3 ethnic groups were similar. Total cholesterol levels were higher for black children than for white and Hispanic children, but dropped during puberty, particularly in white boys. High-density-lipoprotein cholesterol levels were significantly higher in black children than in white or Hispanic children for both boys and girls. However, Hispanic children had higher levels of low-density-lipoprotein cholesterol and triglycerides than white or black children.

Conclusion.—The differences in cardiovascular risk factors among Hispanic, white, and black children are similar to those found in their adult counterparts.

▶ Because adults of different racial and ethnic groups have some variations in risk factors for cardiovascular disease, the investigators asked whether similar differences prevailed among children. To answer this, they applied the same protocol for study to Hispanic children in Texas and to black and white children in Bogalusa, Louisiana. They noted little difference in blood pressure among the 3, but in the other factors studied, they found a change similar to that found in the adult counterparts. If risk factors can be identified, one can hope the early modification might accomplish the desired prevention of premature disability and death.—M.A. Engle, M.D.

Type A Behavior and Its Determinants in Children, Adolescents and Young Adults With and Without Parental Coronary Heart Disease: A Case-Control Study
Räikkönen K, Keltikangas-Järvinen L, Pietikäinen M (University of Helsinki; University of Kuopio, Finland)
J Psychosom Res 35:273–280, 1991   4–24

Background.—Coronary heart disease (CHD) has a strong genetic component, but the familial aggregation of risk factors results at least partly from shared environments and family habits. No previous reports have examined behavioral and psychological characteristics in healthy young persons with and without parental CHD. These characteristics were examined in a case-controlled investigation.

Methods.—Participants were identified from the Finnish Multicenter Study of Cardiovascular Risk in Young Finns. A sample of 3,596 healthy children, drawn from a registry covering the entire population of Finland, including 1,832 girls and 1,764 boys, participated in a baseline survey and then were examined 3 times during the 6-year follow-up period. Groups of 360 children of each sex were drawn from the age cohorts of 3, 6, 9, 12, 15, and 18 years. A group of 78 children whose parents died from CHD, suffered from myocardial infarction, or had CHD and a control group whose parents had no CHD were identified. Variables examined included type A behavior, self-esteem, achievement striving, hyperactivity, and social maladjustment.

Results.—A significant interaction with social maladjustment and hyperactivity by the case-control factor and sex was noted, which was explained by the effect on hyperactivity. Boys with parental CHD appeared to be less hyperactive than boys without parental CHD, and girls with parental CHD appeared to be more hyperactive than those without. This was the only way in which girls with parents with CHD differed from controls. Boys with parental CHD had higher scores for type A behavior, lower self-esteem, and more intense striving for achievement than those without parental CHD.

Conclusion.—High intraindividual stability of variables for type A behavior, self-esteem, achievement striving, hyperactivity, and social maladjustment was noted, suggesting that the risk status of the behavioral characteristics varies as a function of age. It remains unknown whether behavioral and somatic coronary risk indicators are truly independent or share a common origin.

▶ The investigators in Finland took advantage of a unique opportunity to study behavioral characteristics in healthy children, half of whom had parental coronary heart disease. They were identified through the Finnish Multicenter Study of Cardiovascular Risk in Young Finns, which has enrolled 3,596 randomly selected healthy Finnish children. From the register, 360 girls and 360 boys (half of each from rural areas) were chosen for 3 separate examinations, in 1980, 1983, and 1986. Controls were matched from families without evidence of heart disease.

The results indicated that in comparison with controls, that boys with parental heart disease had higher scores on type A behavior, lower self-esteem, and more intense striving for achievement. Girls differed from controls only in a higher level of hyperactivity among those with parents who had heart disease.

This is an excellent start, with intriguing possibilities. We need a crystal ball to look ahead 20, 30, 40, or more years to determine whether the "predictors" of outcome for adult heart disease are valid for studies such as this one from Finland, and those from Bogalusa, Mississippi, and Muscadine, Iowa, in the United States.—M.A. Engle, M.D.

Exercise

Detecting Arrhythmia by Exercise Electrocardiography in Pediatric Patients: Assessment of Sensitivity and Influence on Clinical Management
Weigel TJ, Porter CJ, Mottram CD, Driscoll DJ (Mayo Clin and Found, Rochester, Minn)
Mayo Clin Proc 66:379–386, 1991   4–25

Introduction.—Exercise electrocardiography (EECG) is used to document arrhythmias in children with congenital heart disease, but the usefulness of EECG for inducing or suppressing arrhythmias in children with suspected arrhythmias or for influencing the clinical management of arrhythmias in children with previously documented arrhythmias has never been examined.

Patients.—During an 8-year period, 49 children with suspected arrhythmias and 92 children with previously documented arrhythmias underwent EECG. Before EECG, all patients with suspected arrhythmias had normal sinus rhythm as documented by routine ECG, whereas the other 92 patients had a documented arrhythmia on routine ECG or on 24-hour ambulatory monitoring. All exercise testing was done by cycle ergometry using the James protocol.

Findings.—Of 49 patients with suspected arrhythmias, 10 (20%) had abnormal rhythms on EECG. Treatment was modified in 4 of the 10 patients. Among the 39 patients with normal findings on EECG, further testing with 24-hour ambulatory or transtelephonic ECG monitoring or electrophysiologic study identified another 8 patients with arrhythmias. The sensitivity of EECG was 56% and its negative predictive value was 79%. Of 92 patients with previously documented arrhythmias, 38 had atrial arrhythmias, 31 had ventricular arrhythmias, and 23 had atrioventricular conduction abnormalities before EECG. Sixty-eight (74%) of the 92 patients had abnormal EECG findings. Of 23 patients with normal EECG findings, further testing with 24-hour ambulatory or transtelephonic monitoring or electrophysiologic study identified another 16 patients with arrhythmias. Clinical management was modified based on EECG findings in 27% of patients. Patients with atrial arrhythmias were more likely to have normal EECG findings (42%) than were those with ventricular arrhythmias (23%) or an atrioventricular conduction abnormality (44%).

Conclusion.—Exercise electrocardiography may be an alternative method for inducing an arrhythmia in children suspected of having arrhythmias, but who show no arrhythmias on surface ECG or by 24-hour ambulatory monitoring. Clinical management was changed based on EECG findings in some patients, but the usefulness of EECG for monitoring the effects of anti-arrhythmic therapy could not be confirmed conclusively.

▶ From a study of 49 patients with suspected arrhythmia and 92 with previously documented arrhythmia, the group at Mayo Clinic analyzed the sensitivity and predictive value of EECG in management of patients. They supplemented this technique with Holter monitoring.

In those 49 with suspected arrhythmias, EECG brought out abnormalities in 10, which led to modification of treatment in 4. The sensitivity of EECG in these patients was 56% and its negative predictive value was 79%.

There were 38 patients with atrial arrhythmias, 32 with ventricular arrhythmias, and 23 with atrioventricular conduction abnormalities. Of these patients, 68 (74%) had abnormal EECG. Further testing induced the arrhythmia in 16 patients. Those with atrial arrhythmias were more likely to have a normal EECG than those with ventricular.

Among 35 patients referred to check for suppression of arrhythmia, 25 (71%) did have suppression.

The authors conclude, and I agree, that exercise electrocardiography can help identify a suspected arrhythmia in children.—M.A. Engle, M.D.

The Role of Chronotropic Impairment During Exercise After the Mustard Operation
Paridon SM, Humes RA, Pinsky WW (Wayne State Univ School of Medicine, Detroit)
J Am Coll Cardiol 17:729–732, 1991   4–26

Background.—Prior reports of the exercise performance of children and adolescents who have had the Mustard (atrial switch) operation have demonstrated various levels of exercise limitation and lowered aerobic capacity. Because previous studies have included patients with assorted types of defects, a complete understanding of such exercise limitations has been complicated. The influence of chronotropic impairment on exercise limitation in patients after the Mustard procedure was evaluated by using complete metabolic measurements to determine the achieved maximal heart rate.

Methods.—Fifty-six patients who had surgery between October 1987 and December 1989 were evaluated for the study. Of these 56, 36 were excluded because of other anatomical defects, arrhythmias, or a lack of echocardiogram. The remaining 20 patients had d-transposition of the great arteries as their only congenital heart defect and were receiving no medication at the time of the study. Each patient had a 2-dimensional echocardiogram within 6 months of the exercise testing, which consisted of a 1-minute incremental treadmill protocol. Electrocardiographic, metabolic, and pulmonary measurements were taken at rest and during the exercise.

Results.—For all 20 patients, maximal work rate during exercise was normal. The maximal heart rate for the entire group was 87% of the predicted values for age. Maximal VO_2 was decreased for the study group at 75% of the predicted age and gender values. No correlation was observed between the maximal or resting heart rate and the maximal VO_2 or between the right ventricular volume index and the rest heart rate. An inverse correlation between the right ventricular volume index and the maximal heart rate was documented.

Implications.—These findings indicate that the lower maximal oxygen consumption of patients who have had the Mustard procedure does not result from chronotropic impairment. The right ventricular dilation observed may be a compensatory mechanism for the chronotropic impairment.

▶ The answer to the question of the role of chronotropic impairment during exercise after the Mustard operation, which provides a venous switch for transposed great arteries, is that it plays no role at all. These investigators from Detroit answered their question when they studied response to exercise in 20 patients who had undergone this physiologic palliation at a mean age of .9 years and of 13 years at restudy. The good news is that not only were they asymptomatic but also that their heart rate response was 87% of that predicted for age while their maximum oxygen consumption was 75% of predicted value. Right ventricular volume index, determined by echocardiography, did not correlate significantly with this observation of 13% and 25% reduction over expected exercise performance.—M.A. Engle, M.D.

Lung Function and Pulmonary Regurgitation Limit Exercise Capacity in Postoperative Tetralogy of Fallot
Rowe SA, Zahka KG, Manolio TA, Horneffer PJ, Kidd L (Johns Hopkins Univ, Baltimore)
J Am Coll Cardiol 17:461–466, 1991   4–27

Introduction.—Some patients undergoing the surgical repair of tetralogy of Fallot can have abnormal exercise capacity and are at risk for ventricular arrhythmias. This report presents the analysis of 55 patients who have survived 10–28 years after this surgery. These patients were evaluated by treadmill stress testing, pulmonary function analysis, and rest 2-dimensional and Doppler echocardiography.

Methods.—Of the 144 patients who underwent total repair of tetralogy of Fallot at <11 years of age from January 1958 to December 1975 and survived, 120 were available for follow-up. Only 55 agreed to return for the procedures. Patients were evaluated by exercise and spirometry testing and echocardiography.

Findings.—The average age at the time of operation was 8.1 years, and the average duration of follow-up was 18 years. The age of the subjects at the time of this study ranged from 15–37 years. Exercise testing showed 3 subjects to have a blood oxygen saturation <93% at peak exercise. Thirty patients with expiratory gas collection during their final exercise minute showed maximal oxygen consumption that was 86% of the mean expected. Vital capacity at rest was measured at 82% of the mean expected. No patient exhibited wheezing after exercise or tachycardia during exercise. Echocardiography demonstrated a residual ventricular septal defect during clinical examination that was confirmed by Doppler testing in 8 subjects. A higher right ventricular diastolic area was linked with a longer time since surgery and was statistically associated with lowered exercise duration, decreased maximal heart rate, and decreased vital capacity. A moderate pulmonary regurgitation was statistically associated with lowered vital capacity at rest, a raised respiratory rate, and a small breathing reserve at peak exercise. A history of smoking did not influence any of the outcomes of the tests. Unifocal premature ventricular complexes present during exercise were statistically linked with higher right ventricular diastolic area.

Conclusions.—These findings indicate that the limitation of exercise may be associated with lung function abnormalities at rest and to pulmonary regurgitation after this surgery. Overall, however, these patients appear to have generally good exercise capacity.

▶ Pulmonic regurgitation is a common sequela after surgical valvotomy for valvular pulmonic stenosis, and it is usually mild and of no physiologic consequence. The situation may be different, however, after open repair of tetralogy of Fallot. In that situation, the repair often involves a right ventriculotomy, resection of obstructing infundibular musculature, a pulmonary valvotomy, and an enlarging outflow tract patch that sometimes extends through the anulus. In that setting, pulmonic regurgitation may vary from mild to severe. In addition, some residual left-to-right shunt may add to right ventricular dilatation and to the pulmonary regurgitation.

This study of 55 patients in long-term postoperative follow-up (mean 18 ± 5 years) showed remarkably good exercise duration and heart rate response (about 92% and 94% of normal, respectively) with no stopping of the test for arrhythmia.—M.A. Engle, M.D.

Kawasaki Disease

Failure to Confirm the Presence of a Retrovirus in Cultured Lymphocytes From Patients With Kawasaki Syndrome

Rowley A, Castro B, Levy J, Sullivan J, Koup R, Fresco R, Shulman S (Northwestern Univ Med School, Chicago; Univ of California, San Francisco; Univ of Massachusetts, Worcester; Loyola Univ Med School, Maywood, Ill)
Pediatr Res 29:417–419, 1991   4–28

Background.—Kawasaki syndrome (KS) is an acute febrile illness in children and its cause is unknown. One fifth of untreated patients develop coronary artery aneurysms, and DNA polymerase activity has been described in culture supernatants of peripheral blood mononuclear cells from patients with KS. This activity was studied.

Findings.—Separate characterization studies on 10 stored positive supernatants showed that the polymerase activity is typical of a DNA-dependent DNA polymerase rather than viral reverse transcriptase. Peripheral blood mononuclear cells from 17 other KS patients were negative for reverse transcriptase when analyzed in 3 laboratories.

Conclusion.—These findings fail to support a retroviral cause of KS, but infectious causes still should be considered because of the clinical and epidemiologic features of the disorder.

▶ The cause of the condition that is now being recognized worldwide in young children and is known as Kawasaki syndrome or disease is still unknown. This careful investigation by Dr. Anne Rowley and her associates at 3 other institutions appears to disprove a favored theory—that it is caused by a retrovirus. The search goes on.—M.A. Engle, M.D.

Antiendothelial Cell Antibodies Detected by a Cellular Based ELISA in Kawasaki Disease

Tizard EJ, Baguley E, Hughes GRV, Dillon MJ (Institute of Child Health, London; St Thomas's Hospital, London)
Arch Dis Child 66:189–192, 1991   4–29

Background.—Kawasaki disease is an acute systemic vasculitic illness of childhood that was first described in Japan in 1967. Its cause is unknown, but an infectious cause is suspected. Recent studies have demonstrated the presence of antibodies cytotoxic to cytokine-stimulated endothelial cells during the acute phase of the disease. A cellular-based enzyme-linked immunosorbent assay (ELISA) was used to demonstrate the presence of antiendothelial cell antibodies in the sera from children with Kawasaki disease.

Patients.—Eighteen boys and 14 girls with a mean age of 2.34 years fulfilled the clinical criteria for Kawasaki disease. Ten of the 32 patients (31%) had coronary artery aneurysms and 5 (16%) had coronary artery

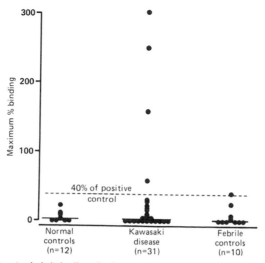

Fig 4–12.—IgG antiendothelial cell antibodies in Kawasaki disease. (Courtesy of Tizard EJ, Baguley E, Hughes GRV, et al: *Arch Dis Child* 66:189–192, 1991.)

dilatation. Serum samples from a control group of normal children with a mean age of 7.41 years undergoing routine surgery and from a control group of children with other acute febrile illnesses with a mean age of 3.05 years were also examined.

Results.—Twenty-one patients with Kawasaki disease had IgM antien-

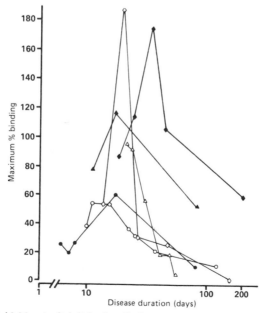

Fig 4–13.—Serial IgM antiendothelial cell antibodies in 6 patients with Kawasaki disease. (Courtesy of Tizard EJ, Baguley E, Hughes GRV, et al: *Arch Dis Child* 66:189–192, 1991.)

dothelial cell antibody titers greater than 40% and 4 also had raised IgG antiendothelial antibody titers (Fig 4–12). The antibody titer paralleled the disease activity in those patients for whom serial serum samples were available (Fig 4–13). No relative increase in binding of antiendothelial cell antibodies was noted after cytokine stimulation. Nine of the 15 patients with cardiac sequelae and 12 patients without cardiac sequelae had raised IgM antiendothelial cell antibody titers. Thus, there was no association between antiendothelial cell antibodies and serious cardiovascular sequelae.

Conclusion.—Although antiendothelial cell antibodies are not specific for Kawasaki disease, they appear to have an important role in the pathogenesis of Kawasaki disease.

▶ Although we have known about Kawasaki disease since 1967, we still know all too little about its cause and pathogenesis. This study from London reports on an association with clinical disease of raised IgM antibody titers (in 21 of 32 children) and of IgG antiendothelial antibody titer in 4. These antibodies were not detected in normal children or in febrile controls. The nature of the antigen is not known, but this test promises possible confirmation of diagnosis as well as a tool for understanding pathogenesis.—M.A. Engle, M.D.

Clinical and Epidemiologic Characteristics of Patients Referred for Evaluation of Possible Kawasaki Disease
Burns JC, Mason WH, Glode MP, Shulman ST, Melish ME, Meissner C, Bastian J, Beiser AS, Meyerson HM, Newburger JW for the US Multicenter Kawasaki Disease Study Group (Univ of California, San Diego)
J Pediatr 118:680–686, 1991   4–30

Introduction.—The early diagnosis of Kawasaki disease (KD) is important because aspirin plus high doses of intravenous gamma-globulin given within the first 10 days of illness reduces cardiovascular sequelae. However, diagnosing KD is difficult because it mimics a number of other infectious and immunologic disorders. Those disorders that most closely mimic KD and the physical or laboratory findings that exclude a diagnosis of KD were identified in a multicenter, case-comparison study.

Patients.—There were 280 children with a mean age of 3 years with a definitive diagnosis of KD and 42 comparison patients with a mean age of 3.8 years in whom an alternative diagnosis was confirmed or suspected. All patients were examined by experienced specialists during the acute phase of illness. The physicians recorded clinical data, patient diagnosis, and disposition. An epidemiologic questionnaire was used to record information on medication use, antecedent illness, allergies, birth order, immunizations, exposure to ill persons, animals, and exposure to recently cleaned carpets.

Results.—The diseases that most closely mimicked KD were measles and group A β-hemolytic streptococcal infection, accounting for 35 (83%) of diagnoses in the comparison group. In all, the clinical diagnostic criteria for KD were fulfilled in 18 (46%) of the 39 comparison patients for whom complete data were available. Thus the clinical criteria for KD alone did not differentiate patients with KD from those with other disorders. Statistical analysis revealed that patients with KD were significantly less likely to have exudative conjunctivitis or pharyngitis, generalized adenopathy, and intraoral lesions. Patients with KD were more likely to have a perineal distribution of their rash, to be anemic, and to have an elevated erythrocyte sedimentation rate. Patients with KD more commonly lived within 200 yards of a body of water. The previously reported association between KD and exposure to recently cleaned carpets was not confirmed in this study.

Conclusion.—Clinical criteria alone are inadequate for reliable differentiation of patients with KD from those with other diagnoses.

▶ Now that we have effective treatment with intravenous gamma-globulin for children with acute KD, what we need is a specific diagnostic test. Lacking that, the pooled experience of a multicenter expert group should help in deciding who has or does not have KD. The 2 most common mimicking febrile illnesses were measles and streptococcal infection. See the following article by Rauch et al. concerning rug shampoo.—M.A. Engle, M.D.

Outbreak of Kawasaki Syndrome in Denver, Colorado: Association With Rug and Carpet Cleaning
Rauch AM, Glode MP, Wiggins JW Jr, Rodriguez JG, Hopkins RS, Hurwitz ES, Schonberger LB (Ctrs for Disease Control, Atlanta; The Children's Hosp, Denver; State of Colorado Dept of Health Services, Denver)
Pediatrics 87:663–669, 1991   4–31

Introduction.—The origin of Kawasaki syndrome, a leading cause of acquired heart disease in infants and young children, remains unknown. A previous case-controlled study of an outbreak of Kawasaki syndrome revealed a statistically significant association between Kawasaki syndrome and rug or carpet cleaning in the home within 30 days of onset of illness. However, subsequent studies did not support this association. A case-controlled study was performed to investigate the largest outbreak of Kawasaki syndrome reported to date in the United States.

Study Design.—Between October 1984 and January 1985, 62 children aged 3 months to 12 years, 8 months had a diagnosis of Kawasaki syndrome; 52 (84%) of the children lived in metropolitan Denver. Cases were not clustered in any part of metropolitan Denver, and no 2 patients lived in the same household, attended the same school or day-care center, or resided in the same neighborhood. Twenty-six patients were enrolled in the case-controlled study. Matched controls were randomly selected from birth certificate records.

Results.—Sixteen of the 26 patients with Kawasaki syndrome (62%) lived in homes where rugs or carpets had been shampooed or spot-cleaned during the 30-day period before the onset of the disease, compared with 10 of 49 matched controls (20%). Ten patients had a single exposure and 6 patients had multiple exposures. Exposure to rug or carpet cleaning outside the home was reported by the parents of 3 additional patients and by none of the parents of controls. In all, 19 of the 26 patients with Kawasaki syndrome (73%) had been exposed to shampooed or spot-cleaned rugs or carpets, compared with 20% of the controls. The difference was statistically significant. None of 23 other factors investigated showed a statistically significant association with Kawasaki syndrome.

Comment.—The overall incidence of Kawasaki syndrome for the 4-month period reported here was 36 cases per 100,000 for children younger than 5 years, the highest incidence reported to date. It is also the third outbreak of Kawasaki syndrome for which a statistically significant association with rug or carpet cleaning was found.

▶ Pathogenesis of this now commonly recognized condition, Kawasaki syndrome or disease, continues to be unknown. In Denver, Colorado, an epidemiologic survey during a remarkable epidemic in the fall and winter of 1984–1985 revealed in yet another study a statistically significant association with recent rug cleaning within 30 days of onset of illness: 62% of Kawasaki patients vs. 20% of controls. This was our experience as well.—M.A. Engle, M.D.

The Changes of Interleukin-2, Tumour Necrotic Factor and Gamma-Interferon Production Among Patients With Kawasaki Disease
Lin C-Y, Lin C-C, Hwang B, Chiang BN (Veterans Gen Hosp, Shih-Pai, Taipei, Taiwan)
Eur J Pediatr 150:179–182, 1991   4–32

Background.—A number of immunoregulatory abnormalities have been seen in patients with Kawasaki disease (KD), although no direct evidence exists that immune complexes are mediators of pathogenesis. The possible roles of interleukin-2 (IL-2), tumor necrosis factor (TNF), and gamma-interferon (IFN-γ) were explored.

Methods.—Serial samples were studied from 43 patients with KD treated with aspirin alone, including 19 who developed coronary aneurysms. Patients ranged in age from 4 months to 5 years. Serum levels and in vitro mononuclear cell production of IL-2, TNF, and IFN-γ were assessed.

Results.—Production of IL-2 peaked during week 2 of the acute phase, with a significantly higher mean peak value in patients in whom coronary aneurysm developed than among those in whom it did not. Serum levels of IL-2 paralleled production from mononuclear cells, with peaks during week 2 or 3 and significantly higher levels in patients with aneurysms. Production of TNF from stimulated monocytes peaked during weeks 3 and 4, with significant differences between patient groups only at 2 months and 4 months. Serum levels of TNF peaked at week 2 and returned to normal levels by 2 months for both groups. In both groups, production of IFN-γ increased for the first 2 to 3 weeks then decreased slowly until 4 months. In sera from 27.9% of febrile patients and from no convalescent patients, IFN-γ was detected, with no differences between groups with and without aneurysm.

Conclusions.—In these patients with KD, production of IL-2, TNF, and IFN by stimulated monocytes corresponded to serum levels of IL-2 and TNF during weeks 2 and 3. Increases in levels of IL-2 and TNF occurred during the period of coronary aneurysm formation. The level or production of IL-2 might be a useful predictor of coronary aneurysm formation. All 3 lymphokines may be involved in the development of vascular injury in KD.

▶ Now that intravenous gamma-globulin has been demonstrated to be effective in the acute stage of Kawasaki disease not only to terminate signs of illness but also to prevent coronary abnormalities, it is unlikely that in the future, patients will be treated with aspirin alone. This report from Taipai can be considered as a study of the "natural history" of Kawasaki disease and also as a study of changes in IL-2, TNF, and IFN-γ in the acute and subacute changes of Kawasaki disease.—M.A. Engle, M.D.

Collateral Circulation in Kawasaki Disease With Coronary Occlusion or Severe Stenosis
Tatara K, Kusakawa S, Itoh K, Honma S, Hashimoto K, Kazuma N, Lee K, Asai T, Murata M (Tokyo Women's Medical College)
Am Heart J 121:797–802, 1991   4–33

Introduction.—Patients with Kawasaki disease and giant coronary aneurysms are likely to have severe coronary sequelae. Previous studies have shown that one third of these patients eventually have coronary occlusion, which may result in myocardial infarction or sudden death. Most patients with coronary occlusion who remain asymptomatic have angiographic evidence of many coronary collateral vessels. Collateral vessels in patients with Kawasaki disease and total coronary occlusion or severe coronary stenosis were investigated, and the effect of collateral vessels on myocardial ischemia was examined by treadmill stress testing and myocardial imaging.

Patients.—Forty patients with Kawasaki disease and at least a 90% reduction in the diameter of the major coronary artery were included in the study. Thirty-three patients had 38 coronary occlusions and 7 patients had 11 stenoses of greater than 90%. Coronary angiography was performed between 13 and 168 months after disease onset. Thirty patients underwent treadmill testing using the Bruce protocol. Thallium 201 cardiac tomography after dipyridamole infusion was performed in 27 patients.

Results.—Collateral vessels were seen in 32 (97%) of the 33 patients with total occlusions (Fig 4–14). In contrast, 6 of the 7 patients with severe stenosis but no total occlusion had no collateral vessels and 1 patient

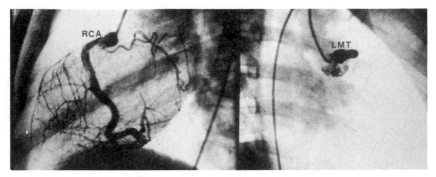

Fig 4–14.—Girl, 8 years, with occlusion of left coronary artery at the left main trunk (*LMT*). Many collateral vessels are seen originating from the right coronary artery (*RCA*). Patient had frequent chest pain, and ischemia was demonstrated by treadmill stress testing and myocardial imaging. (Courtesy of Tatara K, Kusakawa S, Itoh K, et al: *Am Heart J* 121:797–802, 1991.)

had only 1 poorly developed collateral vessel. Patients with and without collaterals had similar results on treadmill stress testing and myocardial imaging. Angiography performed 1 year after surgical bypass showed that the collateral vessels had disappeared when the bypass graft was patent, and that the abnormalities evident on treadmill stress testing and myocardial imaging had normalized or improved.

Conclusion.—As previously demonstrated in adults, the development of angiographically visible coronary collateral vessels in children with severe coronary sequelae after Kawasaki disease depends on whether the coronary arteries are severely stenosed or completely occluded. Collateral vessels afford no protection against myocardial ischemia as measured by treadmill stress testing and myocardial imaging.

▶ We continue to learn from the ongoing follow-up studies by Japanese cardiologists. This paper continues the natural history of coronary artery involvement in Kawasaki disease. In the acute stage we are interested in preventing, through use of intravenous gamma-globulin, the development of coronary aneurysms. In the long-term, we are concerned about stenoses that are acquired over the years after the acute disease.

This paper addresses the adequacy of development of collateral circulation as coronary arteries become occluded. They investigated 40 patients who had at least a 90% reduction in diameter of at least 1 coronary artery. They found collateral vessels in 32 of 33 with total occlusion but poorly developed collaterals in those with severe stenosis but not total occlusion. Neither treadmill testing nor myocardial imaging could distinguish between the 2 groups. They further stated that the presence of collateral circulation "cannot provide protection against stress-induced myocardial ischemia."—M.A. Engle, M.D.

A Single Intravenous Infusion of Gamma Globulin as Compared With Four Infusions in the Treatment of Acute Kawasaki Syndrome

Newburger JW, Takahashi M, Beiser AS, Burns JC, Bastian J, Chung KJ, Colan SD, Duffy CE, Fulton DR, Glode MP, Mason WH, Meissner HC, Rowley AH,

Shulman ST, Reddy V, Sundel RP, Wiggins JW, Colton T, Melish ME, Rosen FS (Harvard Med School, Boston; Northwestern Univ, Chicago; Univ of Colorado, Denver; Univ of Southern California, Los Angeles; Univ of California, San Diego, et al)
N Engl J Med 324:1633–1639, 1991

4–34

Background.—A previous US multicenter trial in children with acute Kawasaki syndrome found that a 4-day course of intravenous gamma-globulin (GG) and concomitant aspirin administration effectively prevented the development of coronary artery lesions and reduced systemic inflammation. A second multicenter trial was designed to determine whether a single, very high dose of intravenous GG would have similar safety and efficacy.

Patients.—During a 3½-year period, 549 children with a diagnosis of acute Kawasaki syndrome were enrolled in the study. Of these 276 were randomly allocated to daily infusion with 400 mg/kg of GG for 4 days and 273 received a single infusion of 2 g/kg of GG given over 10 hours. Both groups were also treated with aspirin 100 mg/kg/day for 14 days and 3–5 mg/kg/day thereafter.

Results.—Children treated with the 4-day intravenous GG regimen had significantly higher maximal temperatures, longer duration and slower resolution of fever, and slower resolution of inflammation than did those treated with the single intravenous GG infusion. At the 2-week follow-up, 24 children (9.1%) in the 4-infusion group and 12 children (4.6%) in the single-infusion group had coronary artery abnormalities. The difference was statistically significant. The overall frequency of adverse effects was 2.7%; the frequency was similar in the 2 treatment groups. Four of 5 children with giant aneurysms were treated with the 4-day regimen, 1 of whom died during the subacute phase of the disease.

Conclusion.—A single large dose of intravenous GG is more effective than the standard 4-day smaller-dose intravenous GG regimen in the treatment of children with acute Kawasaki disease, and is just as safe.

▶ When Newburger and other members of her collaborative study group reported in 1986 (1) on their controlled study of intravenous gamma-globulin over a 4-day period plus aspirin vs aspirin alone, they proved the benefits of gamma-globulin in this disease of still-unknown cause. That was a significant report.

Now comes its sequel, equally significant. Dr. Newburger and her collaborators in 7 centers treated by random assignment 276 children with the 4-day infusion of gamma-globulin plus aspirin and 273 children with a single treatment of 2 gm/kg intravenous GG plus aspirin. They found that in the single-dose regimen, children more quickly became afebrile and that they had about half fewer coronary abnormalities at 2 weeks and 6 weeks. Of the 5 children with giant aneurysms, the most dreaded kind, 4 received the 4-day protocol; 1 died.

Overall, the adverse effects of intravenous GG were rare (2.7%) and were transient. The benefits, it is plain to see, are great. The mechanism of action is still unknown, although gamma-globulin appears to cause a rapid down-regulation of the immune response.—M.A. Engle, M.D.

Reference

1. Newburger JW, et al: *N Engl J Med* 315:341, 1986.

Myocarditis

Immunosuppressive Therapy in the Management of Acute Myocarditis in Children: A Clinical Trial
Chan KY, Iwahara M, Benson LN, Wilson GJ, Freedom RM (Hospital for Sick Children, Toronto)
J Am Coll Cardiol 17:458–460, 1991   4–35

Introduction.—There is evidence that acute myocarditis leads to dilated cardiomyopathy, making effective treatment even more important. Immunosuppressive therapy is controversial, and has never been tested on children.

Methods.—The value of steroid therapy was examined in 13 consecutive infants and children seen from 1984 to 1989 with biopsy-proved acute myocarditis. The mean age was 5½ years. All but 1 of the patients had a structurally normal heart. Prednisone was begun in a dose of 2 mg/kg daily and was tapered to .3 mg/kg over 2 months. One patient received azathioprine as well.

Findings.—Twelve of the 13 patients developed congestive heart failure. Repeat endomyocardial biopsy showed histologic improvement in all 8 patients evaluated. Six lacked an inflammatory infiltrate. Two patients continued receiving prednisone. One patient died of persistent low cardiac output and multisystem dysfunction. In surviving patients, heart failure stabilized and resolved within a week of the start of treatment. Ten patients regained a normal ECG a mean of 4.5 months after start of therapy.

Conclusion.—Immunosuppression effectively reduces myocardial inflammation in these patients and improves cardiac function. Two of the present patients relapsed when treatment was withdrawn and again improved when it was reinstituted.

▶ Myocarditis in children has many causes, including "as yet unknown," and has several outcomes that range from full recovery through chronic debilitation to death. Until recently myocarditis has been a clinical diagnosis unless it was verified by postmortem studies. Now endomyocardial biopsy confirms the clinical diagnosis supported by echocardiographic findings.

Whether any treatment, other than supportive, is helpful or hurtful has long been debated. In this uncontrolled clinical trial of 13 sick patients with bona fide myocarditis, prednisone therapy in moderate dosage with tapering until termination at 2 months appeared beneficial clinically in all but 1 patient who died. Repeat myocardial biopsy in 8 substantiated the benefit.

Preliminary reports require confirmation in larger series and by other investigators before the therapy can be adopted, but this study offers some hope of help.—M.A. Engle, M.D.

Pharmacology

The Pharmacokinetics of Captopril in Infants With Congestive Heart Failure

Pereira CM, Tam YK, Collins-Nakai RL (Univ of Alberta, Edmonton)
Ther Drug Monit 13:209–214, 1991   4–36

Background.—In infants with congestive heart disease, drugs may show altered pharmacokinetics because of altered blood flow and maturational changes. The angiotensin-converting enzyme inhibitor captopril is presently used to treat infants with congestive heart failure, but no studies have determined the relationship between drug concentration and effect in these patients. The pharmacokinetic parameters of this drug were evaluated in infants with congestive heart failure.

Methods.—Ten children aged 2 to 15 months received 1 mg/kg captopril orally every 8 hours for 1 week. All patients had congestive heart failure and were being treated with digoxin during the study. Pharmacokinetic and hemodynamic measurements were taken.

Results.—The mean maximum concentration (C_{max}) was 350 ± 184 ng/mL for unchanged captopril, and for total captopril it was 1.088 ± 621 ng/mL. The times to C_{max} were 1.6 ± .4 h for unchanged and 2.7 ± 1.1 h for total captopril. The mean elimination half-life (t ½) was 3.3 ± 3.3 h for unchanged captopril, and it was 3.4 ± 1.0 h for total captopril. Significant decreases in arterial pressure, pulmonary and systemic resistance, heart rate, and respiratory rate were seen 1 hour after administration of the first dose of captopril, although plasma renin activity was not significantly affected. Echocardiography demonstrated decreases in left ventricular diastolic dimension and ejection time 1 hour after the first dose.

Conclusions.—The pharmacokinetic parameters of captopril in infants with congestive heart failure appear to be similar to those reported in adults with congestive heart failure. The acute hemodynamic changes after captopril administration seem beneficial.

▶ When pediatric cardiologists need more than digoxin and furosemide to get a satisfactory improvement in the infants they are treating for congestive heart failure, they often turn to captopril. This study from Alberta, Canada, reports the pharmacokinetic studies in 10 such infants and demonstrates the acute beneficial effects.—M.A. Engle, M.D.

Psychology

Long-Term Psychologic Implications of Congenital Heart Disease: A 25-Year Follow-Up

Brandhagen DJ, Feldt RH, Williams DE (Mayo Clin and Found, Rochester, Minn)
Mayo Clin Proc 66:474–479, 1991   4–37

Introduction.—Accurate screening tools for evaluating the role of psychological factors or personality traits in acquired cardiovascular disease have only recently become available. The psychological status of 463 adults who survived congenital heart disease was examined after 25 years.

Patients.—In 1989, the survivors of various types of congenital heart disease, who had been examined consecutively for growth and development in 1963 at the Mayo Clinic, were contacted for an update on their health status. Patients were also asked to complete the Symptom Checklist-90-Revised (SCL-90-R) and the dependency scale (Dy) of the Minnesota Multiphasic Personality Inventory (MMPI).

Results.—Of the 463 patients contacted, 168 returned completed forms. Of the responders, 144 (90%) reported that they were in good general health. When the results of the SCL-90-R and the Dy were compared with normative data, statistically significant differences indicating psychological stress were found. The degree of psychological stress was unrelated to the clinical severity of the original heart disease. In addition, the overall achievement and occupational status of the respondents seemed clearly beyond that expected in a normal adult population. Thus, the increased psychological stress seemed unrelated to educational achievement. Forty-six responders (27%) believed that they were overprotected in their youth by their parents, suggesting that parental anxiety and attitudes contributed to the increased generalized and nonspecific distress these patients were experiencing in adulthood.

Conclusion.—Despite current good physical health, survivors of congenital heart disease showed an increased level of psychological stress compared with normal individuals. It is suggested that parental overprotectiveness, rather than the degree of incapacity or severity of the cardiac disorder, is responsible for this increased level of psychological stress.

▶ Pediatric cardiologists in general are aware of the importance of considering the patient as a whole person and as a part of his or her family. That we sometimes fall short of our goal—graduating healthy, wholesome adults after our treatment of them because of their congenital heart disease—is indicated by this study. The Mayo Clinic is famous for long-term follow-ups and keeping in contact with patients through questionnaires. That expertise resulted in a survey of 168 patients, aged 24 to 42 years, 90% of whom considered themselves to be healthy. On the same questionnaire, however, their answers implied stress that did not correlate with severity of illness but perhaps was influenced by parental attitudes.—M.A. Engle, M.D.

Cognitive Development of Children Following Early Repair of Transposition of the Great Arteries Using Deep Hypothermic Circulatory Arrest
Bellinger DC, Wernovsky G, Rappaport LA, Mayer JE Jr, Castaneda AR, Farrell DM, Wessel DL, Lang P, Hickey PR, Jonas RA, Newburger JW (Children's Hosp and Harvard Med School; Massachusetts Gen Hosp, Boston)
Pediatrics 87:701–707, 1991   4–38

Moving?

I'd like to receive my *Year Book of Cardiology* without interruption.

Please note the following change of address, effective: _____

Name: _____

New Address: _____

_____

City: _____ State: _____ Zip: _____

Old Address: _____

_____

City: _____ State: _____ Zip: _____

Reservation Card

Yes, I would like my own copy of the *Year Book of Cardiology*. Please begin my subscription with the current edition according to the terms described below.* I understand that I will have 30 days to examine each annual edition. If satisfied, I will pay just $59.95 plus sales tax, postage and handling (price subject to change without notice).

Name: _____

Address: _____

City: _____ State: _____ Zip: _____

Method of Payment

❑ Visa ❑ Mastercard ❑ AmEx ❑ Bill me ❑ Check (in US dollars, payable to Mosby-Year Book, Inc.)

Card number _____ Exp date _____

Signature _____

LS-0907

---

*Your *Year Book* Service Guarantee:

When you subscribe to the *Year Book*, we'll send you an advance notice of future volumes about two months before they publish. This automatic notice system is designed to take up as little of your time as possible. If you do not want the *Year Book*, the advance notice makes it quick and easy for you to let us know your decision; and you will always have at least 20 days to decide. If we don't hear from you, we'll send you the new volume as soon as it's available. And, of course, the *Year Book* is yours to examine free of charge for 30 days (postage, handling and applicable sales tax are added to each shipment).

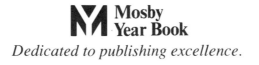

**Mosby
Year Book**

Dedicated to publishing excellence.

Background.—Because mortality rates have declined dramatically for infants who have undergone corrective cardiac surgery, questions about the neurologic and developmental outcome of the survivors have increased. Twenty-eight children who underwent such surgery in early infancy were evaluated to determine whether cardiopulmonary bypass perfusion variables were associated with cognitive function later in life.

Methods.—The children ranged in age from 7 months to 53 months at the time of testing. All had undergone arterial switch operation using deep hypothermic circulatory arrest for the repair of transposition of the great arteries at a median age of 4 days. Circulatory arrest was maintained for a mean duration of 64 minutes. The Bayley Scales were administered to 18 children younger than 30 months of age and the McCarthy Scales were administered to 10 older children.

Results.—Most of the scores were within the normal range, with mean scores of 98.6 on the Mental Development Index of the Bayley Scales and 106.3 on the General Cognitive Index of the McCarthy Scales. There was no correlation between test performance and the duration of deep hypothermic circulatory arrest; however, the duration of core cooling was associated with performance among children whose core cooling periods lasted less than 20 minutes. Shorter cooling periods were associated with lower scores.

Conclusions.—In infants who undergo corrective cardiac surgery, intraoperative events may be associated with subsequent cognitive function. For patients who undergo long periods of deep hypothermic circulatory arrest, some minimum time of cardiopulmonary bypass cooling may be needed to avoid central nervous system injury.

▶ This is a preliminary report on a prospective long-term assessment of cognitive development of children undergoing the arterial switch operation for transposed great arteries. The technique uses cardiopulmonary bypass and deep hypothermic circulatory arrest (DHCA). The group at Boston Children's Hospital is well equipped to carry out this important study. They conclude that, at this time, developmental outcome of the infants may be affected by duration of core cooling before initiation of DHCA.—M.A. Engle, M.D.

Surgery

COARCTATION OF THE AORTA

Repair of Coarctation of the Aorta in Children: Postoperative Morphology
Pinzon JL, Burrows PE, Benson LN, Moës CAF, Lightfoot NE, Williams WG, Freedom RM (Hosp for Sick Children and Univ of Toronto, Toronto)
Radiology 180:199–203, 1991   4–39

Background.—In coarctation of the aorta, resection with end-to-end anastomosis is associated with a significant incidence of re-coarctation. Although modifications have been introduced to avoid this risk, they may be associated with other complications. Therefore, the hemodynamic, clinical, and angiographic data on 215 children who had surgical repair of coarctation of the aorta were reviewed to determine the morphologic sequelae after this operation.

Patients.—The children underwent cardiac catheterization postoperatively during a 13-year period. Two thirds of the 215 patients were boys; the mean age at operation was 1.3 years, and the mean age at catheterization was 5.6 years. The method of repair was resection with end-to-end anastomosis in 45% of the patients, subclavian flap angioplasty in 43%, and synthetic patch repair in 12%. Associated cardiac lesions were diagnosed in 172 of the patients. An aneurysm was defined as a measurement ratio of repair site to diaphragmatic arch that was greater than 1.5.

Results.—Of the patients, 30% had an aneurysm; however, there were no significant differences in the percentage of patients with an aneurysm in the 3 repair groups. Also, 40% of the patients had transverse arch or isthmic hypoplasia or re-coarctation, most often in association with septal defects or obstruction of the left ventricular outflow tract. The patients with transverse arch hypoplasia and re-coarctation had significantly higher pullback systolic pressure gradients at catheterization than those patients who had ratios of transverse arch to diaphragmatic aorta that were greater than .9. Focal aortic enlargement at the site of the repair may commonly be seen at angiography.

Conclusions.—The measurement ratios based on the diameter of the abdominal aorta can predict significant postoperative arch obstructions in children who undergo repair of coarctation of the aorta.

▶ This report of the appearance of the aorta after repair of coarctation of the aorta about a decade earlier by a variety of techniques reminds us of 3 truths. One is that repair of coarctation does not mean "total correction" and normalization. The second is that these patients deserve informed, long-term follow-up. The third is that we should recommend antibiotic prophylaxis at times of potential risk of bacteremia.—M.A. Engle, M.D.

Hypoplastic Transverse Arch and Coarctation in Neonates. Surgical Reconstruction of the Aortic Arch: A Study of Sixty-Six Patients

Lacour-Gayet F, Bruniaux J, Serraf A, Chambran P, Blaysat G, Losay J, Petit J, Kachaner J, Planché C (Paris-Sud University, Le Plessis Robinson, France)
J Thorac Cardiovasc Surg 100:808–816, 1990   4–40

Patients.—Sixty-six consecutive neonates with coarctation of the aorta and marked hypoplasia of the transverse aortic arch underwent resection of the coarctation and arch reconstruction from 1983 to 1988. The mean age at operation was 2 weeks. Associated lesions were present in 80% of patients, and 25 infants had complex intracardiac lesions. More than 80% of the group had hypoplasia of the distal transverse aortic arch (Fig 4–15).

Technique.—The ductus often was divided to gain a better approach to the terminal end of the ascending aorta. The incision of the transverse arch was extended well proximal to origin of the left carotid artery. An extended oblique

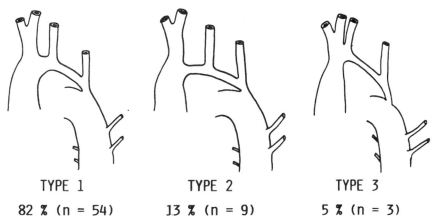

TYPE 1   TYPE 2   TYPE 3

82 % (n = 54)   13 % (n = 9)   5 % (n = 3)

Fig 4–15.—Type 1, hypoplasia of the distal transverse arch; type 2 hypoplasia of both the proximal and distal transverse arches; type 3, absence of the proximal arch and long hypoplastic distal arch. (Courtesy of Lacour-Gayet F, Bruniaux J, Serraf A, et al: *J Thorac Cardiovasc Surg* 100:808–816, 1990.)

anastomosis was performed over the entire aortic arch with 6–0 polypropylene suture material. Pulmonary artery banding was done in 19 infants.

Results.—Postoperative mortality was 14%, but the figure for infants with complex lesions was 28%. There were 6 late deaths, none among infants with simple coarctation. Four surviving infants had prolonged left ventricular dysfunction. Actuarial survival at 5 years was 72%. Recurrent coarctation was diagnosed in 7 patients, 5 of whom underwent reoperation.

Discussion.—This procedure relieves obstruction at the level of the transverse arch. Wide resection of ductus tissue might prevent recurrent coarctation. Preoperative prostaglandin administration is also helpful.

▶ From France comes a good report on the surgical outcome for newborn babies who commonly have cardiac failure with not only coarctation of the aorta but also hypoplasia of the aortic arch. The underdevelopment may occur just proximal to the coarctation or may also involve the transverse aortic arch. More than 75% of the 66 infants had other intracardiac anomalies as well, some quite complex. Considering the severity of the malformation(s), the early mortality rate of 14% is commendable, as is the actuarial survival rate at 5 years of 72% overall but 87% and 88% for simple coarctation and for repair of coarctation plus ventricular septal defect.—M.A. Engle, M.D.

Preoperative and Postoperative "Aneurysm" Associated With Coarctation of the Aorta

Parikh SR, Hurwitz RA, Hubbard JE, Brown JW, King H, Girod DA (Indiana Univ, Indianapolis)
J Am Coll Cardiol 17:1367–1372, 1991   4–41

Introduction.—Postoperative aneurysm formation has been reported as a complication of repair of coarctation of the aorta in 5% to 27% of patients treated surgically and in up to 55% of patients treated by balloon angioplasty. The phenomenon of aneurysm formation after surgical repair for aortic coarctation was better defined by review of the preoperative and postoperative cineangiograms of 65 patients.

Patients.—The mean age of the patients at the time of surgery was 1.5 years. Of the 65 patients, 14 underwent Dacron patch repair, 28 underwent end-to-end anastomosis, and 23 had a subclavian flap repair. Preoperative studies were available for 60 patients. Postoperative studies were obtained a mean of 5.7 years after coarctation repair to evaluate associated cardiac lesions in 46 patients, suspected re-coarctation in 7, and outcome of intracardiac repair for congenital heart disease in 12. Serial postoperative studies were available for 31 patients.

Findings.—Discrete areas of bulging in the anterior aortic wall above the ductus arteriosus were present in 14 (23%) of the 60 preoperative cineangiograms (Fig 4–16). Aneurysmal areas disappeared after end-to-end anastomosis but persisted after Dacron patch or subclavian flap repair. The area of aneurysmal bulging showed no change at follow-up a mean of 4.72 years after operation. Only 3 patients, all of whom had undergone Dacron patch repair, showed significant new changes at the repair site at follow-up. Thus, only 3 (5%) of the 65 patients actually had new aneurysm formation at the surgical repair site.

Conclusion.—The overall incidence of aneurysm formation after long-term follow-up of surgical coarctation repair is only 5%. Aneurysms developed only in patients who had a Dacron patch repair. No new aneurysmal changes were found at the coarctation repair site in the 51 pa-

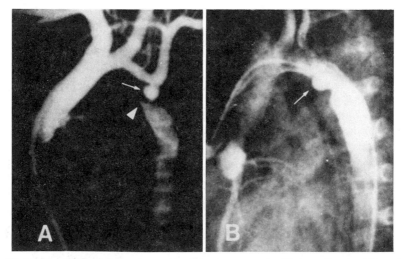

Fig 4–16.—Preductal bulge on preoperative (**A**) and postoperative (**B**) cineangiograms. The preductal bulge is shown by the *arrows* and ductus arteriosus by the *thick arrowhead*. The patient underwent subclavian flap repair; no change was seen in the contour of the preductal bulge postoperatively. (Courtesy of Parikh SR, Hurwitz RA, Hubbard JE, et al: *J Am Coll Cardiol* 17:1367–1372, 1991.)

tients who underwent either an end-to-end repair or a subclavian flap procedure.

▶ Ever since development of the procedure of balloon angioplasty for relief of obstruction in native or recurrent coarctation of the aorta, there has been concern about the occurrence of aneurysm after this controlled damage to the vessel that angioplasty creates. Comparisons with surgical relief of coarctation indicated that sometimes aneurysms were noted in postoperative follow-up. This carefully analyzed report from Indianapolis should do a lot to set the record straight.

The authors compared preoperative and postoperative cineangiograms from 65 young children who underwent surgery that involved end-to-end anastomosis in 28, use of subclavian flap in 23, and use of a prosthetic patch in 14 patients.

Discrete "preductal bulges" were noted in 23% of the preoperative studies (see Fig 4–16) that disappeared after end-to-end anastomosis but not after patch or flap repair. They defined postoperative aneurysm, which was found in 5% of the patients, only after patch repair.

Their review indicated, therefore, that postoperative angiocardiographic evidence of aneurysms was only 5% and that Dacron patch repair was the offender in this series.—M.A. Engle, M.D.

Hʏᴘᴏᴘʟᴀsᴛɪᴄ Lᴇғᴛ Hᴇᴀʀᴛ Sʏɴᴅʀᴏᴍᴇ

Hypoplastic Left Heart Syndrome: Hemodynamic and Angiographic Assessment After Initial Reconstructive Surgery and Relevance to Modified Fontan Procedure
Chang AC, Farrell PE Jr, Murdison KA, Baffa JM, Barber G, Norwood WI, Murphy JD (Children's Hosp of Philadelphia; Univ of Pennsylvania School of Medicine)
J Am Coll Cardiol 17:1143–1149, 1991   4–42

Introduction.—Hypoplastic left heart syndrome, when untreated, is almost always fatal in the first year of life. Techniques of reconstructive surgery for this condition have evolved in recent years, with initial palliation by the Norwood procedure followed by the Fontan procedure. Predictors of outcome in 59 patients with hypoplastic left heart syndrome were reported.

Methods.—During the study period, 135 of 200 infants with hypoplastic left heart syndrome survived the Norwood operation. Fifty-nine of these survivors had elective cardiac catheterization in preparation for a modified Fontan procedure. The hemodynamic and angiographic data for these patients were reviewed, and catheterization data compared for survivors and nonsurvivors of the Fontan procedure.

Results.—The patients had a mean age of 13.8 months at the time of catheterization. All had reconstructive surgery that included either a modified Blalock-Taussig (12) or a central (47) shunt. Most survivors of the Norwood operation had excellent hemodynamic and angiographic findings at the time of postoperative cardiac catheterization. The 50 patients who underwent a Fontan procedure had an early survival rate of 84% and an overall survival rate of 58% (29 survivors). The only factor affecting survival after a modified Fontan procedure appeared to be moderate or severe tricuspid valve regurgitation.

Conclusion.—Initial reconstructive surgery for hypoplastic left heart syndrome should prepare the patient for a successful Fontan procedure. Crucial components of the initial surgery include an unrestrictive interatrial communication, tricuspid valve competence, an unobstructed aortic arch, preservation of right ventricular function, and the establishment of pulmonary blood flow to maintain oxygenation while protecting the pulmonary vascular bed for the subsequent procedure.

▶ From Philadelphia and the group associated with Dr. Norwood comes this follow-up report on the next step for infants with hypoplastic left heart syndrome who survived initial palliation by the Norwood procedure. They analyzed the results of cardiac catheterization in 59 patients before undertaking the next stage in repair. Significant tricuspid regurgitation was the possible predictor of poor outcome that they identified. They concluded that most survivors do have favorable anatomy and function for a subsequent Fontan procedure.—M.A. Engle, M.D.

Transposition of the Great Arteries

Anatomic Correction of Transposition of the Great Arteries With Ventricular Septal Defect: Experience With 118 Cases
Serraf A, Bruniaux J, Lacour-Gayet F, Sidi D, Kachaner J, Bouchart F, Planche C (Marie-Lannelongue Hosp, Le Plessis Robinson, France)
J Thorac Cardiovasc Surg 102:140–147, 1991   4–43

Background.—Infants with transposition of the great arteries (TGA) plus ventricular septal defect (VSD) have had a low rate of survival after a venous switch operation in addition to VSD repair. Improved outcome is reported in a series of 118 patients who underwent combined arterial switch operation and VSD closure.

Patients.—The study group included 75 boys and 43 girls. Their mean age at operation was 3.5 months and mean weight was 4 kg. One hundred had TGA and VSD, and 18 had double-outlet right ventricle (DORV) with subpulmonary VSD (Taussig-Bing heart malformation). The great arteries were in an anteroposterior position or had a mild rightward displacement of the aorta in 95 patients. The great arteries were side by side in 23 patients. Thirty-six of the infants had undergone previous operations.

Results.—The 16 operative deaths (13.5%) were directly related to coronary artery kinking or to the anatomy and size discrepancy of the great arteries. Univariate analysis revealed no significant factor related to early death. All but 2 survivors achieved the mean follow-up of 30.3 months. There were 11 reoperations, 7 for pulmonary stenosis, 2 for residual ventricular septal defect, 1 for recurrent coarctation, and 1 for stenosis of superior vena cava. A permanent pacemaker was necessary in 2 cases. One late death occurred. At 5 years, actuarial survival was 84.5% and freedom from reoperation was 85.7%. All survivors are in New York Heart Association class I, with normal left ventricular function.

Conclusion.—Anatomical repair of complex transposition is a safe method, offering good early and midterm results. If longer follow-up confirms these results, other types of repair may become obsolete. Outcome appears to be better when the repair takes place during the neonatal period.

▶ These authors report a significant experience in France with 118 survivors of the arterial switch operation for transposed great arteries combined with closure of an associated VSD and sometimes repair of other anomalies as well. Not too many years ago, such infants would likely not have survived very long after a venous switch operation plus VSD repair, but the follow-up in this report for 30 ± 24 months is an actuarial survival of 84.5% and freedom from reoperation of 85.7%. Immediate perioperative survival was 86%. Well done!—M.A. Engle, M.D.

TETRALOGY WITH PULMONARY ARTERIES

Pulmonary Artery Morphology and Hemodynamics in Pulmonic Valve Atresia With Ventricular Septal Defect Before and After Repair
Shimazaki Y, Iio M, Nakano S, Morimoto S, Ikawa S, Matsuda H, Kawashima Y
(Osaka University, Osaka, Japan)
Am J Cardiol 67:744–748, 1991   4–44

Introduction.—Patients with tetralogy of Fallot and pulmonary atresia often have structural abnormalities of the pulmonary arteries (PAs). After surgical repair, some of them have pulmonary hypertension and a high pulmonary vascular resistance that cannot be reduced. The purpose of this study was to identify factors predictive of poor postoperative status.

Patients.—Twenty-two patients with pulmonic valve atresia and ventricular septal defect underwent cardiac catheterization and angiography before and after surgical repair. Ten patients had patent ductus arteriosus and 12 had major aortopulmonary collateral arteries, which were ligated in most. All patients had been recommended for restudy because of suspected conduit obstruction or pulmonary hypertension. The patients ranged in age from 1 to 20 years with a mean age of 8.3 years at the time of operation. The mean interval between surgical repair and restudy was 28 months.

Results.—The mean postoperative PA pressure (PAP) ranged from 9 to 92 mm Hg and was greater than 25 mm Hg in 9 patients. Pulmonary vascular resistance ranged from 1.1 to 35.2 units·m² and was greater than 3 units·m² in 11 patients. The number of PA subsegments connected to the central PAs ranged from 22 to 42. Only 55% of patients had all PA subsegments connected to the central PAs. Pulmonary vascular resistance per subsegment ranged from 46 to 774 units·m². Pulmonary vascular resistance correlated with mean PAP. Univariate analysis revealed that the mean postoperative PAP correlated with the number of PA subsegments connected to the central PAs. The incidence of a pulmonary vascular resistance greater than 3 units·m² was significantly higher in patients with more than 36 PA subsegments connected to the central PAs and a preoperative PA area index greater than .5.

Conclusion.—Postoperative PAP and pulmonary vascular resistance in patients with pulmonic valve atresia and ventricular septal defect can be predicted by the PA area at prebranching and by the number of PA subsegments connected to the central PAs as measured before surgical repair. Early palliation to increase PA size and the number of PA subsegments connected to the central PAs to ensure normal postoperative pulmonary hemodynamics is recommended.

▶ From Osaka, Japan, comes a report of cardiac catheterization and angiocardiography in 22 patients. The purpose of the study was to evaluate pulmonary morphology and hemodynamics before and after repair. They found that 12 patients had major aortopulmonary collaterals, with 22 to 42 subsegments connected to central pulmonary arteries. They ligated these collaterals.

The authors found that the postoperative incidence of pulmonary vascular resistance of >3 units/M² was significantly higher in patients who had more than 36 subsegments connected to central pulmonary arteries (PAs). They recommended early palliation to increase pulmonary artery size and the number of subsegments connected to the central PAs (See also Abstract 4–45).—M.A. Engle, M.D.

Analysis of Survival in Patients With Pulmonic Valve Atresia and Ventricular Septal Defect
Hofbeck M, Sunnegårdh JT, Burrows PE, Moes CAF, Lightfoot N, Williams WG, Trusler GA, Freedom RM (Hospital for Sick Children, Toronto; University of Toronto)
Am J Cardiol 67:737–743, 1991   4–45

Introduction.—Pulmonic valve atresia with ventricular septal defect (VSD) is an uncommon congenital cardiac anomaly. Although the results of surgical repair have been well documented, few studies have examined long-term outcome in these patients. The clinical courses and long-term outcomes in 104 patients found in the first year of life to have pulmonic valve atresia and VSD were analyzed.

Patients.—All patients had a large perimembranous outlet VSD. Patients were divided into 2 groups according to the nature of their pulmonary blood supply. Seventy-two patients (69%) had a single ductus arteriosus supplying confluent pulmonary arteries, whereas 32 patients (31%) had collateral pulmonary blood supply provided by systemic collateral arteries (SCAs) alone or in combination with a ductus arteriosus.

Follow-up ranged from 2 days to 13.75 years. Mean follow-up was 4.95 years.

Results.—Atrioventricular discordance was diagnosed in 7 patients. Of the 72 patients with a single patent ductus arteriosus supplying confluent pulmonary arteries, 20 (27.8%) have died, 30 (41.6%) have undergone surgical repair and are alive, 8 (11.1%) are awaiting reparative surgery, 11 (15.3%) are potential candidates for repair, and 3 (4.2%) are inoperable. Of the 32 patients in whom the collateral pulmonary blood supply was provided partially or exclusively by SCAs, 9 (28%) have died, 4 (13%) have undergone surgical repair and are alive, 3 (9%) are awaiting reparative surgery, 8 (25%) are potential candidates, and 8 (25%) are inoperable. The significantly lower chance of undergoing surgical repair in patients with SCAs was attributed to arborization and distribution abnormalities of the pulmonary arteries that were present only in these patients. There was no significant difference in mortality between the 2 groups. The median age of death was 275 days. The estimated overall probability for survival to age 10 years was 69%.

Conclusion.—Patients with pulmonary atresia and VSD have a relatively low risk of death (31%) in the first decade of life. Patients with a ductus-dependent pulmonary circulation have a significantly higher chance of becoming eligible for surgical repair than do patients with SCAs.

▶ This report from the Hospital for Sick Children in Toronto provides valuable information on the diagnosis, surgical management, and follow-up of infants recognized in the first year of life to have this variation of tetralogy of Fallot (pulmonary atresia and ventricular septal defect).

The nature of the pulmonary blood supply influenced the management and the outcome. The larger and the more favorable group (72 of 104 consecutive patients, or 69%) had confluent pulmonary arteries with a single patent ductus arteriosus. The smaller and less favorable group (32 patients) had a pulmonary blood supply dependent partially or exclusively on systemic collateral arteries. Arborization and distribution abnormalities were limited to the latter group, and their chances for successful outcome of reparative surgery were not as good. Overall, the estimated chance of survival to age 10 years for the entire cohort was 69%. (See also Abstract 4–44.)—M.A. Engle, M.D.

Extracardiac Valved Conduits in the Pulmonary Circuit

Sano S, Karl TR, Mee RBB (Royal Children's Hospital, Melbourne)
Ann Thorac Surg 52:285–290, 1991   4–46

Introduction.—Valved conduits in the pulmonary circuit represent one of the weakest aspects in the surgical repair of congenital cardiac malformations because the conduits invariably need to be replaced, either because of growth of the patient or because of valve or conduit failure.

Patients.—During a 10-year period, 141 patients with a mean age of 5.9 years had 169 valved conduits inserted between the heart and the

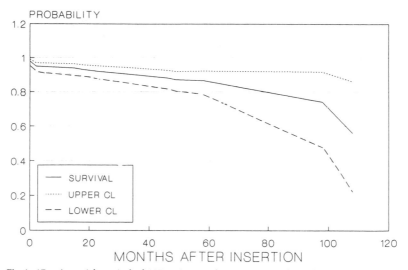

Fig 4–17.—Actuarial survival of 117 patients undergoing extracardiac valved conduit insertion in the pulmonary circuit (including operative mortality). Seventy percent confidence limits (CL) are expressed in broken curves. (Courtesy of Sano S, Karl TR, Mee RBB: *Ann Thorac Surg* 52:285–290, 1991.)

pulmonary artery circuit. Forty-six patients were less than 1 year old. Of 117 patients who had initial conduit placement at this institution, 27 subsequently required 28 conduit replacement. Of 17 patients who had initial conduit placement elsewhere, 15 underwent conduit replacement; arterial continuity could be reestablished without the use of a conduit in the other 2 patients. An additional 9 patients who initially underwent re-

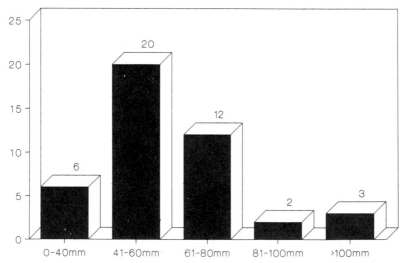

Fig 4–18.—Systolic pressure gradients (mm Hg) across extracardiac valved conduits in 43 patients undergoing conduit replacement. (Courtesy of Sano S, Karl TR, Mee RBB: *Ann Thorac Surg* 52:285–290, 1991.)

pair of tetralogy of Fallot or double-outlet right ventricle elsewhere without use of a conduit were referred for reoperation. All 9 patients had severe pulmonary insufficiency or patch-related aneurysms 51–176 months after operation. Valved conduits were inserted as secondary procedures. The type of valved conduits used varied over the course of the study. Xenografts were used in 126 procedures and cryopreserved aortic and pulmonary homografts were used in 43. Follow-up data were available for 131 patients. The mean follow-up was 41 months.

Results.—There were 6 in-hospital deaths (3.6%) and 7 late deaths (4.1%) out of 169 conduit insertions. All deaths occurred exclusively in the group of 117 patients undergoing primary conduit replacement at this institution. Only 1 of the late deaths was conduit related. Actuarial survival for patients requiring extracardiac valved conduits was 87% at 5 years (Fig 4–17). Forty-five conduits were removed and 43 conduits were reinserted without early or late mortality. The mean systolic right ventricle to pulmonary artery pressure gradient before reoperation in these 43 patients was 52 mm (Fig 4–18). Actuarial freedom from conduit replacement for long-term survivors was 37% at 5 years.

Outcome.—Of the 129 surviving patients, 7 have been lost to follow-up, 6 are alive with mild-to-moderate restrictions, and the remaining 116 patients are alive in New York Heart Association class I or II.

▶ Since the mid 1960s, pediatric cardiologists and cardiac surgeons have been able to recommend a physiologic repair of some complex forms of cyanotic congenital heart disease by use of an external conduit to serve as the pulmonary valve and artery. Early enthusiasm for the procedure was dampened somewhat by the follow-up when it was learned that conduits were outgrown or became obstructed because an internal peel developed and/or the valve deteriorated. The group from Melbourne, Australia, reported on 141 patients in whom 169 conduits were replaced.

Figures 14–17 and 14–18 graphically depict the probability of the patient's survival and the actuarial freedom from conduit replacement more than 80 months after implantation. The authors comment on their current plan of management.

We still have nothing better to offer these patients with their complex cyanotic anomalies, so we will continue to recommend the use of extracardiac valved conduits and take comfort in their good improvement in the early postoperative years and the low operative mortality rate for placement and for replacement of the external valved conduit.—M.A. Engle, M.D.

Fontan

Ventricular Function in the Single Ventricle Before and After Fontan Surgery

Parikh SR, Hurwitz RA, Caldwell RL, Girod DA (Indiana Univ, Indianapolis)
Am J Cardiol 67:1390–1395, 1991   4–47

Background.—Although there have been many modifications of the Fontan principle for the treatment of complex congenital heart disease, there have been no systematic evaluations of the serial changes in ventricular contractile function before and after the Fontan procedure. Therefore, 47 patients with a single ventricle were studied to better define the importance of ventricular function in such patients.

Methods.—The study included 47 patients with a single ventricle who survived beyond infancy and who were followed for more than 20 years. Twenty-four patients underwent a modified Fontan procedure during an 8-year period (age range, 5.5 years–20 years). The other 20 patients were followed for a mean duration of 2.2 years. All patients underwent radionuclide angiocardiography to estimate ejection fraction. The surgical patients were studied at 8 months to 2 years postoperatively. Fifteen patients underwent serial preoperative evaluation of a mean duration of 3.8 years.

Results.—The mean preoperative ejection fraction was .57; this was significantly different from the normal mean left ventricular ejection fraction of .68. There was no significant relationship between ejection fraction and age, ventricular morphology, or the presence of a pulmonary artery band or systemic to pulmonary artery shunt. In the patients who had serial evaluation, there were no significant changes in ejection fraction, although 4 patients did have increased atrioventricular valve regurgitation. Of the 24 surgical patients, 7 died, 1 had undergone cardiac transplantation, and 1 was facing possible transplantation. Survivors and nonsurvivors had no significant differences in postoperative ejection fraction. The functional outcome was unrelated to ventricular morphology, age at operation, and operative factors. The ejection fraction decreased from .52 to .39 at a mean of 1.16 years postoperatively.

Conclusions.—Patients with a single ventricle had a lower ventricular ejection fraction than patients with the normal systemic ventricle. Ejection fraction is unrelated to age or ventricular morphology during childhood, and it frequently decreases after Fontan operation. Until long-term studies of clinical course and ventricular function indicate otherwise, the Fontan operation may still be recommended for these patients.

▶ This sobering study of single ventricular function assessed by radionuclide angiocardiography in 47 such patients and in 24 of them after a Fontan procedure indicates that a single ventricle per se functions less well than a 2-ventricular heart and does not spontaneously change much during childhood. After a Fontan operation, ventricular function frequently tends to decrease.—M.A. Engle, M.D.

Pulmonary Blood Flow After Total Cavopulmonary Shunt
Redington AN, Penny D, Shinebourne EA (Royal Brompton National Heart and Lung Hospital, London)
Br Heart J 65:213–217, 1991   4–48

Background.—The total cavopulmonary shunt procedure is an extracardiac operation for the physiologic correction of the circulation in children with complex congenital heart disease. Anastomosis of the superior vena cava to the pulmonary arteries is usually considered in patients with isomerism of the left atrial appendages and complex associated intracardiac anomalies that preclude biventricular repair. Unlike in the Fontan procedure, the right side of the heart is completely bypassed. Doppler echocardiography was used to study the pattern of pulmonary blood flow at rest in 3 patients who had this operation.

Patients.—The 3 patients ranged in age from 3 years to 14 years at the time of total cavopulmonary anastomosis for left atrial isomerism with complex intracardiac anomalies. All 3 patients had undergone previous surgical procedures. None of the patients had an intrahepatic portion of the inferior vena cava, and the hepatic vein and coronary sinus drained directly to the right-sided left atrium.

Findings.—Doppler studies of the pulmonary circulation at rest revealed a phasic pattern of flow that varied with the respiratory cycle. Pulmonary blood flow increased during normal inspiration and was much augmented by the Müller maneuver, suggesting that blood flow was occurring when a negative intrathoracic pressure was generated. During a brief Valsalva maneuver, blood flowed away from the lungs. A sustained Valsalva maneuver produced a positive intrathoracic pressure, which led to a clinically significant reduction in pulmonary blood flow.

Conclusion.—Respiratory movements after a total cavopulmonary shunt procedure have a major influence on postoperative pulmonary blood flow.

▶ Increasingly, cardiac surgeons are resorting to physiologic repair by total cavopulmonary shunt. This postoperative study by Doppler echocardiography showed how critically dependent pulmonary blood flow is on changes in intrathoracic pressure. For example, flow increases with normal inspiration, and it reverses with sustained Valsalva maneuver. These relationships will be important not only in the early postoperative period, but also in the long-term course.—M.A. Engle, M.D.

Therapeutic/Interventional Catheterization

Radiation Exposure of Pediatric Patients and Physicians During Cardiac Catheterization and Balloon Pulmonary Valvuloplasty
Wu J-R, Huang T-Y, Wu D-K, Hsu P-C, Weng P-S (Kaohsiung Medical College, Kaohsiung, Taiwan; National Tsing Hua University, Hsinchu, Taiwan)
Am J Cardiol 68:221–225, 1991   4–49

Background.—Although the clinical applications and complications of cardiac catheterization have been studied, the radiation hazards have not. The radiation doses to pediatric patients and their physicians during cardiac catheterization and balloon pulmonary valvuloplasty were evaluated.

Methods.—Thermoluminescent dosimeters were applied to various body locations on 61 pediatric patients and their physicians to measure radiation exposure during routine right- and left-sided cardiac catheterizations. Dosimetry also was performed on 4 patients and physicians during balloon pulmonary valvuloplasty. Measurements were taken during chest roentgenography, fluoroscopy, and cineangiography.

Results.—In 22 children, the average skin radiation dose to the chest during precatheterization chest roentgenography was 121 μGy. During 61 catheterizations, the average dose to the chest was 5,182 μGy, and during 4 valvuloplasties, the average dose was 641 μGy. During catheterization, the average radiation to the patient's right lateral chest was equivalent to 83 chest x-rays; the eyes were exposed to .4 chest x-ray equivalents, the thyroid 6, and the gonads .2. Because of long durations of fluoroscopy for balloon pulmonary valvuloplasty, the average skin dose to the right lateral chest was equivalent to 1,037 chest x-rays. The operator performing cardiac catheterization received average radiation doses of 3 μGy to the eyes and 6 μGy to the thyroid. A lead apron reduced body exposure by about 80%, and a thyroid shield allowed a 56% decrease in radiation to the thyroid. The assistant received 1 μGy exposure outside the thyroid shield.

Conclusions.—Balloon pulmonary valvuloplasty of children appears to result in very large doses of radiation. Although all patients had normal leukocyte counts, external appearances, and chromosome studies after 3 to 6 months of follow-up, the number of films or the rate of filming should be reduced whenever possible. The long-term effects of radiation in pediatric patients undergoing valvuloplasty merit further study.

▶ The authors from Taiwan remind us that there are other aspects to new modalities of treatment other than immediate survival and early as well as late hemodynamic improvement. They addressed the matter of radiation received by the patient and the staff while performing the now widely accepted catheterization laboratory intervention of balloon pulmonary valvuloplasty. Based on the risk factor analysis, they concluded that the radiation dose is acceptable, despite the fact that the skin dose to the right lateral chest wall is extremely high—the equivalent of 1,000 chest x-rays!—M.A. Engle, M.D.

Balloon Valvuloplasty for Critical Aortic Stenosis in the Newborn: Influence of New Catheter Technology
Beekman RH, Rocchini AP, Andes A (CS Mott Children's Hosp, Univ of Michigan, Ann Arbor)
J Am Coll Cardiol 17:1172–1176, 1991   4–50

Introduction.—Recent improvements in catheter technology have made successful balloon valvuloplasty feasible in neonates with critical aortic stenosis. The procedure is reported in 8 newborns.

Methods.—The infants all had isolated critical aortic valve stenosis with congestive heart failure and markedly diminished peripheral arterial pulses. Because of technical difficulties, balloon valvuloplasty could not be accomplished successfully in 3 infants who were seen before the improved catheter technology became available. Two of these infants survived after surgical valvotomy. With the new catheter, all 5 infants treated after March 1989 underwent successful transcatheter therapy. A transumbilical approach was used in 4 of the infants. The uninflated balloon has a very low profile and the silicone-coated catheter can easily traverse the umbilical-iliac artery system over a .89-cm guidewire.

Results.—In the latter 5 infants, balloon valvuloplasty resulted in a decrease in valve gradient and improvement in left ventricular function and cardiac output. There were mean reductions in peak systolic gradient (from 69 to 25 mm Hg), left ventricular systolic function (from 128 to 95 mm Hg), and in left ventricular end-diastolic pressure (from 20 to 11 mm Hg). The time from first catheter insertion to valve dilation averaged 57 minutes; median hospital stay was 4 days. At follow-up of 2–16 months, all 5 infants were doing well with no recurrence of severe stenosis.

Conclusion.—Surgical therapy for critical aortic stenosis is associated with considerable morbidity and mortality in newborns. Balloon valvuloplasty using newly available balloon catheters can be performed quickly, safely, and effectively. Should significant stenosis recur, the femoral arteries are preserved for transcatheter intervention.

▶ When any new technique is introduced, later improvements reduce the failures and improve the successes. So it is for balloon valvuloplasty for infants with critically severe aortic stenosis. Credit is given to improved catheter technology that permitted the valvuloplasty to be accomplished quickly and successfully in all 5 infants so treated. Quite remarkably, 4 procedures were accomplished by a transumbilical approach.—M.A. Engle, M.D.

Percutaneous Transluminal Balloon Angioplasty of Stenotic Standard Blalock-Taussig Shunts: Effect on Choice of Initial Palliation in Cyanotic Congenital Heart Disease

Marks LA, Mehta AV, Marangi D (Temple Univ School of Medicine, Philadelphia; East Tennessee State Univ, Kingsport)
J Am Coll Cardiol 18:546–551, 1991   4–51

Background.—Results of balloon dilation of stenotic standard (classical) Blalock-Taussig shunts have been disappointing, possibly because the balloons used have been of insufficient diameter. The procedure was attempted using relatively large balloons in 5 patients with cyanotic heart disease.

Methods.—The patients, who ranged in age from 11 to 67 months, were becoming progressively cyanotic and polycythemic as a result of discrete stenosis of the shunt at the pulmonary anastomosis. Mean hemoglobin was 17.9 g/dL. Balloon dilation of the shunt was attempted using a balloon equal to or within 1 mm of the diameter of the unobstructed proximal shunt.

Results.—Mean diameter of the stenotic site increased from 2.8 mm before the procedure to 5.7 mm afterward. Mean increase was 2.8 mm, or 108.2%, for a range of 2 to 3.5 mm. Systemic oxygen saturation increased from 72.8% to 83.6%. Mean increase in blood oxygen saturation was 10.8%, and all patients had a satisfactory increase. At a mean follow-up of 5.8 months after the balloon dilation procedure, oxygen saturation by pulse oximetry was 85.8% and hemoglobin was 15.6 g/dL.

Conclusions.—Stenotic standard Blalock-Taussig shunts can be satisfactorily relieved by balloon dilation if a balloon of adequate size is used. When the initial shunt is selected, its dilatability should be considered. By prolonging the life of the shunt, this procedure can avoid the complications of replacement shunt surgery.

▶ Palliation is still needed for many cyanotic infants and for some older children with critically decreased pulmonary blood flow. Since 1944 the Blalock-Taussig (BT) operation (subclavian-to-pulmonary artery anastomosis) has been the most effective shunt. In recent years a modification of this shunt has been popular, using a Gortex tube between the subclavian and the pulmonary artery. Most BT shunts, whether classical or modified, become inadequate over time. This paper reports success in dilating the classical BT shunt when it becomes stenotic by use of large balloon catheters equal to or within 1 mm of the diameter of the unobstructed proximal artery. The authors suggest that dilatability of native arteries in a classic BT anastomosis should be considered when a Blalock-Taussig shunt is to be used and a choice is made between classical or modified BT.—M.A. Engle, M.D.

Left Ventricular Mid-Cavity Obstruction After Balloon Dilation in Isolated Aortic Valve Stenosis in Children

Ludomirsky A, O'Laughlin MP, Nihill MR, Mullins CE (Baylor College of Medicine, Texas Children's Hospital, Houston)
Cathet Cardiovasc Diagn 22:89–92, 1991   4–52

Introduction.—The percutaneous transluminal balloon dilation procedure has provided a therapeutic alternative to surgery for obstruction of the left ventricular outflow in cases of congenital aortic valve stenosis. However, a hyperdynamic left ventricle in children can lead to a midcavitary blockage after the balloon procedure. The incidence and clinical course of the postdilation midcavitary blockage was assessed.

Methods.—Thirty-three patients ranging in age from 3 days to 18 years underwent balloon dilation of the aortic valve. A postdilation left ventricular angiogram evaluated each patient for the presence or absence of postdilation midcavitary obstruction, which was then quantitated by echocardiography and Doppler testing. A complete 2-dimensional echocardiogram, with Doppler study, and color flow Doppler examination, was performed 1 day before, immediately after, and 1–3 months after the dilation in all patients.

Findings.—Patients experienced a peak-to-peak systolic gradient across the aortic valve that varied from 55–120 mm Hg before the procedure, and dropped to 0–20 mm Hg immediately after the dilation.

Three children (9%) under the age of 2 years did develop a midcavitary obstruction immediately after the balloon procedure. Color flow Doppler study demonstrated 2 areas of turbulent flow during systole, 1 in the left ventricle and the other in the aortic valve region. The Doppler spectral display of the midcavitary blockage represented a typical dynamic obstruction with a late systolic peak (estimated gradients were between 42–66 mm Hg). The patients had a complete regression of the midcavitary blockage within 3–5 months after the balloon procedure.

Conclusions.—These findings suggest that postdilation left ventricular midcavitary obstruction can occur in children under 2 years of age after undergoing the balloon dilation procedure for severe aortic valve stenosis. The obstruction appears to resolve spontaneously, however, over a period of months after the procedure.

▸ It is well known that after relief of severe valvular pulmonic stenosis, a subvalvular pressure gradient resulting from hyperdynamic, hypertrophied right ventricular musculature may develop and gradually decrease and disappear. These therapeutic cardiologists at Texas Children's Hospital asked whether midcavitary obstruction could develop in the left ventricle after balloon aortic valve dilation. They found that it could, and that it did resolve in 3 (all under 2 years of age) of 35 patients treated in this way and evaluated by echocardiography with Doppler before the ballooning and in follow up immediately and 1 to 3 months later.—M.A. Engle, M.D.

Preoperative Transcatheter Closure of Congenital Muscular Ventricular Septal Defects
Bridges ND, Perry SB, Keane JF, Goldstein SAN, Mandell V, Mayer JE Jr, Jonas RA, Casteneda AR, Lock JE (Children's Hosp; Harvard Med School, Boston)
N Engl J Med 324:1312–1317, 1991   4–53

Introduction.—Surgical repair of muscular ventricular septal defects is riskier than the repair of membranous defects. This is especially true for muscular ventricular septal defects associated with complex heart lesions. Approaching the defect through an incision in the systemic ventricle can produce late ventricular dysfunction. The preoperative transcatheter closure of muscular ventricular septal defects remote from the atrioventricular and semilunar valves, followed by the surgical repair of associated defects, was described.

Patients.—Twelve patients, aged 10 months to 20 years, were selected jointly by a cardiologist and cardiac surgeon for this treatment. Preoperative transcatheter umbrella closure of 21 defects was attempted. Half the patients had associated complex heart lesions. The rest of the patients had undergone pulmonary-artery banding to decrease the amount of left-to-right shunting. Severe ventricular septal deficiency was present in half the cases.

Results.—All defects were closed successfully. There were no major complications. Subsequent cardiac procedures for associated conditions in 11 cases resulted in a mean pulmonary-to-systemic flow ratio of 1.1, which indicates minimal residual left-to-right shunting. The last patient was still awaiting surgery. After a follow-up of 7 to 20 months, none of the patients had died, needed reoperation, or suffered late complications.

Discussion.—These findings confirm the usefulness of a prospective, collaborative approach between pediatric interventional cardiologists and pediatric cardiac surgeons in the treatment of complex congenital heart disease. Such an approach using transcatheter closure followed by surgical repair may reduce the rates of operative mortality, reoperation, and left ventricular dysfunction in children with muscular ventricular septal defects.

▶ Muscular ventricular septal defects that are small cause little physiologic derangement and frequently close spontaneously. Those defects that are large, especially when they are associated with other complex anomalies, are a different situation altogether. Surgical closure, when needed, is difficult and sometimes incomplete. The group at Boston Children's Hospital attempted transcatheter umbrella closure in 12 patients, jointly selected by cardiologists and cardiac surgeons. Happily, they reported that all 21 defects were closed successfully and that subsequent surgery on the associated malformations succeeded in 11 of the 12 patients.—M.A. Engle, M.D.

5 Cardiovascular Function and Noninvasive Testing

Introduction

In this chapter, 60 recently published articles provide clinically relevant information on 13 major subjects concerned with cardiovascular function. Various types of cardiovascular pathophysiology, including experimental cardiac disease and vascular biology, commonly used noninvasive techniques, and new diagnostic and therapeutic approaches are reviewed. A total of 167 additional references are provided at the end of various sections.

In the first section, Myocardial Contractility and Experimental Cardiomyopathy, 8 published articles are discussed and 22 additional references are provided. These concern the estimation of myocardial contractility from end-systolic pressure-volume relations, left ventricular performance resulting from "hibernating" myocardium, the effects of alcohol on left ventricular function, and the pathophysiology of tachycardia-induced cardiomyopathy.

The second section on Left Ventricular Hypertrophy and Diastolic Dysfunction includes comments on 4 abstracted manuscripts and 8 additional references. The pathophysiology of experimental renovascular hypertension is discussed as well as the long-term effects of renal hypertension and genetic hypertension on left ventricular hypertrophy and diastolic ventricular performance. Studies concerning the regression of hypertrophied myocardium with angiotensin-converting enzyme inhibition in rats with genetic hypertension are highlighted.

Ten abstracted articles on Vascular Smooth Muscle and Coronary Vascular Tone and 20 additional references comprise section 3. Abstracted articles discuss the effects of angiotensin II and of cocaine on vascular smooth muscle, the effects of endothelin on mammlian atrial and ventricular muscle, and the effects of various agents on coronary arterial endothelium. The effects of several coronary vasoconstrictors and vasodilators are discussed in the last 3 articles in this section.

In section 4, 4 manuscripts on myocardial ischemia-infarction are reviewed and 28 additional references on this topic are provided. The effects of pacing-induced ischemia on regional myocardial blood flow and left ventricular diastolic properties are discussed and the potential usefulness of troponin T measurements in acute myocardial infarction is detailed. Ventricular remodeling after experimental myocardial infarction

261

and the reduction of infarct size by an oxygen metabolite scavenger are also discussed in this section.

Section 5, dealing with Cardiac Electrophysiology, includes 4 abstracts and 22 additional references. Subjects discussed include the effects of thrombin on cardiac impulse initiation, the mechanism of the pro-arrhythmic effects of flecainide, the relation between sympathetic stimulation and cardiac cycle length, and the electrophysiologic effects of cocaine.

Sections 6 through 12 concern the use of noninvasive diagnostic techniques. Section 6 contains 6 abstracts on myocardial perfusion imaging and 15 additional references on this well published topic. Considerable information concerning thallium reinjection after stress test redistribution imaging, the usefulness of dipyridamole thallium 201 scintigraphy for risk stratification, and the use of intravenous adenosine as a pharmacologic stress test in association with thallium perfusion imaging are discussed.

In the next section, 2 manuscripts on Positron Emission Tomography with four additional references are included. The usefulness of oxygen 15-labeled carbon dioxide inhalation for measuring regional myocardial blood flow is discussed as is the measurement of regional blood flow by nitrogen 13 ammonia in patients with hypertrophic cardiomyopathy.

Section 8 concerns transthoracic 2-dimensional and Doppler echocardiography and consists of 4 abstracted articles plus 15 additional references. The accuracy of the Doppler pressure half-time for quantitating mitral stenosis is discussed, as is the usefulness of 2-D echocardiography for prognostication in emergency room patients with cardiac-related symptoms. The experience necessary to obtain expertise in both stress echocardiography and abnormal echo measurements of left ventricular dimensions in patients with syncope induced by head-up tilt are delineated.

Section 9 includes 4 abstracts and 2 additional references on transesophageal echocardiography. In this section the safety of transesophageal echocardiography is discussed as is its value in detecting noninfective cardiac masses, left atrial appendage function and thrombi, and blood flow in the left anterior descending coronary artery.

Three articles are discussed in section 10, which concerns Intravascular Ultrasound Imaging. The results and possible advantages of intravascular ultrasound as compared with digital angiography of the coronary arteries and peripheral arteries are discussed in this section. One additional reference is provided.

Section 11 concerns exercise and exercise testing and includes 3 abstracted articles and 15 additional references. The discussion includes information concerning the relative sensitivity and specificity of exercise-induced angina versus ST segment depression in the detection of coronary artery disease, the variable thresholds in individual patients on differed occasions for exercise-induced ischemia, and the persistent depression of diastolic function after transient episodes of myocardial ischemia.

The signal averaged electrocardiogram is the subject of section 12 in this chapter. It includes 2 abstracts on the topic and 4 additional references. A comparison of the time domain and the frequency domain analysis of the signal averaged electrocardiogram is discussed, as is a Task Force Report concerning the current status of the high resolution ECG for determining risk in postinfarction patients.

The final section of 4 Miscellaneous topics contains 4 abstracts and 4 additional references. The usefulness of ultrafast CT for assessing right ventricular function is discussed, the nephrotoxicity of nonionic versus ionic contrast angiography is compared, the altered β-adrenergic receptor function in subjects with symptomatic mitral valve prolapse is documented, and the identification of a ouabainlike compound from human plasma is described in this section.

Robert A. O'Rourke, M.D.

Myocardial Contractility and Experimental Myocardial Infarction

Single-Beat Estimation of the Slope of the End-Systolic Pressure— Volume Relation in the Human Left Ventricle

Takeuchi M, Igarashi Y, Tomimoto S, Odake M, Hayashi T, Tsukamoto T, Hata K, Takaoka H, Fukuzaki H (Kobe University, Kobe, Japan)

Circulation 83:202–212, 1991   5–1

Background.—A new method for estimating the slope (Ees) of end-systolic pressure-volume relation (ESPVR) for a single beat of the human heart was assessed. The goal was to provide a reliable single-beat analysis of Ees that could help estimate contractile changes in a less invasive, simpler, and less time-consuming way than conventional methods.

Methods.—Study patients included 25 with coronary artery disease, 2 with dilated cardiomyopathy, and 2 with chest-pain syndrome. Left ventricular pressure was recorded during left ventriculography and peak isovolumic pressure at the end-diastolic volume was estimated by a curve-fitting technique from an isovolumic left ventricular pressure curve. The ESPVR line extended from the estimated peak isovolumic pressure-volume point tangential to the left upper corner of the pressure-volume loop. The slope of this estimated line from the single-beat analysis was compared with the slope of the ESPVR line obtained from 3 pressure-volume loops in 16 patients given angiotensin II or nitroglycerin infusion (Fig 5–1).

Results.—The estimated Ees was 5 ± 2.2 and the conventional Ees was 4.9 ± 2.7. In the 13 patients given dobutamine infusion, the estimated Ees increased from 5.6 ± 1.4 to 7.4 ± 2. The estimated Ees approximated conventional Ees and was sensitive to positive inotropic intervention.

Discussion.—This single-beat method is effective in estimating the slope of ESPVR throughout a physiologic range. Because the estimated Ees was reasonably close to the conventional Ees, the single-beat analysis facilitates assessment of the beat-by-beat ESPVR and the ventricular contractile state of the human heart.

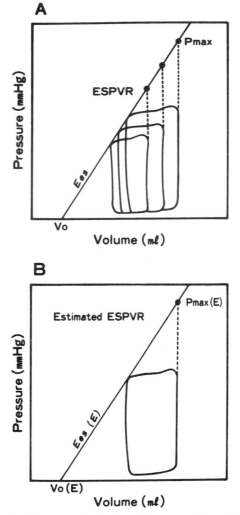

Fig 5-1.—**A**, schematic of the conventional end-systolic pressure-volume relation (ESPVR) line determined by a set of 3 pressure-volume loops. Pmax is the peak isovolumic pressure at end-diastolic volume. Ees is the slope of ESPVR. **B**, schematic of a method for determining the ESPVR line from a single ejecting beat. Pmax(E) at end-diastolic volume was estimated by a curve-fitting technique. End-systolic pressure-volume relation (estimated ESPVR) line was drawn from the Pmax(E)-volume point tangential to the left upper corner of the pressure-volume loop. Slope of this line is the estimated Ees [Ees(E)], and the volume axis intercept of the estimated ESPVR line is the estimated Vo [Vo(E)]. (Courtesy of Takeuchi M, Igarashi Y, Tomimoto S, et al: *Circulation* 83:202–212, 1991.)

▶ During the past decade, the slope of the end-systolic pressure-volume relation (ESPVR) has been used as an index of left ventricular contractility in man and experimental animals that is relatively independent of loading conditions and heart rate. In the above article, the authors obtained the slope of the ESPVR from a single pressure-volume loop in patients and the results obtained during cardiac catheterization correlated well with the conventional ESPVR line that was determined from a set of 3 pressure-volume loops. Also, the estimated ESPVR slope increased appropriately in response to an infusion of a positive inotropic agent. This analysis from a single beat is a simpler method for assessing contractility, with comparable results.—R.A. O'Rourke, M.D.

Nonlinearity and Load Sensitivity of End-Systolic Pressure–Volume Relation of Canine Left Ventricle in Vivo
van der Velde ET, Burkhoff D, Steendijk P, Karsdon J, Sagawa K, Baan J (Leiden University Hospital, The Netherlands)
Circulation 83:315–327, 1991   5–2

Background.—How the end-systolic pressure–volume relation (ESPVR) is used to assess left ventricular contractile performance depends on the shape of the relation and its sensitivity to altered cardiac loading conditions.

Objective.—This study was designed to determine the shape of the left ventricular ESPVR in vivo in anesthetized dogs, and to determine its sensitivity to steady-state changes in arterial impedance induced by an increase or reduction in peripheral resistance. Left ventricular volume was varied by adjusting the height of a reservoir connected to the left atrium, and measured by the conductance catheter method. Nine open-chest dogs were studied, 3 of them before and after the administration of β-adrenergic blockade.

Observations.—In the unblocked state, a second-order polynomial equation gave a better fit for ESPVR than did a linear relation. The volume intercept changed significantly with impedance. The local slope of the relation usually was increased at high impedance, which was produced by occluding the descending aorta, and decreased at low impedance, which was produced by a subclavian–left atrial shunt. Nonlinearity was somewhat less under β-blockade, but load dependency of the ESPVR persisted. The relation between dP/dt_{max} and end-diastolic volume and that between stroke work and end-diastolic volume generally behaved the same as the ESPVR.

Discussion.—The ESPVR is influenced by arterial impedance and therefore is not an ideal index of myocardial contractility. The finding that a positive inotropic effect of shortening, compared with isovolumic contraction is present in the isolated heart suggests that the mechanism involved resides at least partly within the myocardium.

▶ This important study, like several others, indicates that the ESPVR over a wide volume range is affected by changes in loading conditions and that indices of contractility derived from these relations are such that an increase in aortic impedance may be misinterpreted as an increase in contractility.—R.A. O'Rourke, M.D.

Left Ventricular-Arterial Coupling in Conscious Dogs

Little WC, Cheng C-P (Wake Forest Univ, Winston-Salem, NC)
Am J Physiol 261:H70–H76, 1991   5–3

Introduction.—Interaction of the left ventricle (LV) with the arterial system determines stroke work and also significantly influences determinants of myocardial oxygen demand. This study of conscious instrumented dogs was designed to determine the effect of altering coupling between the LV and arterial system on LV stroke work and pressure-volume area.

Methods.—The dogs were instrumented to measure LV pressure and to determine LV volume from 3 ultrasonically estimated dimensions. The LV end-systolic pressure-volume relationship was determined by caval occlusion, and its slope was compared with arterial elastance. The ratio of the end-systolic pressure-volume stroke to arterial elastance (E_{ES}/E_A) was varied by infusing graded doses of phenylephrine and nitroprusside before and during dobutamine administration.

Observations.—Left ventricular stroke work was maximal when the E_{ES}/E_A equaled .99. At constant end-diastolic volume and contractile state, the stroke work was within 20% of maximum when the E_{ES}/E_A was between .56 and 2.29. Conversion of the LV pressure-volume area to stroke work increased as the ratio increased.

Conclusions.—It appears useful to analyze LV-arterial coupling in the pressure-volume plane. In conscious dogs with intact reflexes, stroke work falls substantially only when arterial elastance greatly exceeds the slope of the LV end-systolic pressure-volume relation.

▶ This investigation in conscious, closed-chest dogs demonstrates that the left ventricle and arterial system operate in the range that maximizes left ventricular stroke work. Only when the effective arterial end-systolic elastance greatly exceeds the slope of the ESPVR does the stroke volume fall substantially; also, the conversion of the pressure-volume area to stroke work increases as the relationship between the slope and the effective arterial end-systolic elastance increases.—R.A. O'Rourke, M.D.

Effect of Graded Reductions of Coronary Pressure and Flow on Myocardial Metabolism and Performance: A Model of "Hibernating" Myocardium

Keller AM, Cannon PJ, Wolny AC (Columbia Univ, New York)
J Am Coll Cardiol 17:1661–1670, 1991   5–4

Introduction.—"Hibernating" myocardium is the downward reduction of mechanical function in hearts with chronic left ventricular dysfunction. It is reversible by increasing coronary blood flow. Despite arteriographically significant coronary artery lesions, patients do not manifest angina pectoris, ischemic electrocardiographic changes, or release of lactate into the coronary sinus at rest. A study was undertaken to investigate the relation between coronary blood flow and ventricular function.

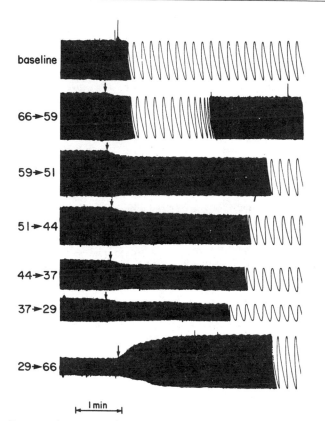

Fig 5–2.—Representative response of myocardial developed pressure to stepwise reductions in perfusion pressure in a paced rat heart. Tracings of function at 25 mm/min (**left**) and 25 mm/s (**right**) of baseline pressure (66 mm Hg) (**top**) and then at each transition of perfusion pressure show that with each change in pressure (*vertical arrows*), an abrupt decrease in function was observed. At medium and low perfusion pressures, an additional delayed (1 to 2 min) decrease in function was seen. After perfusion at the lowest pressure (29 mm Hg), function recovered completely when the pressure returned to its baseline level (66 mm Hg). (Courtesy of Keller AM, Cannon PJ, Wolny AC: *J Am Coll Cardiol* 17:1661–1670, 1991.)

Method.—Experiments were performed in male Wistar rats. Graded reductions in coronary artery pressure were produced in the animals' isolated, perfused hearts. Phosphorus-31 nuclear magnetic resonance (NMR) spectroscopy was used to measure contractile performance and metabolic variables.

Results.—Significant reductions in myocardial oxygen consumption and contractile performance were noted when coronary pressure and flow were reduced. These reductions were reversed to control levels when coronary artery pressure and flow were restored to baseline levels (Fig 5–2). Myocardial hibernation appeared to be associated with 2 metabolic patterns. Modest reductions in coronary artery pressure and flow caused only minimal metabolic abnormality, little or no reduction in creatine phosphate levels, and no significant change in adenosine triphosphate (ATP), pH, or lactate formation. Greater reductions brought about a greater decrease in creatine phosphate and ATP levels and in pH.

Conclusion.—The animal model mimicked the syndrome of hibernating myocardium in vitro, providing evidence in normal hearts for the resetting of myocardial contractile behavior and oxygen consumption in the presence of reduced coronary flow. Contractility and metabolic abnormalities returned to control values when coronary artery pressure and flow returned to initial values, suggesting that the coupling of myocardial contractility and oxygen consumption might be related to oxygen delivery to the tissue.

▶ There has been considerable recent interest in the concept of the "hibernating" myocardium. Various methods have been used to identify patients with markedly depressed left ventricular performance in whom the surgical or mechanical improvement in coronary blood flow results in better left ventricular function. The results of these experiments in isolated perfused hearts, in which heart rate and ventricular volume were controlled, demonstrate that sustained and reversible reduction in ventricular contractility can be produced by reducing coronary artery pressure and blood flow. This study in isolated perfusion rat hearts has considerable clinical relevance.— R.A. O'Rourke, M.D.

Left Ventricular Dysfunction Induced by Chronic Alcohol Ingestion in Rats
Capasso JM, Li P, Guideri G, Anversa P (New York Med College, Valhalla, NY)
Am J Physiol 261:H212–H219, 1991   5–5

Background.—Systematic ingestion of ethanol often is associated with cardiomyopathy, characterized by ventricular dysfunction and heart failure. In vitro animal studies demonstrated depressed contractile performance and marked changes in transmembrane electrical characteristics after alcohol exposure.

Study Design.—Hemodynamic performance of the left and right sides of the heart was monitored in rats that were maintained on a 30% oral ethanol intake for 8 months. Animals were 4 months of age at the outset and were evaluated hemodynamically and morphometrically at age 12 months.

Observations.—Heart weight and left ventricular (LV) weight declined in parallel with reduced body growth in alcoholic rats, but right ventricular (RV) weight remained fairly constant. At end-diastole, RV pressure was increased significantly after 8 months of ethanol ingestion, and LV end-diastolic pressure also increased. The major intracavitary axis increased 25% in alcoholic rats. The ventricular chamber was significantly dilated, and the ratio of diastolic wall thickness to chamber radius ratio was reduced. Overall stress on the myocardium increased substantially. Myocardial structure was preserved, but there were scattered foci of damage in alcohol-treated animals.

Conclusions.—These findings suggest that the constant ingestion of even modest amounts of alcohol may produce myocyte injury and loss, fibrosis, and LV dysfunction. All of these are components of alcoholic heart failure.

▶ With chronic alcohol ingestion, structural and hemodynamic alterations resulted in a 571% increase in the volume of diastolic circumferential LV wall stress. Myocardial damage and ventricular wall remodeling precipitated LV dysfunction. This experimental animal study indicates the sequence by which alcohol ingestion leads to deterioration of myocardial structure and function, leading to heart failure.—R.A. O'Rourke, M.D.

Ethanol Acutely and Reversibly Suppresses Excitation-Contraction Coupling in Cardiac Myocytes

Danziger RS, Sakai M, Capogrossi MC, Spurgeon HA, Hansford RG, Lakatta EG
(National Inst on Aging, Baltimore)
Circ Res 68:1660–1668, 1991   5–6

Introduction.—Ethanol is known to depress myocardial contractility, but the mechanism of its negative inotropic effect is incompletely understood. Advances in isolating Ca-tolerant adult cardiocytes and the acqui-

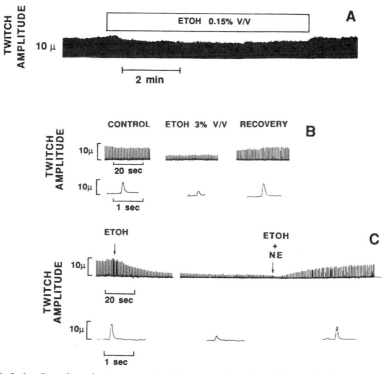

Fig 5–3.—Recordings showing examples of the suppression of the twitch amplitude in single ventricular myocytes by rats of .15% (vol/vol) ethanol (ETOH) (**A**) and 3% (vol/vol) ETOH (**B**) Ethanol was present in the bath during the time indicated. Recovery of contractile function occurs on ETOH washout. C, reversal of ETOH twitch depression by 10 μM norepinephrine (NE). The ETOH concentration was 4% (vol/vol), and it was present during the period between the arrows. (Courtesy of Danziger RS, Sakai M, Capogrossi MC, et al: *Circ Res* 68:1660–1668, 1991.)

sition of Ca-sensitive fluorescent probes provide a means for investigating the cardiac depressant effect of ethanol.

Methods.—The acute effects of .1% to 5% ethanol were examined in adult rat cardiac myocytes. The cytosolic Ca^{++} transient was measured by the fluorescence method during electrical stimulation of single cells. In addition, the Ca^{++} content of sarcoplasmic reticulum was measured in cell suspensions.

Findings.—Ethanol depressed contraction amplitude in low concentration without lowering the Ca transient initiating contraction. Higher concentrations profoundly depressed contraction and also lowered the Ca transient (Fig 5–3). The effects of ethanol were reversed by adding norepinephrine or by increasing the Ca concentration. Ethanol depleted the sarcoplasmic reticulum of Ca^{++} in unstimulated myocyte suspensions.

Interpretation.—Ethanol reversibly depresses contraction in single cardiac myocytes, as it does in intact isolated myocardium and in the heart in situ. It may be that ethanol decreases Ca^{++} binding to myofilaments. The effect of norepinephrine may explain how reflex adrenergic stimulation of the heart compensates for ethanol-induced depression of cardiac function.

▶ This important study using adult rat cardiac myocytes indicates that acute ethanol exposure reversibly depresses contraction in single cardiac myocytes, just as in the intact isolated myocardium and in the heart in situ. At clinically relevant ethanol concentrations, the depressed effects on myocardial function appear to occur as a result of a depression of the myofilament response to calcium.—R.A. O'Rourke, M.D.

Tissue-Specific Activation of Cardiac Angiotensin Converting Enzyme in Experimental Heart Failure

Hirsch AT, Talsness CE, Schunkert H, Paul M, Dzau VJ (Brigham and Women's Hosp, Boston)
Circ Res 69:475–482, 1991   5–7

Introduction.—Recent studies have suggested that tissue renin-angiotensin systems may have a role in the regulation of local tissue function. However, the relative activities of the circulating and tissue renin-angiotensin systems in disease states have not yet been studied. This experimetnal animal study was done to examine the status of plasma and tissue angiotensin-converting enzyme (ACE) activities in compensated heart failure.

Methods.—Compensated experimental heart failure (HF) was induced by coronary artery ligation in 11 rats. Five nonoperated rats and 5 sham-operated rats were also studied. The rats were studied for an average of 85 days after ligation.

Results.—Mean infarct size in HF rats was 37% of left ventricular circumference. Plasma renin concentrations and serum ACE activities did not differ among nonoperated, sham-operated, and HF animals. Cardiac

ACE activities in the right ventricle of nonoperated and sham-operated rats was 50% greater than that in the septum. There was no significant difference in cardiac ACE activity between sham-operated and nonoperated controls. Cardiac ACE activities in HF rats were significantly increased. Right ventricular ACE activity and interventricular septal ACE activity were increased approximately twofold in HF animals compared with nonoperated and sham-operated rats. In contrast to the ACE activities in the heart, pulmonary, aortic, and renal ACE activities remained unaltered in HF rats as compared with nonoperated and sham-operated rats. There was a positive correlation between myocardial infarct size and right ventricular ACE activity. A similar correlation was seen between interventricular septal ACE activity and infarct size. Such a relation was not observed between infarct size and serum or noncardiac tissue ACE activities. Because of the relative paucity of ACE mRNA in cardiac tissue and the small sample size, routine Northern blotting or poly(A) purification of this mRNA was not possible. Harvested RNA was therefore amplified by 25 cycles of polymerase chain reaction. Subsequent quantitation showed a twofold increase in ACE mRNA level that also correlated with myocardial infarct size.

Conclusion.—Compensated experimental HF is associated with tissue-specific activation of cardiac ACE activity, but not plasma or other tissue ACE activities. This finding has potential clinical relevance because increased cardiac ACE activity and increased local angiotensin II concentrations may contribute to the compensatory ventricular remodeling that ultimately causes cardiac dilatation and progressive heart failure.

▶ These data indicate that compensated experimental heart failure in a rat model is associated with tissue-specific activation of cardiac tissue angiotensin-converting enzyme activity, but not with plasma or other tissue angiotensin-converting enzyme activities. The beneficial effects of ACE inhibition may be related to the inhibition of tissue angiotensin II production. Furthermore, increased cardiac ACE activity and increased local angiotensin II concentrations may be responsible for compensatory ventricular remodeling that is eventually responsible for cardiac dilatation and progressive heart failure.—R.A. O'Rourke, M.D.

Effects of Quinapril, a New Angiotensin Converting Enzyme Inhibitor, on Left Ventricular Failure and Survival in the Cardiomyopathic Hamster: Hemodynamic, Morphological, and Biochemical Correlates

Haleen SJ, Weishaar RE, Overhiser RW, Bousley RF, Keiser JA, Rapundalo SR, Taylor DG (Warner-Lambert Co, Ann Arbor, Mich)
Circ Res 68:1302–1312, 1991   5–8

Background.—Angiotensin-converting enzyme (ACE) inhibitors have not been proven beneficial in animal studies of heart failure involving cardiomyopathy. Cardiomyopathic (CM) hamsters have been shown to progress to dilated congestive heart failure. The new ACE inhibitor quinapril was evaluated for its effect on the temporal progression of left ventricular failure and survival in this model.

Methods.—The experimental animals were 146 age-matched CM hamsters and Golden Syrian (GS) hamsters with congestive heart failure. Hamsters were randomized to receive quinapril or vehicle. The treated animals received quinapril in their drinking water in average daily doses of 10.2, 112.4, and 222.4 mg/kg/day. The death of more than 75% of the hamsters in the CM-quinapril group marked the endpoint of the study. Animals were evaluated by isolated perfused heart studies and biochemical measurements.

Results.—Beginning at about 180 days, untreated CM hamsters had progressive deterioration of in vitro left ventricular performance with increasing age. An accompanying decrease in coronary flow and an increase in left ventricular volume were also seen. Quinapril prevented the decline of in vitro left ventricular contractile performance and coronary flow when administered from 180 to 300 days of age. The age-dependent decreases in left ventricular volume were also reduced. Quinapril doses of 112.4 and 222.4 mg/kg/day, but not 10.2 mg/kg/day, exerted the cardioprotective effect. At all dose levels and in both GS and CM hamsters, quinapril significantly inhibited lung ACE activity at 240 and 300 days of age. Significant inhibition of ventricular ACE activity was seen only with the 2 higher doses. From 180 to 390 days of age, 78.3% of the vehicle-treated hamsters died, compared with 27.7% of the quinapril-treated hamsters.

Conclusions.—In an idiopathic animal model of congestive heart failure, chronic quinapril therapy provides significant cardioprotection and markedly prolongs survival. It avoids the decline in in vitro left ventricular contractile performance and coronary flow and reduces the increases in left ventricular volume. Quinapril appears to prolong survival by preventing progression of left ventricular failure.

▶ The results of this study indicate that the chronic administration of an ACE inhibitor prevents the reduction of in vivo left ventricular contractility and coronary blood flow developing in cardiomyopathic hamsters and reduces the usually progressive increase in left ventricular volume. Importantly, chronic ACE inhibition prolonged median survival by approximately one third in this idiopathic model of congestive heart failure.—R.A. O'Rourke, M.D.

Tachycardia-Induced Cardiomyopathy: Effects on Blood Flow and Capillary Structure
Spinale FG, Zellner JL, Tomita M, Tempel GE, Crawford FA, Zile MR (Med Univ of South Carolina, Charleston)
Am J Physiol 261:H140–H148, 1991   5–9

Background.—In both animals and human beings chronic supraventricular tachycardia (SVT) produces a dilated cardiomyopathy characterized by reduced wall thickness and increased left ventricular (LV) wall

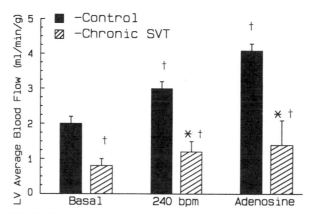

Fig 5–4.—Under basal resting heart rate, rapid atrial pacing, and adenosine infusion, average LV myocardial blood flow was significantly lower in chronic SVT group than in sham controls. (*P<.05). Rapid atrial pacing increased LV myocardial blood flow in both groups from basal heart rate values (†P<.05). However, when LV myocardial blood flow significantly increased again with adenosine in control group (P<.05), there was no significant change in chronic SVT animals. (Courtesy of Spinale FG, Zellner JL, Tomita M, et al: *Am J Physiol* 261:H140–H148, 1991.)

stress. If myocardial blood flow fails to increase to meet the increased demand, ischemic injury may ensue.

Objective.—Myocardial blood flow was estimated during acute pacing-induced tachycardia and during adenosine-mediated coronary vasodilation in conscious pigs. In addition to relating altered LV function to myocardial flow, changes in capillary structure were monitored.

Methods.—Atrial pacing continued for 3 weeks to produce SVT at a rate of 240 beats/minute. Ventricular function was examined by echocardiography and catheterization, and myocardial blood flow was studied by using microspheres. Adenosine was infused at a rate of 1.5 μM/kg/min without pacing.

Observations.—Left ventricular fractional shortening was less in animals with SVT, and left atrial pressure was significantly greater than in control animals. Myocardial blood flow was significantly less in the setting of SVT under resting conditions, with rapid atrial pacing, and with adenosine infusion (Fig 5–4). Under all conditions coronary vascular resistance was higher in the SVT group. Although capillary density was unchanged with SVT, luminal diameter was reduced and the capillary-myocyte distance was increased.

Conclusions.—Myocardial blood flow and coronary reserve are reduced in chronic SVT despite increased oxygen demand. In addition, the capillary structure is altered. These changes may contribute to SVT-induced cardiomyopathy.

▶ In this first of 2 studies on tachycardia-induced cardiomyopathy, the authors demonstrated that an increase in myocardial oxygen demand, a reduction in myocardial blood flow and coronary reserve, and significant alterations in capillary structure may be responsible for the development of tachycardia-induced cardiomyopathy in this animal model.—R.A. O'Rourke, M.D.

Relation Between Ventricular and Myocyte Remodeling With the Development and Regression of Supraventricular Tachycardia-Induced Cardiomyopathy

Spinale FG, Zellner JL, Tomita M, Crawford FA, Zile MR (Med Univ of South Carolina, Charleston)
Circ Res 69:1058–1067, 1991   5–10

Background.—In both humans and animals, chronic supraventricular tachycardia (SVT) produces dilated cardiomyopathy. Recent evidence suggests that hypertrophy and ventricular dysfunction persist after recovery.

Objective.—The precise nature of the remodeling that occurs as ventricular dysfunction caused by chronic SVT develops and after the tachyarrhythmia ends, was studied in swine. Groups of animals underwent atrial pacing at a rate of 240 beats per minute for 3 weeks, pacing followed by a 4-week recovery period, or sham surgery.

Observations.—Supraventricular tachycardia led to reduced left ventricular fractional shortening and increased end-diastolic dimension, with no change in ventricular mass. Myocyte length increased significantly. The ratio of nuclear to myocyte areas increased significantly, but nuclear number did not change with SVT. Both the volume percent of myocytes in the ventricular wall and that of myofibrils within myocytes decreased with SVT compared with controls. In the 4-week recovery from SVT group, dilatation persisted and left ventricular hypertrophy occurred. Myocyte length and width were increased, and the number of nuclei per myocyte increased (Fig 5–5). Total myocyte volume was significantly greater than in the atrial pacing for 3 weeks group and control group, but the volume percent of myocytes and myofibrils returned to baseline after the recovery period.

Conclusions.—Significant myocyte remodeling attends both SVT and . the post-SVT recovery process. Regression of SVT-induced cardiomyopa-

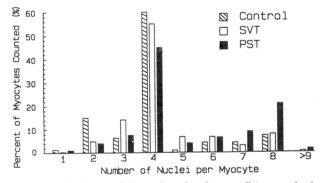

Fig 5–5.—Frequency distribution of the number of nuclei per cell in control, after 3 weeks of chronic supraventricular tachycardia (SVT), and after SVT followed by a 4-week recovery period (PST). Nuclear hyperplasia was observed in the PST group, as evidenced by a significant increase in the number of cells with greater than 4 nuclei ($P<.05$). (Courtesy of Spinale FG, Zellner JL, Tomita M, et al: *Circ Res* 69:1058–1067, 1991.)

thy is associated with both chamber and myocyte hypertrophy as well as with nuclear hyperplasia.

▶ In this study of tachycardia-induced cardiomyopathy, Spinale and associates demonstrate a significant change in myocyte structure and myocardial composition in pigs with left ventricular dysfunction resulting from chronic tachycardia. Termination of supraventricular tachycardia improved left ventricular function but was accompanied by ventricular myocyte hypotrophy. Also, this is the first study reporting that nuclear hyperplasia occurs during the recovery from dilated cardiomyopathy.—R.A. O'Rourke, M.D.

Additional recent publications concerning myocardial contractility and experimental cardiomyopathy are listed as follows:

1. Shoucri RM: Theoretical study of pressure-volume relation in left ventricle. *Am J Physiol* 260:H282–H291, 1991.
2. Santamore WP, Peterson JT, Johnston WE, et al: Variable nonlinearity in end systolic pressure-volume relationships results from interaction between end diastolic and developed pressure-volume relations. *Cardiovasc Res* 25:36–41, 1991.
3. Kass DA, Beyar R: Evaluation of contractile state by maximal ventricular power divided by the square of end-diastolic volume. *Circulation* 84:1698–1708, 1991.
4. Beyar R, Burkhoff D, Sideman S: Force interval relationship (FIR) related to the global function of the left ventricle: A computer study. *Med Biol Eng Comput* 28:446–456, 1990.
5. Toombs CF, Vinten-Johansen J, Yokoyama H, et al: Nonlinearity of indexes of left ventricular performance: effects on estimation of slope and diameter axis intercepts. *Am J Physiol* 260:H1802–H1809, 1991.
6. Adler D, Nikolic S, Sonnenblick EH, et al: Mechanism of sustained mechanical alternans. Effect of variations in ventricular filling volume. *Circ Res* 69:26–38, 1991.
7. Gulick T, Pieper SJ, Murphy MA, et al: A new method for assessment of cultured cardiac myocyte contractility detects immune factor-mediated inhibition of β-adrenergic responses. *Circulation* 84:313–321, 1991.
8. Klitzner TS: Maturational changes in excitation-contraction coupling in mammalian myocardium, in Katz A (ed): *Basic Concepts in Cardiology. J Am Coll Cardiol* 17:218, 1991.
9. Isaaz K, Pasipoularides A: Noninvasive assessment of intrinsic ventricular load dynamics in dilated cardiomyopathy. *J Am Coll Cardiol* 17:112–121, 1990.
10. Hayashida W, Kumada T, Nohara R, et al: Left ventricular regional wall stress in dilated cardiomyopathy. *Circulation* 82:2075–2083, 1990.
11. Kingma I, Harmsen E, ter Keurs, HEDJ, et al: Cyclosporine-associated reduction in systolic myocardial function in the rat. *Int J Cardiol* 31:15–22, 1991.

12. Bauer JA, Fung, H-L: Concurrent hydralazine administration prevents nitroglycerin-induced hemodynamic tolerance in experimental heart failure. *Circulation* 84:35–39, 1991.
13. Danziger RS, Sakai M, Capogrossi MC, et al: Ethanol acutely and reversibly suppresses excitation-contraction coupling in cardiac myocytes. *Circ Res* 68:1660–1668, 1991.
14. Yamada T, Matsumori A, Watanabe Y, et al: Pharmacokinetics of indium-111-labeled antimyosin monoclonal antibody in murine experimental viral myocarditis. *J Am Coll Cardiol* 16:1280–1286, 1990.
15. Zhou X-P, Zhong X-L, Zhu X-X, et al: Electronmicroscopic observation of chronic cardiopathy in spontaneous diabetic biobreeding rats. *Chinese Med J* 103:359–362, 1990.
16. Kagiya T, Hori M, Iwakura K, et al: Role of increased α_1-adrenergic activity cardiomyopathic Syrian hamster. *Am J Physiol* 260:H80–H88, 1991.
17. Wainai Y: Adaptive mechanisms of the aorta and left ventricle to volume overloading following abrupt aortic regurgitation in rabbits. *Cardiovasc Res* 25:463–467, 1991.
18. Carabello BA, Nakano K, Ishihara K, et al: Coronary blood flow in dogs with contractile dysfunction due to experimental volume overload. *Circulation* 83:1063–1075, 1991.
19. Nakano K, Swindle MM, Spinale F, et al: Depressed contractile function due to canine mitral regurgitation improves after correction of the volume overload. *J Clin Invest* 87:2153–2161, 1991.
20. Arnold L, McGrath BP, Johnston CI: Vasopressin and angiotensin II contribute equally to the increased afterload in rabbits with heart failure. *Cardiovasc Res* 25:68–72, 1991.
21. Hano O, Mitsuoka T, Matsumoto Y, et al: Arrhythmogenic properties of the ventricular myocardium in cardiomyopathic Syrian hamster, BIO 14.6 strain. *Cardiovasc Res* 25:49–57, 1991.
22. Cumming DVE, Pattison CW, Lovegrove CA, et al: Biochemical and structural adaptation of autologous skeletal muscle used for counterpulsation. *Int J Cardiol* 30:181–190, 1991.

Left Ventricular Hypertrophy and Diastolic Function

Changes in Diastolic Cardiac Function in Developing and Stable Perinephritic Hypertension in Conscious Dogs

Gelpi RJ, Pasipoularides A, Lader AS, Patrick TA, Chase N, Hittinger L, Shannon RP, Bishop SP, Vatner SF (Harvard Med School; Brigham and Women's Hosp, Boston; New England Regional Primate Research Ctr, Southborough, Mass)
Circ Res 68:555–567, 1991   5–11

Introduction.—Recent studies of the development of hypertension have focused on the passive diastolic properties of the myocardium during this time. Early and late diastolic function in hypertension development was investigated in dogs to determine whether these 2 stages differ.

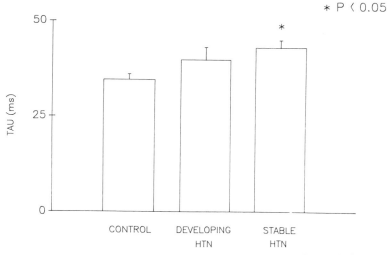

Fig 5–6.—Bar graph shows isovolumic relaxation time constant (TAU) in the 3 studied groups: control, dogs studied before the induction of perinephritic hypertension (HTN); developing HTN, dogs from the control group studied early (2–4 weeks) in the development of perinephritic hypertension; stable HTN, separate group of dogs studied later (at about 14 weeeks) in the development of perinephritic HTN. Compared with controls, tau increased significantly only in stable hypertension. (Courtesy of Gelpi RJ, Pasipoularides A, Lader AS, et al: *Circ Res* 68:555–567, 1991.)

Methods.—Aortic and left atrial blood pressures were assessed with implanted catheters and measured with strain-gauge manometers. Regional myocardial blood flow was recorded with isotopically labeled microsphere in 5 sham-operated dogs, in 7 animals before and after hypertension development, and in 5 animals during stable hypertension (late hypertension, about 14 weeks). The dogs were monitored 2–3 weeks after instrumentation and 2–4 weeks after nephrectomy. Nine dogs were studied with graded doses of phenylephrine while normotensive and then 2–4 weeks after nephrectomy.

Results.—Significant increases were found in left ventricular (LV) plus septum mass or in body weight ratios in animals with developing or stable hypertension. During developing hypertension, significant increases occurred in LV end-diastolic pressure and in LV end-diastolic stress. Peak filling rate and passive myocardial stiffness rose significantly. The isovolumic relaxation time constant also rose, but not significantly (Fig 5–6). In animals with stable hypertension, the LV end-diastolic pressure and end-diastolic stress, as well as the peak filling rate, returned to normal, but the isovolumic relaxation time constant was significantly elevated. Hypertension did not affect the endocardial and epicardial blood flows per unit of myocardial weight. Histologic studies showed that stainable connective tissue did not increase in dogs with stable hypertension compared with controls, and hydroxyproline levels did not rise in the subendomyocardium, the midmyocardium, or the subepimyocardium of animals afflicted with chronic perinephritic hypertension.

Conclusions.—These findings indicate that major changes in diastolic function, which are related to changes in LV systolic and diastolic wall stresses, occur during the development of hypertension. Stable hypertension produced normalization of the myocardial and chamber stiffness.

▶ This study is a logical extension of this laboratory's previous work in conscious dogs with left ventricular hypertrophy caused by 1-wrap, 1 kidney renal hypertension. Interestingly, the authors demonstrated major alterations in diastolic function during the development of hypertension that could be attributed to changes in systolic and diastolic left ventricular wall stresses. However, with more stable hypertension, myocardial and chamber stiffness normalized, and only the isovolumic relaxation time was modestly prolonged. Interestingly, quantitative histopathologic evaluation and hydroxyproline determination in 8 dogs with stable hypertension compared with control dogs did not demonstrate increased connective tissue in the myocardium. The failure to detect significant increases in collagenous connective tissue in these dogs differs from studies of hypertensive primates previously reported by other investigators and abstracted in the 1989 YEAR BOOK OF CARDIOLOGY (1).—R.A. O'Rourke, M.D.

Reference

1. Weber KT, et al: *Circ Res* 62:757–765, 1988.

Hypertrophy, Fibrosis and Diastolic Dysfunction in Early Canine Experimental Hypertension
Douglas PS, Tallant B (Hosp of the Univ of Pennsylvania, Philadelphia)
J Am Coll Cardiol 17:530–536, 1991   5–12

Introduction.—Left ventricular hypertrophy from pressure overload is related to diastolic abnormalities of relaxation and compliance. Such functional problems have been associated with increased fibrosis and pathologic hypertrophy. The relationship between fibrosis, hypertrophy, and diastolic performance was examined in early hypertension as observed in a canine model.

Methods.—Thirty mongrel dogs were studied: 18 controls and 12 animals who had experimental left ventricular (LV) hypertrophy. After institution of perinephritic hypertension, blood pressure increased from 148 to 235 mm Hg, accompanied by raises in every index of hypertrophy such as posterior wall thickness, LV mass, and relative wall thickness. Two-dimensional guided M-mode echocardiograms and ultrasonograms were performed on the left ventricle. All 12 hypertensive dogs and 10 controls underwent midline sternotomy for invasive testing.

Results.—Serial Doppler sonograms of LV filling showed that the hypertensive dogs had a significant increase in the rapid filling velocity/ atrial filling velocity ratio. The hypertensive dogs had significantly higher subendocardial and subepicardial muscle fiber diameters than did controls. The percent of fibrosis did not differ significantly between the 2 groups of animals, however. A significant inverse correlation was observed between the peak filling rate and the overall fiber size.

Conclusions.—These findings show that diastolic dysfunction can develop in dogs with early pressure overload hypertrophy without significant fibrosis. The increased size of myocytes was related to the abnormalities of relaxation and filling but not compliance.

▶ In this group of dogs with perinephritic hypertension and experimental left ventricular hypertrophy studied at 12 weeks after nephrectomy, diastolic function was impaired but neither chamber stiffness nor passive elastic stiffness was increased. At postmortem examination, there was no increase in left ventricular fibrosis as compared with control dogs, although there was an increase in myocyte size.—R.A. O'Rourke, M.D.

Impaired Diastolic Function and Coronary Reserve in Genetic Hypertension: Role of Interstitial Fibrosis and Medial Thickening of Intramyocardial Coronary Arteries
Brilla CG, Janicki JS, Weber KT (Univ of Missouri-Columbia)
Circ Res 69:107–115, 1991   5–13

Background.—In rats with genetic hypertension, abnormalities in myocardial stiffness and impaired coronary reserve may involve a structural remodeling of the myocardium that includes an interstitial and perivascular fibrosis, myocyte hypertrophy, or medial wall thickening of the intramyocardial coronary arteries. The cause of these functional defects is unknown.

Methods.—Rats with established hypertension and left ventricular hypertrophy (LVH) were treated for 12 weeks with low-dose orally administered lisinopril (the SLO group) to sustain hypertension and LVH or

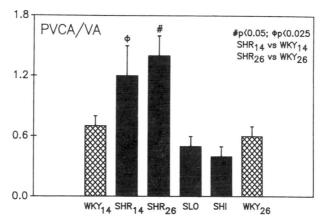

Fig 5–7.—Bar graph showing perivascular collagen area of intramyocardial coronary arteries normalized to vessel luminal area (PVCA/VA). Perivascular collagen was significantly increased in untreated 14- and 26-week-old spontaneously hypertensive rats (SHR$_{14}$ and SHR$_{26}$, respectively). In spontaneously hypertensive rats treated with either low or high doses of lisinopril (SLO and SHI, respectively), perivascular collagen was restored to levels seen in 14- and 26-week-old normotensive Wistar-Kyoto rats (WKY$_{14}$ and WKY$_{26}$, respectively). (Courtesy of Brilla CG, Janicki JS, Weber KT: *Circ Res* 69:107–115, 1991.)

high-dose orally administered lisinopril (the SHI group) to normalize arterial pressure and myocardial mass.

Results.—Compared with controls, the SHI group showed normalization of blood pressure and complete regression of LVH, and the SLO group showed no significant blood pressure or LVH reduction. Both the SHI and the SLO groups showed complete regression of myocardial interstitial and perivascular fibrosis associated with normalization of diastolic stiffness. Regression of the medial wall thickening of intramyocardial coronary arteries with accompanying normalization of coronary vasodilator reserve to adenosine was found only in the SHI group (Fig 5–7).

Conclusion.—In genetic hypertension, interstitial fibrosis and not LVH is responsible for abnormal myocardial diastolic stiffness. Coronary vasodilator reserve is dependent on the medial wall thickening of intramyocardial resistance vessels, which is influenced by arterial pressure.

▶ In this study of 14-week-old spontaneously hypertensive rats with established hypertension, the investigators were able to normalize arterial pressure and myocardial mass in those treated with a high-dose oral angiotensin-converting enzyme (ACE) inhibitor (lisinopril). This was associated with complete regression of myocardial interstitial and perivascular fibrosis and with regression of medial wall thickening of intramyocardial coronary arteries. The authors conclude that interstitial fibrosis and not left ventricular hypertrophy is responsible for abnormal myocardial diastolic stiffness, whereas medial wall thickening of intramyocardial resistance is associated with impaired coronary reserve. In this animal model, regression in left ventricular hypertrophy did not occur until left ventricular systolic pressure had been reduced by high-dose ACE inhibitor.—R.A. O'Rourke, M.D.

Cardioreparative Effects of Lisinopril in Rats With Genetic Hypertension and Left Ventricular Hypertrophy
Brilla CG, Janicki JS, Weber KT (Univ of Chicago)
Circulation 83:1771–1779, 1991   5–14

Background.—Genetic and acquired hypertension are characterized by structural remodeling of the nonmyocyte compartment of the myocardium. This constitutes a major determinant of pathologic hypertrophy that leads to ventricular dysfunction. The usefulness of angiotensin-converting enzyme inhibition in reversing such interstitial and vascular remodeling was assessed in rats.

Methods.—Fourteen-week-old male rats with genetic spontaneous hypertension and established left ventricular hypertrophy were treated with orally administered lisinopril for 12 weeks. Average dose was 15 mg/kg/day. Fourteen-week-old baseline and 26-week-old untreated genetic spontaneous hypertension and age- and sex-matched Wistar-Kyoto rats were also studied as controls. In the isolated heart, myocardial stiffness and coronary vascular reserve to adenosine were studied. Morphometric analysis of myocardial collagen and intramural coronary artery architecture was also done.

Results.—Left ventricular hypertrophy regressed and blood pressure normalized in rats treated with lisinopril. Interstitial collagen fraction decreased from 7% to 3.2%, reflecting complete regression of interstitial fibrosis. Myocardial stiffness constant normalized from 19.5 to 13.7, and intramural coronary artery remodeling reversed, with the ratio of perivascular fibrosis to vessel lumen size decreasing from 1.4 to .4 and medial thickening decreasing from 12.3 to 7.4 μm. Coronary vasodilator response to adenosine was also restored.

Conclusions.—Angiotensin-converting enzyme inhibition by lisinopril has cardioreparative properties that may reverse left ventricular dysfunction in hypertensive heart disease. The nature of the cardioreparative process will vary according to the cause of the remodeling and hypertrophy. Further study is therefore needed to discover the pathogenetic mechanisms.

▶ This article provides additional information by the authors of Abstract 5–13 concerning ACE inhibition in rats with genetic hypertension resulting in left ventricular hypertrophy. With control of hypertension they were able to regress completely myocardial fibrosis and restore interstitial and perivascular collagen to that in a nonhypertensive control group. This response is somewhat different from that reported in rats with renal vascular hypertension (1). The results of therapy with the ACE inhibitor has clinical implications for patients who develop symptomatic heart failure secondary to left ventricular hypertrophy resulting from chronic systemic hypertension.—R.A. O'Rourke, M.D.

Reference

1. Sens DA, et al: *Am J Physiol* 240:H408–H412, 1981.

Additional important studies concerning left ventricular hypertrophy and its effect on diastolic function published recently are listed below:

1. Mann DL, Urabe Y, Kent RL, et al: Cellular versus myocardial basis for the contractile dysfunction of hypertrophied myocardium. *Circ Res* 68:402–415, 1991.
2. Takemura G, Fujiwara H, Mukoyama M, et al: Expression and distribution of atrial natriuretic peptide in human hypertrophic ventricle of hypertensive hearts and hearts with hypertrophic cardiomyopathy. *Circulation* 83:181–190, 1991.
3. Chen L, Vatner DE, Vatner SF, et al: Decreased mRNA levels accompany the fall in $G_{s\alpha}$ and adenylyl cyclase activities in compensated left ventricular hypertrophy. *J Clin Invest* 87:293–298, 1991.
4. Shannon RP, Gelpi RJ, Hittinger L, et al: Inotropic response to norepinephrine is augmented early and maintained late in conscious dogs with perinephritic hypertension. *Circ Res* 68:543–554, 1991.
5. Bache RJ, Homans DC, Dai X-Z: Adrenergic vasoconstriction limits

coronary blood flow during exercise in hypertrophied left ventricle. *Am J Physiol* 260:H1489–H1494, 1991.

6. Frohlich ED, Sasaki O: Dissociation of changes in cardiovascular mass and performance with angiotensin-converting enzyme inhibitors in Wistar-Kyoto and spontaneously hypertensive rats. *J Am Coll Cardiol* 16:1429–1499, 1990.

7. Fein FS, Cho S, Malhotra A, et al: Beneficial effects of diltiazem on the natural history of hypertensive diabetic cardiomyopathy in rats. *J Am Coll Cardiol* 18:1406–1407, 1991.

8. Dumesnil JG, Gaudreault G, Honos GN, et al: Use of Valsalva maneuver to unmask left ventricular diastolic function abnormalities by Doppler echocardiography in patients with coronary artery disease or systemic hypertension. *Am J Cardiol* 68:515–519, 1991.

Vascular Smooth Muscle and Coronary Vascular Tone

Mechanisms of Angiotensin II- and Arginine Vasopressin-Induced Increases in Protein Synthesis and Content in Cultured Rat Aortic Smooth Muscle Cells: Evidence for Selective Increases in Smooth Muscle Isoactin Expression

Turla MB, Thompson MM, Corjay MH, Owens GK (Univ of Virginia, Charlottesville)
Circ Res 68:288–299, 1991   5–15

Background.—Studies of arteries from humans and animals with hypertension show that they have a greater amount of smooth muscle cell (SMC) mass than those who are normotensive. Previous research indicates that angiotensin II (Ang II) and arginine vasopressin (AVP) act as hypertrophic agents in cultures of rat aortic smooth muscle cells. The major proteins that result from Ang II-induced and AVP-induced hypertrophic cells and the results of the initial molecular mechanism experiments were examined.

Methods.—Rat thoracic aortic SMCs were isolated and cultured. Protein and actin content studies were conducted by SDS-polyacrylamide gel electrophoresis (SDS-PAGE). Isoactins and vimentin were detected using IEF-PAGE, the SM α-actin mRNA was measured using specific probes and Northern blot hybridization.

Findings.—Induction of smooth muscle cell hypertrophy by Ang II and/or AVP led to large raises in many cellular proteins resolved on 1- and 2-dimensional gel electrophoresis. Many of these increases were much greater than those expected by the overall cellular protein content and included a twofold to threefold increase in actin, a 2.5-fold to sevenfold increase in vimentin, a threefold to sixfold increase in tropomyosin, and an overall increase in myosin heavy chain. The smooth muscle α-actin mRNA also increased by 5–8 times the normal amount.

Implications.—These results indicate that Ang II-induced and/or AVP-induced SMC hypertrophy is related to a selective but large increase in the cellular proteins; thus agonist-induced hypertrophy may not be caused by translation alone. The findings suggest that agonists may initiate general alterations in protein synthesis by control of the translation process, leading to an overall increase in smooth muscle-specific contractile proteins.

▶ This mechanistic study indicates that Ang II-induced and/or arginine vasopressin-induced smooth muscle cell hypertrophy, as occurs in arteries from hypertensive patients, is associated with large increases in many cellular proteins. This study demonstrates the usefulness of molecular biology techniques to determine the sequence of events responsible for pathologic changes observed in patients with naturally occurring disease.—R.A. O'Rourke, M.D.

Angiotensin II Causes Vascular Hypertrophy in Part by a Non-Pressor Mechanism
Griffin SA, Brown WCB, MacPherson F, McGrath JC, Wilson VG, Korsgaard N, Mulvany MJ, Lever AF (Western Infirmary, Glasgow, Scotland; University of Glasgow, Scotland; Aarhus University, Aarhus, Denmark)
Hypertension 17:626–635, 1991   5–16

Background.—In low doses, angiotensin II (Ang II) slowly increases blood pressure. Both mitogenic and trophic effects are seen on in vitro testing on vascular smooth muscle cells, but it is unknown whether these effects occur in vivo. Experiments were done in rats to determine whether slow pressor infusion of angiotensin results in vascular hypertrophy and whether hypertrophy is induced by pressure.

Methods.—Male Sprague-Dawley rats had subcutaneous infusion of Ang II, 200 ng/kg/minute by minipump for 10–12 days. Three experiments were done. The first was designed to determine the effects on arterial pressure and plasma concentrations of Ang II and renin. In the second experiment, changes in the isolated-perfused mesenteric circulation after Ang II infusion were assessed. In the third experiment, vessel myography was done after Ang II infusion with and without a pressor response.

Results.—In experiment 1, systolic blood pressure gradually rose from 143 to 208 mm Hg after Ang II infusion. Plasma renin was significantly suppressed and plasma Ang II was nonsignificantly increased. In experiment 2, rats that received a slow pressor infusion of Ang II had enhanced vasoconstrictor responses to norepinephrine, vasopressin, and potassium chloride. Response sensitivity was unaltered. These findings suggested that vascular hypertrophy developed. In experiment 3, systolic blood pressure and heart weight were increased by Ang II. Myographic changes of vascular hypertrophy in the mesenteric circulation and increasing media width, media cross-sectional area, and media/lumen ratio were also seen. The pressure increase but not the vascular changes were prevented by hydralazine. Independent of hydralazine, Ang II significantly increased media width, media cross-sectional area, and media/lumen ratio.

Conclusions.—Given in low doses for 10 days, Ang II raises arterial pressure in rats, resulting in changed structure of the resistance vessels and increased cardiac weight. Increased pressure probably causes the cardiac effect, but the structural vascular alteration probably results at least partly from a nonpressor action.

▶ This study, relevant to the previous topic, indicates that a slow pressor infusion of Ang II produces hypertrophy of smooth muscle cells in the mesentery circulation. Although not completely elucidated, the structural vascular changes appear to result at least partially from a nonpressor action of Ang II, and this mechanism needs further definition.—R.A. O'Rourke, M.D.

Effects of Cocaine on Excitation-Contraction Coupling of Aortic Smooth Muscle From the Ferret
Egashira K, Morgan KG, Morgan JP (Beth Israel Hosp; Harvard Med School, Boston)
J Clin Invest 87:1322–1328, 1991   5–17

Background.—Cocaine alters vascular tone by a mechanism that is not completely understood. Isolated ferret aorta was used in a study to determine the effects of cocaine on excitation-contraction coupling.

Methods.—Tissue strips from the thoracic aorta of adult male ferrets were attached to a force transducer. Some animals received pretreatment with reserpine before killing. Transmural nerve stimulation was done in selected tissues, and intracellular calcium was measured with aequorin.

Results.—Cocaine induced a dose-dependent contractile response in concentrations of 10^{-4} M or less. Control muscle had a significantly greater response than that from ferrets pretreated with reserpine. Endothelial factors had no effect on cocaine-induced contraction, but pretreatment with prazosin, 10^{-7} M, significantly inhibited contraction. Intracellular calcium rose with cocaine-induced contraction. Contraction decreased after cocaine concentrations of 10^{-3} M or greater, and aequorin luminescence remained above the levels before 10^{-6} M of cocaine. In control muscles, but not in muscle from ferrets who receive reserpine, the dose-response relationships of norepinephrine and sympathetic nerve stimulations were enhanced by 10^{-6} M of cocaine.

Conclusions.—In studies of ferret aortic smooth muscle, cocaine concentrations of 10^{-4} M or less cause vascular contraction, probably because of its presynaptic action and consequent rise in intracellular calcium. Concentrations of 10^{-3} M or greater reduce muscle tone by decreasing the calcium sensitivity of the contractile proteins. The drug's action on adrenergic nerve endings mediates supersensitivity to norepinephrine.

▶ There is increasing interest and experience with the cardiovascular complications associated with the use of cocaine, including acute myocardial ischemia and/or infarction. In this study, cocaine-induced increases in vascular tone do not differ in vessels with or without endothelial cells, indicating that cocaine-induced contraction is not dependent on endothelial factor(s). It also indicated that cocaine-induced supersensitivity to norepinephrine is the result solely of cocaine's action on adrenergic nerve endings. Although not directly transferable to patients using cocaine for recreational use, this study provides information on the mechanisms underlying cocaine-induced changes in vascular tone and provides experimental information that partially explains the pathophysiology of cocaine-related cardiovascular complications.—R.A. O'Rourke, M.D.

Endothelin and Increased Contractility in Adult Rat Ventricular Myocytes: Role of Intracellular Alkalosis Induced by Activation of the Protein Kinase C-Dependent Na$^+$-H$^+$ Exchanger

Krämer BK, Smith TW, Kelly RA (Brigham and Women's Hosp, Boston; Harvard Med School)
Circ Res 68:269–279, 1991   5–18

Introduction.—The contractile nature of the myocardium under normal conditions has been thought to be governed by the mechanical loading capabilities of the muscle fibers and the amount of autonomic nervous system activation. Endothelin, the 21-amino acid vasoactive peptide, is one of the most potent positive inotropic agents. However, endothelin's activation mechanism that produces a positive inotropic effect in cardiac myocytes is unknown. Whether the apparent sensitization of cardiac myofilaments to intracellular calcium is related to an increase in intracellular pH (pH$_i$) in adult rat cardiac myocytes or to an increase in sarcoplasmic pH was investigated.

Methods.—Calcium-tolerant isolated ventricular cells were extracted from the hearts of male Sprague-Dawley rats and cultured. Contractility measurements were made on an inverted phase-contrast microscope. Freshly isolated adult ventricular myocytes underwent loading with a pH-sensitive fluorescent dye, so that any changes in these cells' pH could be measured with a dual excitation spectrofluorometer.

Results.—Then endothelin increased contractility in isolated rat ventricular myocytes, with a maximal response occurring after 7 minutes. The EC$_{50}$ was at about 50 pM in all cells. The maximal increase in pH in the ventricular myocytes bathed in superfusion buffer at pH 7.4 correlated with the maximal increase in contractility at 1 nM. Extracellular alkalinization resulted in a marked rise in contractile amplitude but with little or no decrease in the contractility at a pH$_o$ of 6.9. Amiloride applied alone did not influence the pH$_i$ of the cells, thus reducing the inotropic response by 45%. Myocyte contractility in amiloride-pretreated cells increased when combined with intracellular alkalinization that had been induced by a superfusion with buffer containing NH$_4$Cl. After washout of the NH$_4$Cl, the contractile amplitude decreased in the amiloride-pretreated cells, both with or without endothelin. High concentrations of ouabain alone produced initial rises in the myocyte contractile amplitude. Pretreatment of the myocyte cells with pertussis toxin partially lowered the intracellular alkalinization induced by the peptide.

Conclusions.—These findings indicate a positive inotropic action by endothelin, which is produced partially from stimulation of the sarcolemmal Na^+-H^+ exchanger by a protein kinase C-mediated pathway. This results in the increase in pH_i and in the sensitization of myofilaments in the heart to intracellular Ca^{2+}.

▶ Endothelin, a potent vasoconstrictor peptide derived from media-bathing endothelial cell cultures, is a strong positive inotropic agent on mammalian atrial and ventricular muscle. This study indicates that the positive inotropic effect of endothelin is at least in part the result of sensitization of cardiac myofilaments to intracellular calcium, which results from a rise in pH.—R.A. O'Rourke, M.D.

Inhibitory Role of the Coronary Arterial Endothelium to α-Adrenergic Stimulation in Experimental Heart Failure
Main JS, Forster C, Armstrong PW (University of Toronto and St Michael's Hospital, Toronto, Ontario, Canada)
Circ Res 68:940–946, 1991   5–19

Background.—The effects of congestive heart failure on adrenergic control of coronary arterial tone is unclear; but many peripheral neurohumoral adjustments take place in congestive heart failure, including ac-

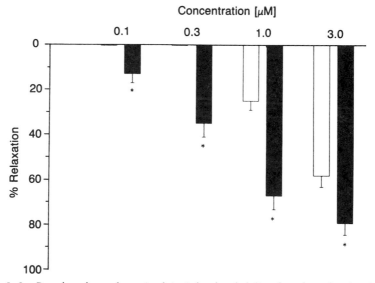

Fig 5–8.—Dose dependency of norepinephrine-induced, endothelium-dependent relaxations in control and congestive heart failure vessels that displayed biphasic responses. The percent change in tension evoked by various concentrations of norepinephrine was calculated such that the reference point for 0% relaxation was the active force developed by a vessel immediately before the administration of a dose that elicited a relaxation. Return to baseline tension represents 100% relaxation. *Open and solid bars* depict vessels from control and heart failure dogs, respectively. *Asterisk* indicates $P < .05$, heart failure vs. control. Data are from 3 control and 8 heart failure dogs (n = 17–36). (Courtesy of Main JS, Forster C, Armstrong PW: *Circ Res* 68:940–946, 1991.)

tivation of the sympathetic nervous system. Previous studies have not addressed the role of endothelium-derived relaxing factor (EDRF) in the coronary vasculature in congestive heart failure.

Methods.—The influence of the endothelium on α-adrenoceptor–mediated coronary artery contractions was examined in dogs with congestive heart failure produced by rapid ventricular pacing. Organ bath studies also were carried out.

Findings.—The peak contractile response to methoxamine was attenuated by more than 40% in both intact and denuded congestive heart failure coronary artery rings. Norepinephrine-induced contractions were reduced 58% in intact arterial vessels and 39% in denuded congestive heart failure vessels. Norepinephrine produced rapid, transient relaxations preceding slow, sustained contractions in both intact control and congestive heart failure coronary arteries. The relaxation phase was endothelium dependent. The norepinephrine concentration at which endothelium-dependent relaxation first appeared was 10-fold lower in congestive heart failure than in control vessels (Fig 5–8). Relaxation responses to a selective α₂-adrenoceptor agonist also were dependent on the presence of endothelium.

Discussion.—Alpha-adrenergic tone appears to be reduced by pacing-induced congestive heart failure in dogs. Constriction responses are impaired, and the endothelium is better able to antagonize direct vascular smooth muscle responses to norepinephrine because of enhanced endothelium-dependent relaxation.

▶ The data, derived from isolated coronary arteries from dogs with pacing-induced congestive heart failure, indicates an attenuation of α-1 adrenoceptor mediated contractions and an enhancement of endothelium-dependent α-2 adrenoceptor mediated relaxations. Such an alteration may be an important protective response of the coronary vasculature in the setting of congestive heart failure. Whether or not these animal studies are applicable to man remains to be defined.— R.A. O'Rourke, M.D.

Endothelial Dysfunction in Response to Psychosocial Stress in Monkeys
Strawn WB, Bondjers G, Kaplan JR, Manuck SB, Schwenke DC, Hansson GK, Shively CA, Clarkson TB (Bowman Gray School of Medicine, Winston-Salem, NC, University of Göteborg, Göteborg, Sweden, Univ of Pittsburgh)
Circ Res 68:1270–1279, 1991   5–20

Background.—To examine the theory that psychosocial factors contribute to the development of atherosclerosis, the effects of a disrupted social environment on the endothelial integrity of various vascular segments were evaluated in 20 male cynomolgus monkeys. During a 10-week baseline period, each single-caged monkey ate a diet comparable to a person's 240 mg cholesterol per day diet. This produced total plasma cholesterol concentrations typical of North American humans not at risk for coronary heart disease.

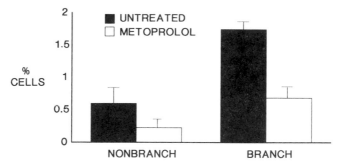

Fig 5–9.—*Bar graph* shows the percent of endothelial cells (mean ± SEM) with evidence of immunoglobulin G incorporation (injury) at nonbranched and branched sites within the thoracic portion of the aorta in monkeys. (Courtesy of Strawn WB, Bondjers G, Kaplan JR, et al: *Circ Res* 68:1270–1279, 1991.)

Methods.—After the baseline period, each experimental monkey was introduced as a stranger into a 4-member social group for 3 days, then returned to an individual cage. This pattern was repeated each week, with different host monkeys each time. Half the experimental monkeys received subcutaneous metoprolol throughout the experiment, the other half received saline solution. Heart rates (HR) and plasma lipid concentrations were measured during the baseline and experimental periods.

Results.—Whereas metoprolol-treated and untreated monkeys showed no difference in HR during the baseline period, HR was elevated significantly in untreated monkeys during social manipulation. Postmortem evaluation of the thoracic aorta assessed endothelial incorporation of immunoglobin G, endothelial cell replication, the presence of adherent leukocytes, and arterial low density lipoprotein permeability and concentration. Endothelial cell replication and immunoglobulin G incorporation were significantly greater at branching sites in untreated monkeys than in metoprolol-treated monkeys, and nonbranch sites showed no difference (Fig 5–9). Coronary arteries exhibited greater endothelial cell replication among untreated monkeys. Arterial low density lipoprotein permeability and leukocyte adherence were similar in both treatment groups. Estimates of arterial low density lipoprotein concentrations were higher only in the abdominal portion of the aorta of untreated monkeys than among metoprolol-treated ones.

Discussion.—Monkeys subjected to psychological distress show evidence of endothelial cell injury that can be suppressed by treatment. This is consistent with the hypothesis that endothelial injury may, at least initially, mediate atherosclerosis exacerbated by psychological stress.

▶ This interesting study in the nonhuman primates indicates that social disruption is associated with both sympathetic nervous system arousal and some evidence of endothelial dysfunction; these effects may be prevented by treatment with a β-adrenergic blocking agent. These data are consistent with previous studies in other animal models that have lead to the speculation that sympathetically induced elevations in heart rate may initiate early events in atherogenesis. The concept that psychosocial stress is an important factor in the development of atherosclerosis in coronary artery disease is intriguing and deserves further investigation.— R.A. O'Rourke, M.D.

Heterogeneity of Endothelium-Dependent and Endothelium-Independent Responses to Aggregating Platelets in Porcine Pulmonary Arteries

Zellers TM, Shimokawa H, Yunginger J, Vanhoutte PM (Mayo Clin and Mayo Found, Rochester, Minn)
Circ Res 68:1437–1445, 1991   5–21

Background.—In canine and porcine coronary arteries, the endothelium inhibits contractions to aggregating platelets. This is not the case in canine pulmonary arteries, where aggregating platelets cause contractions in vessels with and without endothelium. Experiments in porcine pulmonary arteries were done to determine the endothelium-dependent and endothelium-independent responses to aggregating platelets.

Methods.—Large, 5 to 7 mm in diameter, and small, 2 to 3 mm in diameter, pulmonary arteries were taken from male swine. Isolated rings, with and without endothelium, were suspended in modified Krebs-Ringer bicarbonate solution bubbled with 95% O_2 and 5% CO_2 in the presence of indomethacin. Concentration-response curves to concentrations of various agents and platelets were obtained.

Results.—In response to aggregating platelets, rings with endothelium relaxed and those without endothelium contracted. Both of these responses were greater in small than in large rings. Serotonin and ADP resulted in relaxations that depended on concentration and were augmented by endothelium. Platelet-induced endothelium-dependent relax-

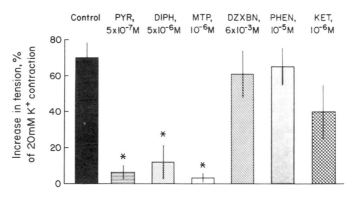

Fig 5–10.—Effects of methiothepin (*MTP*, 10^{-6}M), ketanserin (*KET*, 10^{-6} M), pyrilamine (*PYR*, 5×10^{-7} M), diphenhydramine (*DIPH*, 5×10^{-6} M), phentolamine (10^{-5} M) plus propranolol (5×10^{-6} M) on platelet-induced concentrations in quiescent rings without endothelium from small (2 to 3 mm in diameter) porcine pulmonary arteries. Indomethacin (10^{-5} M) was present in all experiments. Changes in tension are expressed as percent of the contraction evoked by 20 mM kCl in the same ring. Data are shown as mean ± SEM. Platelets = 75,000 μL. *Asterisk* indicates $P < .05$ compared with controls. (Courtesy of Zellers TM, Shimokawa H, Yunginger J, et al: *Circ Res* 68:1437–1445, 1991.)

ations were significantly reduced by methiothepin but not apyrase. When rings were incubated with methiothepin, apyrase, and theophylline, the residual relaxation was abolished; however, it was unaffected when apyrase was absent, suggesting that ADP was responsible for the residual relaxation. Quiescent rings showed dose-dependent contraction in response to norepinephrine and histamine but not serotonin or vasopressin. Methiothepin, pyrilamine, and diphenhydramine blocked the contraction to aggregating platelets, but it was unaffected by phentolamine, ketanserin, or incubation of platelets with dazoxiben (Fig 5–10).

Conclusions.—In both large and small porcine pulmonary arteries, the major contributors to the endothelium-dependent relaxation caused by aggregating platelets appear to be serotonin and ADP. For contractions in rings without endothelium, histamine appears to be responsible. Endothelium may be important in protecting lung vessels against the mechanical blockade of platelet aggregates.

▶ The data from this study indicate that the endothelium reduces the contraction of pulmonary vascular smooth muscle evoked by the vasoconstrictor mediators released from aggregating platelets; when the endothelium is absent, platelets cause contraction of porcine pulmonary arteries and platelet-derived histamine contributes importantly to the contraction. Thus, the endothelium may be important in protecting the lung vessels against the mechanical blockade of platelet aggregates, resulting in less ventilation and perfusion abnormalities.—R.A. O'Rourke, M.D.

Circadian Variation in Vascular Tone and Its Relation to α-Sympathetic Vasoconstrictor Activity
Panza JA, Epstein SE, Quyyumi AA (Natl Heart, Lung, and Blood Inst, Bethesda, Md)
N Engl J Med 325:986–990, 1991   5–22

Background.—Several cardiovascular events, including AMI, sudden death, and stroke, are more frequent in the early morning hours. Because there is a similar circadian pattern for blood pressure and other physiologic variables, circadian variations in vascular tone may have a role in the onset of acute events.

Study Plan.—Baseline blood flow and vascular resistance in the forearm and responses to phentolamine and sodium nitroprusside were examined in 12 normal individuals of both sexes aged 35–53 years at 7 AM, 2 PM, and 9 PM. Drugs were infused into the brachial artery, and responses were measured by strain-gauge plethysmography.

Findings.—The mean forearm vascular resistance was significantly higher in the morning than in the afternoon or evening, and blood flow was significantly lower in the morning (Fig 5–11). This pattern was evident in 10 of the 12 subjects evaluated. Phentolamine-induced reductions in vascular resistance were most marked in the morning in 11 subjects.

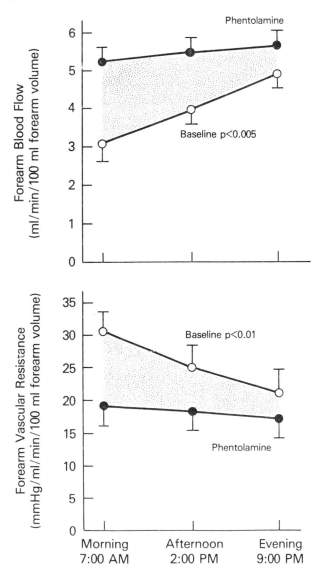

Fig 5–11.—Mean forearm blood flow and vascular resistance at 3 times during the day in 12 healthy subjects. Values shown were obtained at baseline (*open circles*) and after α-sympathetic blockade with the infusion of phentolamine (*filled circles*). The *stippled areas* indicate the vascular tone contributed by α-sympathetic vasoconstrictor forces. *P* values refer to the slope of the curve and were obtained by analysis of variance. *Vertical bars* indicate standard errors. (Courtesy of Panza JA, Epstein SE, Quyyumi AA: N Engl J Med, 325:986–990, 1991.)

The degree of sodium nitroprusside-induced vasodilation did not differ significantly at different times of the day.

Conclusions.—Circadian change in the degree of α-sympathetic–mediated vasoconstriction has an important role in varying arterial tone throughout the day. The findings may well relate to the higher blood pressure and increased number of cardiovascular events that occur in the early morning.

▶ The authors demonstrated a significantly higher basal forearm vascular resistance and reduced systemic arterial blood flow in the morning as compared to the afternoon and evening in a group of normal patients. The vasodilator effect of an α-adrenergic antagonist drug was also significantly greater in the morning. This circadian rhythm in basal vascular tone, which is at least partially the result of increased α-sympathetic vasoconstrictor activity during the morning, is consistent with multiple clinical observations concerning the increased likelihood of cardiac events and elevated blood pressure during this time interval. Interestingly, several studies have shown that treatment with β-blockers decreases the frequency of silent ischemia and angina pectoris during the time interval between 6 AM and 12 noon as well as during the other 18 hours of the day. This suggests that a positive β-adrenergic response during the early morning is also an important mediator of cardiovascular events.—R.A. O'Rourke, M.D.

Coronary Vasodilator Reserve: Comparison of the Effects of Papaverine and Adenosine on Coronary Flow, Ventricular Function, and Myocardial Metabolism
Christensen CW, Rosen LB, Gal RA, Haseeb M, Lassar TA, Port SC (Univ of Wisconsin Med School, Sinai Samaritan Med Ctr, Milwaukee)
Circulation 83:294–303, 1991   5–23

Background.—Intracoronary adenosine and papaverine have been used clinically to assess coronary flow reserve during cardiac catheterization. Papaverine is effective in maximizing coronary blood flow, but has induced several toxic effects that reduce its desirability as a coronary dilator. The subselective intracoronary administration of papaverine was compared with that of adenosine in an animal model.

Methods.—Thirty-four dogs were studied. The effects of each agent on hemodynamics, regional myocardial blood flow, contractility, metabolism, and electrocardiographic parameters were noted. A left thoractomy was done, and an arterial shunt was created from the left carotid artery to the left anterior descending coronary artery. One group of 16 dogs was studied for regional myocardial blood flow and mechanical function, and a group of 18 dogs was studied for biochemical measures.

Results.—Both adenosine and papaverine infused into the left anterior descending coronary artery produced similar increases in total and regional coronary blood flows. Papaverine induced significant changes in subendocardial ST segment electrocardiogram, QT prolongation, myocardial creatinine phosphate, and coronary sinus serum lactate when compared with control values. Intracoronary papaverine also produced an abnormal contractile pattern. There were no significant changes in ST segment, QT prolongation, myocardial creatinine phosphate level, or lactate level with intracoronary adenosine infusion (Fig 5–12).

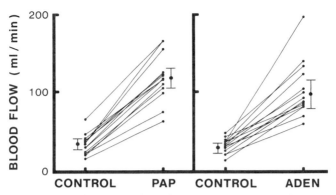

Fig 5–12.—Plots of individual coronary blood flow reserve measurements before (*CONTROL*) and during either intracoronary papaverine (*PAP*) (6 ± 1mg/min) or intracoronary adenosine (*ADEN*) (67 ± 2 μg/min) infusion into left anterior descending coronary artery. (Courtesy of Christensen CW, Rosen LB, Gal RA, et al: *Circulation* 83:294–303, 1991.)

Conclusions.—Intracoronary adenosine may be comparable to papaverine in producing a maximal coronary flow response in patients. The significant difference between the 2 is that papaverine may induce deleterious metabolic, electrocardiographic, and regional wall motion changes, whereas adenosine apparently does not.

▶ In this dog study, there was a greater decrease in the perfusion pressure with intracoronary papaverine as compared to intracoronary adenosine. Both drugs produce comparable coronary vasodilatation that exceeded the hyperemia observed after a 20-second total coronary artery occlusion. As in previous studies, intracoronary papaverine produced more electrocardiographic changes, had a longer hemodynamic effect, and was associated with higher coronary sinus lactate concentrations. Preliminary reports by others suggest a similar difference in adenosine as compared to papaverine on the coronary circulation in humans.—R.A. O'Rourke, M.D.

5-Hydroxytryptamine Mediates Endothelium Dependent Coronary Vasodilatation in the Isolated Rat Heart by the Release of Nitric Oxide
Mankad PS, Chester AH, Yacoub MH (Natl Heart and Lung Inst, London)
Cardiovasc Res 25:244–248, 1991   5–24

Background.—5-Hydroxytryptamine (5-HT) is a potent vasoconstrictor in large coronary arteries but not in coronary resistance vessels. Its direct action is opposed by a dilator response mediated by the endothelium. A study was done in rats to investigate this endothelium-dependent vasodilator action of 5-HT on the coronary circulation.

Methods.—The hearts of 56 rats were excised and perfused with a modified Langendorff preparation. Saponin, 30 μg·mL^{-1}, to remove the endothelium, and L-N^G-monomethyl-arginine (L-NMMA), the selective inhibitor of nitric oxide formation, were used. This allowed study of the role of endothelium and nitric oxide in causing 5-HT vasodilation. Eight rats were pretreated with L-NMMA, 100 mg·kg^{-1}. These hearts and 8 normal hearts were later perfused with L-arginine, 10^{-4} M.

Results.—A dose-dependent increase in coronary flow was seen with 5-HT at 10^{-9} to 10^{-5} M and with glyceryl trinitrate at 10^{-5} to 10^{-3} M. Removal of the endothelium eliminated the vasodilatory effect of 5-HT but had no effect on the response to glyceryl trinitrate. Pretreatment with L-NMMA unmasked a strong vasoconstrictor effect of 5-HT and had no effect on glyceryl trinitrate–induced vasodilation. L-arginine perfusion restored the vasodilation induced by 5-HT in hearts pretreated with L-NMMA. However, in normal hearts, L-arginine had no effect on the extent of 5-HT– or glyceryl trinitrate–induced vasodilation.

Conclusions.—In the isolated rat heart, the vasodilator effect of 5-HT is mediated by endothelium-dependent release of nitric oxide. This model may be useful for studies of agents or procedures believed to have a deleterious effect on endothelial function.

▶ This study indicates that 5-hydroxytryptamine induces a dose-dependent increase in coronary blood flow in the isolated perfused rat heart that is dependent on an intact endothelium and the release of nitric oxide from the endothelium. This is one of many studies performed in experimental animals in which endothelium dependent versus endothelium independent effects on vascular tone have been assessed before and after pretreatment with other drugs. Thus, mechanisms of action on the endothelium and endothelium dependent release of various substances can be evaluated. Different results may also occur with normal endothelium as compared to the endothelium present in diseased arteries (e.g., atherosclerosis).—R.A. O'Rourke, M.D.

Additional recent publications concerning vascular smooth muscle and coronary vasculature are listed as follows:

1. Chen C, Wagoner PK: Endothelin induces a nonselective cation current in vascular smooth muscle cells. *Circ Res* 69:447–454, 1991.
2. Li K, Stewart DJ, Rouleau J-L: Myocardial contractile actions of endothelin-1 in rat and rabbit papillary muscles. Role of endocardial endothelium. *Circ Res* 69:301–312, 1991.
3. Itoh S, van den Buuse M: Sensitization of baroreceptor reflex by central endothelin in conscious rats. *Am J Physiol* 260:H1106–H1112, 1991.
4. Suzuki S, Kajikuri J, Suzuki A, et al: Effects of endothelin-1 on endothelial cells in the porcine coronary artery. *Circ Res* 69:1361–1368, 1991.
5. Gupta S, Ruderman NB, Cragoe EJ Jr, et al: Endothelin stimulates NA$^+$-K$^+$-ATPase activity by a protein kinase C-dependent pathway in rabbit aorta. *Am J Physiol* 261:H38–H45, 1991.
6. Tschudi M, Richard V, Bühler FR, et al: Importance of endothelium-derived nitric oxide in porcine coronary resistance arteries. *Am J Physiol* 260:H13–H20, 1991.

7. Chu A, Chambers DE, Lin C-C, et al: Effects of inhibition of nitric oxide formation on basal vasomotion and endothelium-dependent responses of the coronary arteries in awake dogs. *J Clin Invest* 87:1964–1968, 1991.

8. Ahlner J, Ljusegren ME, Grundström N, et al: Role of nitric oxide and cyclic GMP as mediators of endothelium-independent neurogenic relaxation in bovine mesenteric artery. *Circ Res* 68:756–762, 1991.

9. Mügge A, Peterson T, Harrison DG: Release of nitrogen oxides from cultured bovine aortic endothelial cells in not impaired by calcium channel antagonists. *Circulation* 83:1404–1409, 1991.

10. Archer SL, Cowan NJ: Measurement of endothelial cytosolic calcium concentration and nitric oxide production reveals discrete mechanisms of endothelium-dependent pulmonary vasodilatation. *Circ Res* 68:1569–1581, 1991.

11. Egashira K, Pipers FS, Morgan JP: Effects of cocaine on epicardial coronary artery reactivity in miniature swine after endothelial injury and high cholesterol feeding. *J Clin Invest* 88:1307–1314, 1991.

12. Kuhn FE, Johnson MN, Gillis RA, et al: Effect of cocaine on the coronary circulation and systemic hemodynamics in dogs. *J Am Coll Cardiol* 16:1481–1491, 1990.

13. Vargas R, Gillis RA, Ramwell PW: Propranolol promotes cocaine-induced spasm of porcine coronary artery. *J Pharmacol Exper Ther* 257:644–646, 1991.

14. Kushwaha SS, Crossman DC, Bustami M, et al: Substance P for evaluation of coronary endothelial function after cardiac transplantation. *J Am Coll Cardiol* 17:1537–1544, 1991.

15. Schini VB, Vanhoutte PM: L-Arginine evokes both endothelium-dependent and -independent relaxations in L-arginine-depleted aortas of the rat. *Circ Res* 68:209–216, 1991.

16. Sung C-P, Arleth AJ, Feuerstein GZ: Neuropeptide Y upregulates the adhesiveness of human endothelial cells for leukocytes. *Circ Res* 68:314–318, 1991.

17. Mügge A, Elwell JH, Peterson TE, et al: Chronic treatment with polyethylene-glycolated superoxide dismutase partially restores endothelium-dependent vascular relaxations in cholesterol-fed rabbits. *Circ Res* 69:1293–1300, 1991.

18. Angus JA, Ward JE, Smolich JJ, et al: Reactivity of canine isolated epicardial collateral coronary arteries: Relation to vessel structure. *Circ Res* 69:1340–1352, 1991.

19. de Lanerolle P, Strauss JD, Felsen R, et al: Effects of antibodies to myosin light chain kinase on contractility and myosin phosphorylation in chemically permeabilized smooth muscle. *Circ Res* 68:457–465, 1991.

20. Ma X-l, Tsao PS, Viehman GE, et al: Neutrophil-mediated vasoconstriction and endothelial dysfunction in low-flow perfusion-reperfused cat coronary artery. *Circ Res* 69:95–106, 1991.

Myocardial Ischemia/Infarction

Regional Myocardial Blood Flow and Left Ventricular Diastolic Properties in Pacing-Induced Ischemia

Momomura S-I, Ferguson JJ, Miller MJ, Parker JA, Grossman W (Beth Israel Hosp, Boston; Harvard Med School)

J Am Coll Cardiol 17:781–789, 1991

5–25

Background.—Coronary heart disease patients with angina often experience elevated left ventricular (LV) diastolic pressure and an LV diastolic pressure-volume that shifts upward. In addition, transmural redistribution of myocardial blood flow has been reported during exercise and pacing tachycardia in animal studies. Transmural myocardial blood flow and LV diastolic relaxation and distensibility were measured in 8 open-chest dogs with critical stenoses of the proximal left anterior descending and circumflex coronary arteries.

Technique.—Eight mongrel dogs were anesthetized and pretreated with propranolol. A pair of pacing electrodes was sutured to the left atrial appendage to assess rapid atrial pacing, and a high fidelity micromanometer was inserted into the left ventricle. Ultrasonic crystals were inserted into the inner third of the myocardium. Pacing tachycardia with and without coronary stenosis was measured. The microsphere assessed blood flow.

Results.—Left ventricular systolic pressure without coronary stenosis remained unchanged after pacing tachycardia, whereas LV minimal and end-diastolic pressure were also unchanged during and after the induced tachycardia. With coronary stenoses, the LV minimal and end-diastolic pressure increased during pacing tachycardia and stayed elevated for more than 30 seconds after stopping. The end-systolic and end-diastolic segment lengths in both ischemic sections were greater after the pacing tachycardia. Peak negative dP/dt decreased, but peak positive dP/dt remained the same after pacing tachycardia. With coronary stenoses, anterograde coronary flow decreased significantly in the left anterior descending artery and in the circumflex artery during pacing. Mean perfusion pressure and vascular resistance also decreased significantly with stenoses during pacing, whereas subendocardial blood flow fell to 65% of prepacing levels and subepicardial flow increased. Diastolic abnormalities were inversely related with myocardial perfusion assessments during the pacing-induced ischemia.

Conclusions.—These findings indicate that pacing tachycardia causes impaired relaxation and decreases regional myocardial distensibility in animals with critical coronary stenoses. The reduction of subendocardial flow probably results from aggravation by the extrinsic compression of the subendocardium and its heart vasculature as a result of increased LV end-diastolic pressure.

▶ In a study reported in the 1991 YEAR BOOK OF CARDIOLOGY (1) pacing-induced ischemia led to marked reductions in regional epicardial and endocardial blood flow and even more severe flow reductions after complete bilateral coronary artery occlusion. Thus, the reduction in subendocardial blood flow observed in pacing-induced ischemia in the current study is not surprising. It likely occurs for the reasons elucidated by the authors. The increase in subepicardial flow was less expected; however, and in any experimental study, measurements of blood flow and cardiac function depend on the duration, extent, and severity of myocardial ischemia, which may vary in different animal models.—R.A. O'Rourke, M.D.

Reference

1. Applegate RJ, et al: *Circulation* 81:1380–1392, 1990.

Diagnostic Efficiency of Troponin T Measurements in Acute Myocardial Infarction
Katus HA, Remppis A, Neumann FJ, Scheffold T, Diederich KW, Vinar G, Noe A, Matern G, Kuebler W (University of Heidelberg, Germany)
Circulation 83:902–912, 1991   5–26

Objective.—A new troponin T enzyme immunoassay was evaluated for detecting AMI in a series of 388 patients with chest pain and 101 others in whom both skeletal muscle and myocardial cell damage were sus-

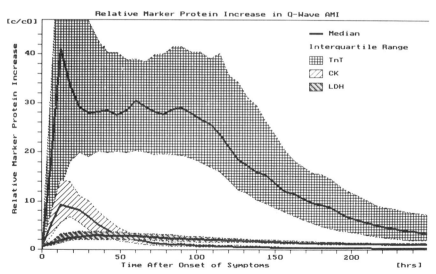

Fig 5–13.—Plot of median and 25th–75th percentile range of relative increase of serum CK and lactate dehydrogenase (LDH) activity and troponin T (TnT) concentrations in 121 patients with Q wave AMI. Relative increase of marker protein in serum corresponds to the ratio of patients' serum activity to the upper limit of normal for CK and LDH and the ratio of patients' serum concentration to the analytical sensitivity of the test for TnT. (Courtesy of Katus HA, Remppis A, Newmann FJ, et al: *Circulation* 83:902–912, 1991.)

pected. The assay exhibits only 1% to 2% cross-reactivity with troponin T of mixed skeletal muscle.

Findings.—All patients with infarction, even non–Q-wave infarction, had troponin T levels more than twice the lower limit of detection (.5 μg/L). Troponin T was seen in serum as early as 3 hours after pain began and remained elevated for longer than 5 days. Troponin T levels were increased in all patients with unstable angina, and the levels correlated with the presence of reversible ST-segment and T-wave changes on the ECG, as well as with in-hospital complications. Correlation between troponin T and creatine kinase (CK) levels is illustrated in Figure 5–13. Troponin T estimates were substantially more discriminatory than CK-MB determinations in patients with skeletal muscle damage.

Conclusions.—Troponin T is a cardiospecific antigen that, being a subcellularly compartmented protein, is released into serum long after AMI. It is especially helpful in detecting minor degrees of myocardial cell necrosis and myocardial damage in patients who also have skeletal muscle damage.

▶ This study of almost 500 patients indicates that the newly developed immunoassay for the troponin T enzyme may be a useful additional and/or alternative test to CK-MB measurements for detecting AMI. Its sensitivity appears to be excellent, but false positive results do occur. Additional clinical and experimental tests will be necessary to clearly define its role in the serologic detection of subacute myocardial infarction. See also the article by Ellis (1).—R.A. O'Rourke, M.D.

Reference

1. Ellis AK: *Circulation* 83:1107–1109, 1991.

Cellular Basis of Chronic Ventricular Remodeling After Myocardial Infarction in Rats
Olivetti G, Capasso JM, Meggs LG, Sonnenblick EH, Anversa P (University of Parma, Italy; New York Med College, Vahalla; Albert Einstein College of Medicine, Bronx, NY)
Circ Res 68:856–869, 1991   5–27

Introduction.—After AMI, some patients have reduced pump function directly related to the amount of the lost myocardium, particularly with infarcts affecting 40% of the left ventricle. Whether the hypertrophic response of the remainder of the postinfarct myocardium can lead to normalization of the ventricular hemodynamics and wall stress was studied in a rat model.

Methods.—A total of 55 male, 3-month-old Wistar-Kyoto rats underwent left coronary artery ligation. Before the induction of cardiac arrest, the 28 surviving animals underwent internal monitoring of arterial blood pressure and left-ventricular pressures. One month after the

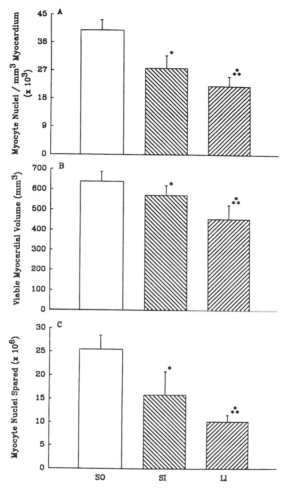

Fig 5–14.—*Abbreviations: SO,* sham-operated rats; *SI,* rats with small infarcts; *LI,* rats with large infarcts. *Bar graph*s showing the effects of coronary artery occlusion on the number of myocyte nuclei in the viable ventricle. The results are presented as mean ± SD. *Asterisk* indicates significantly different at $P < .05$ compared with sham-operated control rats. Double asterisk indicates significantly different at $P < .05$ compared with rats with small infarcts. (Courtesy of Olivetti G, Capasso JM, Meggs LG, et al: *Circ Res* 68:856–869, 1991.)

infarct induction, the animals were killed and the heart perfused for further analysis.

Results.—Of the 28 infarcted hearts, 15 ventricles had infarcts composed of up to 12% of the wall with a 7.48% scar, and 13 ventricles had infarcts involving more than 12% of the wall with a 17.3% scar. The 30% reduction of the myocyte nuclei numerical density and the 11% lowering of the free-wall myocardial mass produced a significantly lower (38%) total number of myocyte nuclei in rats with small infarcts (Fig 5–14). The large infarcts also significantly reduced the nuclear numerical density and myocardial volume, leading to a significant decrease in the aggregate number of myocyte nuclei in the affected ventricle. The left-ventricular end-diastolic pressure increased, the left ventricular dP/dt decreased, and the diastolic wall stress rose by 2.4-fold. The recovery of viable myocardium demonstrated a 10% deficit. The ventricular function was greatly reduced and the diastolic wall stress had risen by ninefold. Chamber dilation resulted from the alteration of gross anatomy and cellular parameters.

Implications.—These findings suggest that decompensated eccentric ventricular hypertrophy usually develops chronically after infarction. It appears that the growth of myocytes cannot normalize the wall stress, especially when the myocyte reduction reaches 40% or more. Constant raised myocardial and cellular loads may even cause the disease to progress to end-stage congestive heart failure.

▶ There is now considerable interest in the use of cardiovascular drugs (e.g., ACE inhibitors) to alter ventricular remodeling and decrease "infarct expansion" in patients with recent AMI, particularly anterior Q wave infarction. This study in an experimental rat model of myocardial infarction indicates that the hypertrophic response of myocytes in the region bordering the scar tissue is greater than the areas remote from the infarct and that the difference is greater with larger infarcts. Moreover, the decrease in capillary density involves the peri-infarcted region more than it does the tissue away from the scar. Also, the diffusion distance for oxygen increases to a greater extent in the border zone. Interaction of the area of infarction with the viable myocardium may alter series elasticity and increase tension, with these superimposed on augmentation of load associated with increased ventricular diameter and diastolic filling pressure. As indicated by the authors, the protective effect of ACE inhibitors may be the result of an increase in the myocardial mass/chamber volume ratio, augmentation of the wall thickness/chamber radius ratio, preservation of the transverse chamber diameter/longitudinal axis ratio, or a combination of these 3 factors.—R.A. O'Rourke, M.D.

Reduction of Canine Myocardial Infarct Size by a Diffusible Reactive Oxygen Metabolite Scavenger: Efficacy of Dimethylthiourea Given at the Onset of Reperfusion

Carrea FP, Lesnefsky EJ, Repine JE, Shikes RH, Horwitz LD (Univ of Colorado, Denver)

Circ Res 68:1652–1659, 1991   5–28

Objective.—To be clinically useful, an agent intended to reduce myocardial injury resulting from reactive oxygen metabolites produced during reperfusion after infarct must be effective when regional myocardial perfusion is already reduced; it must enter cells swiftly to counteract the initial eruption of oxidant production and remain active for several hours. Dimethylthiourea (DMTU) is exceedingly diffusible, has an exceptionally long half-life of 43 hours, and is a powerful scavenger of hydrogen peroxide, hydroxyl radical, and hypochlorous acid. Its efficacy in preventing reperfusion damage after a period of ischemia, which is sufficiently long to permit injured cells to become necrotic, was tested in an animal model.

Study Design.—Sixteen anesthetized dogs were randomly given 100 mL of intravenously administered saline or 500 mg/kg of intravenously administered DMTU in saline during the final 15 minutes of a 90-minute period of occlusion of the left anterior descending coronary artery and during the first 15 minutes of reperfusion. Regional myocardial blood flow was quantified by injecting radioactive microspheres at baseline, 75 minutes after occlusion of the left anterior descending coronary artery, and after 60 minutes and 48 hours of reperfusion. Infarct size was determined histologically after 48 hours of reperfusion; the ability of 2,3,5-triphenyltetrazolium chloride (TTC) to distinguish infarcted from viable tissue after dual perfusion with Evan's blue dye in the presence of the antioxidant DMTU was tested by blinded evaluation of the study tissue samples, and in vitro by measuring conversion of TTC to formazan in homogenized myocardium with or without added DMTU.

Results.—Infarcted tissue comprised 42% of the weight of tissue at risk for damage in the DMTU group, a highly significant 17% reduction compared with saline controls. At no time did blood flow, ischemic injury, or left ventricular mass differ significantly between DMTU and saline-treated dogs. Evan's blue and TTC staining was not altered by DMTU and accurately indicated infarct size.

Conclusion.—Dimethylthiourea reduction of infarction size by 40% after only 3 hours of reperfusion reported in a previous study was an overestimate; damage probably continues from 24 to 48 hours, and TTC staining after a 3-hour reperfusion may pick up tissue that is irrevocably damaged but still viable at that time point. In the present study, DMTU given after the onset of reperfusion afforded significant protection to myocardial tissue; although DMTU does not scavenge oxygen free radicals, its oxygen metabolite scavenging, swift delivery to the critical area and protracted efficacy give it considerable potential clinical usefulness.

▶ In this carefully designed dog study, DMTU was administered after regional myocardial ischemia was well established, and a 30% reduction in infarct size was demonstrated with 48 hours of reperfusion. Whether or not agents such as DMTU, an extremely diffusible potent scavenger of hydroxyradical, provide additive myocardial salvage when combined with thrombolytic therapy remains to be determined.—R.A. O'Rourke, M.D.

The following references pertain to important articles appearing in the cardiology literature concerning myocardial ischemia and myocardial infarction during the past year:

1. Ohgoshi Y, Goto Y, Futaki S, et al: Increased oxygen cost of contractility in stunned myocardium of dog. *Circ Res* 69:975–988, 1991.

2. Kitakaze M, Hori M, Sato H, et al: Beneficial effects of α_1-adrenoceptor activity on myocardial stunning in dogs. *Circ Res* 68:1322–1339, 1991.
3. Whittaker P, Boughner DR, Kloner RA, et al: Stunned myocardium and myocardial collagen damage: Differential effects of single and repeated occlusions. *Am Heart J* 121:434–441, 1991.
4. Safwat A, Leone BJ, Norris RM, et al: Pressure-length loop area: Its components analyzed during graded myocardial ischemia. *J Am Coll Cardiol* 17:790–796, 1991.
5. Takahashi T, Levine MJ, Grossman W: Regional diastolic mechanics of ischemic and nonischemic myocardium in the pig heart. *J Am Coll Cardiol* 17:1203–1212, 1991.
6. Litwin SE, Litwin CM, Raya TE, et al: Contractility and stiffness of noninfarcted myocardium after coronary ligation in rats. Effects of chronic angiotensin converting enzyme inhibition. *Circulation* 83:1028–1037, 1991.
7. Connelly CM, McLaughlin RJ, Vogel WM, et al: Reversible and irreversible elongation of ischemic, infarcted, and healed myocardium in response to increases in preload and afterload. *Circulation* 84:387–399, 1991.
8. Segar DS, Moran M, Ryan T, et al: End-systolic regional model of normal, ischemic and reperfused myocardium. *J Am Coll Cardiol* 17:1651–1660, 1991.
9. Kloner RA, Giacomelli F, Alker KJ, et al: Influx of neutrophils into the walls of large epicardial coronary arteries in response to ischemia/reperfusion. *Circulation* 84:1758–1772, 1991.
10. Dreyer WJ, Michael LH, West MS, et al: Neutrophil accumulation in ischemic canine myocardium. Insights into time course, distribution, and mechanism of localization during early reperfusion. *Circulation* 84:400–411, 1991.
11. Jondeau G, Sullivan ML, Eng C: Reciprocal strains in the normal and ischemic myocardium and their relation to the size of the ischemic region. *J Am Coll Cardiol* 18:1388–1396, 1991.
12. Pauly DF, Kirk KA, McMillin JB: Carnitine palmitoyltransferase in cardiac ischemia. A potential site for altered fatty acid metabolism. *Circ Res* 68:1085–1094, 1991.
13. Schneider CA, Taegtmeyer H: Fasting in vivo delays myocardial cell damage after brief periods of ischemia in the isolated working rat heart. *Circ Res* 68:1045–1050, 1991.
14. Kahn NN, Mueller HS, Sinha AK: Restoration by insulin of impaired prostaglandin E_1/I_2 receptor activity of platelets in acute ischemic heart disease. *Circ Res* 68:245–254, 1991.
15. Koretsune Y, Coretti MC, Kusuoka H, et al: Mechanism of early ischemic contractile failure. Inexcitability, metabolite accumulation, or vascular collapse? *Circ Res* 68:255–262, 1991.
16. Villarreal FJ, Lew WYW, Waldman LK, et al: Transmural myocardial deformation in the ischemic canine left ventricle. *Circ Res* 68:368–381, 1991.

17. Santamore WP, Yelton BW Jr, Ogilby JD: Dynamics of coronary occlusion in the pathogenesis of myocardial infarction. *J Am Coll Cardiol* 18:1397–1405, 1991.
18. Geenen DL, Malhotra A, Liang D, et al: Ventricular function and contractile proteins in the infarcted overloaded rat heart. *Cardiovasc Res* 25:330–336, 1991.
19. Vanhaecke J, Van de Werf F, Ronaszeki A, et al: Effect of superoxide dismutase on infarct size and postischemic recovery of myocardial contractility and metabolism in dogs. *J Am Coll Cardiol* 18:224–230, 1991.
20. Carrea FP, Lesnefsky EJ, Repine JE, et al: Reduction of canine myocardial infarct size by a diffusible reactive oxygen metabolite scavenger. Efficacy of dimethylthiourea given at the onset of reperfusion. *Circ Res* 68:1652–1659, 1991.
21. Werns SW, Grum CM, Ventura AN, et al: Xanthine oxidase inhibition does not limit canine infarct size. *Circulation* 83:995–1005, 1991.
22. Iwamoto T, Miura T, Adachi T, et al: Myocardial infarct size-limiting effect of ischemic preconditioning was not attenuated by oxygen free-radical scavengers in the rabbit. *Circulation* 83:1015–1022, 1991.
23. Cohen MV, Liu GS, Downey JM: Preconditioning causes improved wall motion as well as smaller infarcts after transient coronary occlusion in rabbits. *Circulation* 84:341–349, 1991.
24. Liu GS, Thornton J, Van Winkle DM, et al: Protection against infarction afforded by preconditioning is mediated by α_1 adenosine receptors in rabbit heart. *Circulation* 84:350–356, 1991.
25. Rousseau G, St-Jean G, Latour J-G, et al: Diltiazem at reperfusion reduces neutrophil accumulation and infarct size in dogs with ischaemic myocardium. *Cardiovasc Res* 25:319–329, 1991.
26. Litwin SE, Raya TE, Anderson PG, et al: Induction of myocardial hypertrophy after coronary ligation in rats decreases ventricular dilatation and improves systolic function. *Circulation* 84:1819–1827, 1991.
27. Axford-Gatley RA, Wilson GJ: Reduction of experimental myocardial infarct size by oral administration of α tocopherol. *Cardiovasc Res* 25:89–92, 1991.
28. Haskel EJ, Prager NA, Sobel BE, et al: Relative efficacy of antithrombin compared with antiplatelet agents in accelerating coronary thrombolysis and preventing early reocclusion. *Circulation* 83:1048–1056, 1991.

Cardiac Electrophysiology

Thrombin Modulates Phosphoinositide Metabolism, Cytosolic Calcium, and Impulse Initiation in the Heart

Steinberg SF, Robinson RB, Lieberman HB, Stern DM, Rosen MR (Columbia Univ, New York)

Circ Res 68:1216–1229, 1991

5–29

Background.—In several different types of cells, thrombin stimulates hydrolysis of phosphoinositide and increases cytosolic calcium. The effects of thrombin on several biochemical and electrophysiologic parameters in animal tissues were studied to determine whether similar actions occur in the heart and whether this mechanism is related to changes in cardiac electrical activity.

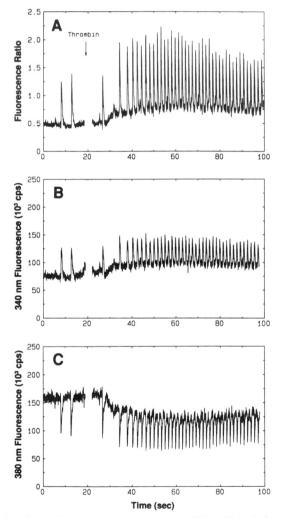

Fig 5–15.—Effect of thrombin on automatic rate and intracellular calcium. **A**, fura-2 fluorescence ratio from a single, spontaneously contracting myocyte in a monolayer culture. This ratio is derived from fluorescence records at 340 nm (**B**, where fluorescence increases with calcium and 380 nm (**C**, where fluorescence decreases with calcium). The ratio is proportional to cytosolic calcium and is not distorted by motion artifact because records at the isosbestic excitation wavelength (360 nm) were flat (not shown). The cell was observed to contract at a rate of approximately 6 beats/min for 2 minutes before this record (data not shown). Thrombin (1 unit/mL) was added to the superfusate in the prechamber at the *arrow*. The figure depicts results obtained in a single cell that are representative of the group of 7 cells studied according to this protocol. Note that in this particular cell, a rise in diastolic calcium preceded the onset of enhanced automaticity. Increases in calcium that preceded increases in automaticity occurred in 3 of the cell studies. (Courtesy of Steinberg SF, Robinson RB, Lieberman HB, et al: *Circ Res* 68:1216–1229, 1991.)

Results.—Thrombin induced rapid phosphoinositide breakdown in neonatal rat ventricular myocyte cultures freed of fibroblast contamination by irradiation. Detectable inositol triphosphate formed in 5 seconds, followed by sequential accumulation of inositol biphosphate and inositol monophosphate. Hirudin inhibited stimulation of phosphoinositide hydrolysis by thrombin, but propranolol, prazosin, and pretreatment with pertussis toxin did not. There was no association between inositol phospholipid response and changes in intracellular cAMP levels. In dog Purkinje fibers, microelectrode techniques were used to study thrombin's electrophysiologic effects. Beating rate of depolarized fibers was increased by thrombin but not that of fibers at normal maximal diastolic potential. In fibers driven at a constant cycle length, thrombin prolonged the action potential duration. Hirudin and nisoldipine inhibited this response, but propranolol, prazosin, and pretreatment with pertussis toxin did not. Early afterdepolarizations were also augmented by thrombin. Thrombin increased beating rate, diastolic calcium, and peak systolic calcium of spontaneously contracting cultured ventricular myocytes. In rat ventricular myocytes and canine Purkinje myocytes that were electrically driven at a constant basic cycle length, cytosolic calcium also increased. Thrombin thus appeared to modulate cellular calcium metabolism independent of its actions to enhance automaticity (Fig 5–15).

Conclusions.—Among the stimulatory effects of thrombin in the mammalian heart is inositol triphosphate formation, which is associated with increased cytosolic calcium and enhanced automaticity. The various actions of thrombin may be functionally related and contribute to the electrical abnormalities seen in myocardial ischemia and infarction.

▶ This basic electrophysiologic study is of great interest and leads to several hypotheses concerning the role of thrombin in patients with myocardial ischemia and/or infarction. Thrombin exerts a range of stimulatory effects in many kinds of mammalian cells through its action to activate phosphoinositide hydrolysis. Observation in the current study concerning the effects of thrombin on electrophysiologic properties of Purkinje fibers indicate that thrombin could act as a plasma-derived humoral mediator of electrophysiologic events. Thrombin could modify the propagation of premature depolarizations and be either anti-arrhythmic, but it could be arrhythmogenic, if early after depolarizations observed were of sufficient magnitude to attain threshold and induce triggered activity. Hence, thrombin formed locally during myocardial infarction could have important arrhythmogenic consequences. Additional studies concerning the potential clinical role of thrombin in altered electrophysiology properties in patients with acute myocardial ischemia may have great clinical relevance.—R.A. O'Rourke, M.D.

Proarrhythmic Effects of Flecainide: Experimental Evidence for Increased Susceptibility to Reentrant Arrhythmias
Brugada J, Boersma L, Kirchhof C, Allessie M (University of Limburg, Maastricht, The Netherlands)
Circulation 84:1808–1818, 1991

Background.—Class Ic anti-arrhythmic drugs (e.g., flecainide and encainide) have a high degree of proarrhythmic effects. No data directly address the electrophysiologic mechanism of these effects. The proarrhythmic effects of flecainide were studied in Langendorff-perfused rabbit hearts.

Methods.—Sixteen Flemish rabbits were used in this study. After removal of the hearts and Langendorff perfusion, a thin layer of epicardium was obtained by an endocardial cryotechnique from 10 hearts. The remaining 6 hearts were left intact. Programmed electrical stimulation was performed, with 1–3 closely coupled premature stimuli and burst pacing. This was done to evaluate the inducibility of arrhythmias, both under control conditions and during administration of 1 µg/mL of flecainide.

Results.—In the epicardial specimens, under control conditions, premature stimuli induced nonsustained ventricular tachycardia in 1 of 10 hearts. On administration of burst pacing, nonsustained ventricular tachycardia occurred in 4 hearts, and sustained ventricular tachycardia occurred in 2. With flecainide, premature stimuli induced sustained ventricular tachycardia in 5 hearts and burst pacing causes sustained ventricular tachycardia in 9. On epicardial mapping, all of the tachycardias were shown to be based on circus movement of the impulse around arcs of functional block. The same heart showed different locations of the arc of block; this resulted in different reentrant circuits and different cycle lengths. Premature stimuli induced ventricular fibrillation in all of the intact hearts, both with and without flecainide administration.

Conclusions.—The proarrhythmic effects of flecainide appear to result from altered propagation of impulses in thin layers of surviving myocardium. This occurs in such a way as to favor induction of functionally determined reentry. In patients who have had myocardial infarction, flecainide could result in rapid ventricular tachycardias and sudden death through this mechanism.

▶ Investigations concerning the proarrhythmic effects of class Ic antiarrhythmic agents have been stimulated since the initial CAST preliminary report showing an increased cardiac mortality in postinfarction patients treated with encainide and flecainide (1). This experimental animal study suggests that the mechanism of ventricular arrhythmias causing the proarrhythmic effect in flecainide is functionally determined reentry. Although a possible substrate for reentrant ventricular tachycardia is present in at least 40% of patients after myocardial infarction, the possible implications of this animal study must be made with caution. The pathophysiologic substrate after infarction is much more complex than in the thin layers of normal epicardium used in this present investigation.—R.A. O'Rourke, M.D.

Reference

1. CAST Investigators: *N Engl J Med* 321:406–412, 1989.

Sympathetic Modulation of the Relation Between Ventricular Repolarization and Cycle Length

Zaza A, Malfatto G, Schwartz PJ (Università degli Studi di Milano, Italy)
Circ Res 68:1191–1203, 1991   5–31

Background.—Despite their relevance to arrhythmogenesis, the sympathetic influences on ventricular repolarization have not been fully explained. A study was done in cats to investigate the sympathetic control of repolarization, measured from an endocardial monophasic action potential duration (APD) and the QT interval.

Methods.—Twenty-four anesthetized cats were studied. One experiment was done to study the effects of right and left stellectomy and subsequent bilateral stellectomy or β-blockade on the relation between APD or QT and cycle length (CL), and another to study kinetics of adaptation of APD to a sudden change in CL. Atrial pacing at different CLs was done to determine relations between steady-state APD/CL or QT/CL. The APD kinetics were evaluated for a sudden 100 ms decrease in pacing CL. The hyperbolic function APD = $CL/[(a \cdot CL)+b]$ fitted the steady-state relation, and 2 parameters were computed from this: APD (QT) extrapolated at infinite CL, APD_{max} or QT_{max}; and CL at which 50% of the change in APD or QT occurred, $CL_{50} = b/a$.

Results.—Right stellectomy reduced APD_{max} and CL_{50}, and this effect was reversed by left stellectomy or β-blockade. Left stellectomy prolonged APD_{max} and CL_{50}. In both groups, bilateral stellectomy resulted in further increases. The QT/CL relation gave similar results. The sum of 2 exponentials described the adaptation kinetics of ADP to cycle length, the first time constant was unchanged by any intervention and the second was shortened by right stellectomy and prolonged by left stellectomy. The second time constant increased in both groups on further removal of the remaining stellate ganglion.

Conclusions.—Both steady-state dependence on CL and kinetics of adaptation to sudden rate changes of ventricular repolarization are modulated by sympathetic innervation, with asymmetrical effects. The APD_{max} and QT_{max} are shortened, CL_{50} is reduced, and APD adaptation to a new steady state is accelerated by right stellectomy. These effects are reversed by β-blockade or left stellectomy; therefore, they probably result from a reflexly enhanced sympathetic outflow to the ventricles through the left-sided nerves.

▶ Adrenergic mechanisms are thought to play a major role in the genesis of the rhythm disturbances associated with QTc prolongation in various clinical conditions, including the idiopathic long QT syndrome. The importance of the present studies to the long QT syndrome depends on the validity of right stellectomy as a model for its pathogeneses. In any case the techniques used in these studies can be applied clinically in patients with a long QT syndrome; the sympathetic modulation of the time course by which action potential duration adapts after a change in heart rate could be relevant to the initiation of arrhythmias.—R.A. O'Rourke, M.D.

Hemodynamic and Electrophysiological Actions of Cocaine: Effects of Sodium Bicarbonate as an Antidote in Dogs

Beckman KJ, Parker RB, Hariman RJ, Gallastegui JL, Javaid JI, Bauman JL
(Univ of Illinois at Chicago; Illinois State Psychiatric Inst, Chicago)
Circulation 83:1799–1807, 1991

5–32

Background.—Cocaine abusers may die because of sudden cardiac arrest, but there have been reports of ventricular arrhythmias and sudden death in the absence of acute myocardial infarction. The effects of high-dose cocaine, as well as the potential of intravenously administered sodium bicarbonate as an antidote, were investigated in dogs.

Methods.—Fifteen anesthetized mongrel dogs were given cocaine in repeated 5 mg/kg intravenous boluses, as well as in a continuous infusion of .2 mg/kg/minute. In 11 dogs, sodium bicarbonate, 40 mEq was given intravenously, and the remainder received 5% dextrose intravenously.

Results.—The hemodynamic and electrophysiologic effects of cocaine occurred in dose-dependent fashion. It significantly decreased blood pressure, coronary blood flow, and cardiac output. It increased PR, QRS, QT, and QTc intervals and sinus cycle length; and it increased ventricular effective refractory period and dispersion of ventricular refractoriness. Monophasic action potential recording showed no afterdepolarizations. Two animals had spontaneous nonsustained monomorphic ventricular tachycardia. In 5 of 11 dogs, programmed stimulation at the end of the dosing protocol induced sustained ventricular tachycardia. Cocaine-induced QRS prolongation was quickly reduced to near baseline with sodium bicarbonate, but none of the other ECG or hemodynamic variables were affected. Sodium bicarbonate did revert ventricular tachycardia to sinus rhythm in 1 animal.

Conclusions.—Given in high doses, cocaine appears to have negative inotropic and potent type I electrophysiologic effects. The resulting QRS prolongation is selectively reversed by sodium bicarbonate, which may have a place in the treatment of cocaine-induced ventricular arrhythmias with slowed ventricular conduction. Further study of the mechanism of this reversal, especially at the cellular level, is needed.

▶ Cocaine abuse has been implicated as a cause of sudden cardiac death and ventricular arrhythmias, even in the absence of acute myocardial infarction or myocardial ischemia. In this dog study, intravenous cocaine in a dose-dependent manner significantly decreased blood pressure, coronary blood flow, and cardiac output while increasing QT and QTc intervals, and sinus cycle length; the ventricular effective refractory period and the dispersion of ventricular refractoriness also increased. Sustained ventricular tachycardia could be induced in 5 of 11 animals; sodium bicarbonate decreased cocaine-induced QRS prolongation but had no effect on other variables. These animal studies indicate that high-dose cocaine poses potent type 1 electrophysiologic effects and that sodium bicarbonate may be useful in treating ventricular arrhythmias associated with slow ventricular conduction in the setting of cocaine overdose. This is not surprising, considering the effectiveness of sodium bicarbonate in reversing ventricular arrhythmias caused by high doses of quinidine.—R.A. O'Rourke, M.D.

Additional recent publications concerning cardiac electrophysiology are listed as follows:

1. Luo C-h, Rudy Y: A model of the ventricular cardiac action potential. Depolarization, repolarization and their interaction. *Circ Res* 68:1501–1526, 1991.
2. Roth BJ: Action potential propagation in a thick strand of cardiac muscle. *Circ Res* 68:162–173, 1991.
3. Lorente P, Delgado C, Delmar M, et al: Hysteresis in the excitability of isolated guinea pig ventricular myocytes. *Circ Res* 69:1301–1315, 1991.
4. Delmar M, Ibarra J, Davidenko J, et al: Dynamics of the background outward current of single guinea pig ventricular myocytes. Ionic mechanisms of hysteresis in cardiac cells. *Circ Res* 69:1316–1326, 1991.
5. Tranum-Jensen J, Wilde AAM, Vermeulen JT, et al: Morphology of electrophysiologically identified junctions between Purkinje fibers and ventricular muscle in rabbit and pig hearts. *Circ Res* 69:429–437, 1991.
6. Page RL, Tang ASL, Prystowsky EN: Effect of continuous enhanced vagal tone on atrioventricular nodal and sinoatrial nodal function in humans. *Circ Res* 68:1614–1620, 1991.
7. Sicouri S, Antzelevitch C: A subpopulation of cells with unique electrophysiological properties in the deep subepicardium of the canine ventricle. The M Cell. *Circ Res* 68:1729–1741, 1991.
8. Opthof T, Misier ARR, Coronel R, et al: Dispersion of refractoriness in canine ventricular myocardium. Effects of sympathetic stimulation. *Circ Res* 68:1204–1215, 1991.
9. Kihara Y, Morgan JP: Intracellular calcium and ventricular fibrillation. Studies in the aequorin-loaded isovolumic ferret heart. *Circ Res* 68:1378–1389, 1991.
10. Du X-J, Dart AM, Riemersma RA, et al: Sex difference in presynaptic adrenergic inhibition of norepinephrine release during normoxia and ischemia in the rat heart. *Circ Res* 68:827–835, 1991.
11. Furukawa T, Moroe K, Mayrovitz HN, et al: Arrhythmogenic effects of graded coronary blood flow reductions superimposed on prior myocardial infarction in dogs. *Circ Res* 84:368–377, 1991.
12. Rosen S, Lahorra M, Cohen MV, et al: Ventricular fibrillation threshold is influenced by left ventricular stretch and mass in the absence of ischaemia. *Cardiovasc Res* 25:458–462, 1991.
13. Hagar JM, Hale SL, Kloner RA: Effect of preconditioning ischemia on reperfusion arrhythmias after coronary artery occlusion and reperfusion in the rat. *Circ Res* 68:61–68, 1991.
14. Miyamoto MI, Rockman HA, Guth BD, et al: Effect of α-adrenergic

stimulation on regional contractile function and myocardial blood flow with and without ischemia. *Circulation* 84:1715–1724, 1991.

15. Fujita M, Nagamoto Y, Furuno Y, et al: Effect of preexisting four hour coronary stenosis on ventricular arrhythmias during a subsequent 10 minutes occlusion in dogs. *Cardiovasc Res* 24:896–902, 1990.

16. Vanoli E, De Ferrari GM, Stramba-Badiale M, et al: Vagal stimulation and prevention of sudden death in conscious dogs with a healed myocardial infarction. *Circ Res* 68:1471–1481, 1991.

17. Cerbai E, Ambrosio G, Porciatti F, et al: Cellular electrophysiological basis for oxygen radical-induced arrhythmias. A patch-clamp study in guinea pig ventricular myocytes. *Circulation* 84:1773–1782, 1991.

18. Allessie M, Kirchhof C, Scheffer GJ, et al: Regional control of atrial fibrillation by rapid pacing in conscious dogs. *Circulation* 84:1689–1697, 1991.

19. Johnson NJ, Marchlinski FE: Arrhythmias induced by device antitachycardia therapy due to diagnostic nonspecificity. *J Am Coll Cardiol* 18:1418–1425, 1991.

20. Vos MA, Gorgels APM, Leunissen JDM, et al: Significance of the number of stimuli to initiate ouabin-induced arrhythmias in the intact heart. *Circ Res* 68:38–44, 1991.

21. Swartz JF, Jones JL, Jones RE, et al: Conditioning prepulse of biphasic defibrillator waveforms enhances refractoriness to fibrillation wavefronts. *Circ Res* 68:438–449, 1991.

22. Auteri JS, Jeevanandam V, Bielefeld MR, et al: Effect of AICD patch electrodes on the diastolic pressure-volume curve in pigs. *Ann Thorac Surg* 52:1052–1057, 1991.

Myocardial Perfusion Imaging

Thallium Reinjection After Stress-Redistribution Imaging: Does 24-Hour Delayed Imaging After Reinjection Enhance Detection of Viable Myocardium?

Dilsizian V, Smeltzer WR, Freedman NMT, Dextras R, Bonow RO (Natl Heart, Lung, and Blood Inst, Bethesda, Md; Natl Inst of Health, Bethesda, Md)
Circulation 83:1247–1255, 1991   5–33

Introduction.—It is vital to distinguish ischemic myocardium that is capable of recovery from myocardium that is irreversibly scarred, especially when invasive procedures are being considered for salvage of myocardial tissue. Re-injection of thallium and re-imaging 10 minutes after customary 3- to 4-hour redistribution imaging yields greater estimates of tissue viability because of thallium uptake at sites thought to have permanent damage. To determine whether further redistribution would take place during a 24-hour interval, 40 men and 10 women with stable coronary artery disease were studied.

Methods.—All patients underwent cardiac diagnostic tests, including exercise thallium single-photon emission computed tomography (SPECT) with 2 mCi ^{201}Tl injected at the peak of exercise. They were included in the study only if partially reversible or irreversible thallium defects were evident on visual evaluation of the 3- to 4-hour redistribution images. Those who met this criterion received an immediate extra dose of 1 mCi ^{201}Tl and were re-imaged 10 to 15 minutes and 24 hours later.

Results.—Of 127 myocardial regions qualitatively graded as abnormal on the stress images, 10% normalized completely, 46% were partially reversed, and 43% were judged irreversibly abnormal from the standard redistribution images. Images made immediately after re-injection showed that uptake at 80% of the partially reversed sites improved, 64% to normal levels. No further changes occurred in these areas after 24 hours. Just after re-injection, thallium uptake improved in 45% of the sites considered irreversibly damaged at the 3- to 4-hour redistribution, but an additional 24-hour redistribution did not further enhance uptake in 92% of these areas. Likewise, 97% of the 30 areas considered irreversibly damaged at re-injection remained so at the 24-hour evaluation.

Discussion.—Re-injection of thallium after the conventional 3 to 4 hours of redistribution resulted in normal images of tissues earlier considered to have irreversible thallium uptake defects. No additional benefit accrued from allowing an extra 24-hour redistribution.

▶ Recently there has been great enthusiasm for the clinical detection of under-perfused but viable myocardium that will improve its contractility after myocardial revascularization by coronary artery bypass surgery or mechanical dilatation of coronary artery stenoses. Metabolic and blood flow imaging with positron emission tomography has been used to demonstrate areas of viability that have continuing uptake of glucose despite marked diminution of uptake of radionuclides that reflect myocardial perfusion.

Thallium myocardial perfusion imaging has also been used to identify the probability of viable myocardium. Two techniques for the better identification of likely viable myocardium are (1) delayed imaging at 24 hours after the initial injection of thallium during exercise showing that a greater number of reperfused segments show a late reuptake of thallium than segments present 3–4 hours after the initial intravenous injection of thallium and/or (2) the re-injection of thallium at rest after images taken 3–4 hours after the initial intravenous injection at the end of exercise testing.

Previous study by the same authors (1) demonstrated enhanced thallium uptake within apparently "irreversible" thallium defects, which is compatible with viable myocardium. In as many as 50% of myocardial regions interpreted as having irreversible thallium, images abnormalities on the conventional redistribution images were identified as viable by thallium re-injection.

The authors studied 50 patients with stable coronary artery disease with exercise thallium SPECT immediately after injection of thallium at the peak of exercise, 3–4 hours after exercise, and 15 minutes and 24 hours after a second extra dose of thallium, which was administered intravenously after the initial 3- to 4-hour redistribution images. Again re-injection was followed by an improved thallium uptake in 45% of the sights considered irreversibly damaged at 3- to

4-hour redistribution. However, an additional 24-hour redistribution did not further enhance uptake in 92% of these areas, indicating that an extra 24-hour redistribution series of images was unnecessary in those having a re-injection of thallium when defects were present on the images made 3–4 hours after exercise.—R.A. O'Rourke, M.D.

Reference

1. Dilsizian V, et al: *N Engl J Med* 323:141–146, 1990.

Dipyridamole Thallium-201 Scintigraphy as a Preoperative Screening Test: A Reexamination of Its Predictive Potential
Mangano DT, London MJ, Tubau JF, Browner WS, Hollenberg M, Krupski W, Layug EL, Massie B, the Study of Perioperative Ischemia Research Group (Univ of California, San Francisco)
Circulation 84:493–502, 1991   5–34

Background.—Recent myocardial infarction and current congestive heart failure are consistently identified as predictors of perioperative cardiac morbidity, although the importance of other predictors remains controversial. Whether dipyridamole thallium-201 (^{201}Tl) scintigraphy is useful in preoperative screening for perioperative myocardial ischemia and infarction was investigated in 59 men and 1 woman who were undergoing elective vascular surgery.

Methods.—All patients underwent ^{201}Tl scintigraphy before their operation. The surgeon was blinded to the scintigraphy results. Intraoperatively, myocardial ischemia was monitored by continuous 12-lead ECG and transesophogeal echocardiography (TEE) and postoperatively by continuous 2-lead ECG.

Results.—Redistribution effects—defects that improved or were reversed on delayed scintigrams—were seen in 37% of patients, persistent defects were seen in 30%, and no defects were seen in 33%. Fifty-four percent of adverse outcomes occurred in patients who did not have redistribution defects. Patients with such defects had no significant increase in the risk of an adverse outcome. Fifty-four percent of perioperative ECG and TEE episodes of ischemia and 58% of severe ischemic episodes occurred in patients who did not have redistribution defects. The ^{201}Tl scintigraphy had a sensitivity of 40% to 54%, specificity of 65% to 71%, positive predictive value of 27% to 47%, and negative predictive value of 61% to 82%.

Conclusions.—In patients undergoing vascular surgery, routine screening use of ^{201}Tl scintigraphy does not appear to be warranted. The procedure has limited sensitivity for detecting perioperative ischemia or adverse cardiac outcome, and its negative predictive value appears lower than previously thought. This result contrasts with the findings of previous studies.

▶ These results in only 60 patients undergoing elective vascular surgery suggest that the value of dipyridamole ^{201}Tl scintigraphy as a preoperative screening test for perioperative cardiac events in patients with peripheral vascular disease has been overrated. However, various results concerning the usefulness of dipyridamole thallium imaging may differ related to patient population, and the presence or absence of other high-risk features such as age more than 70, operation for abdominal aortic aneurysm, presence of diabetes mellitus as well as the presence of prior myocardial infarction or congestive heart failure. In patients with several risk factors, a normal ^{201}Tl scintigram study likely indicates a much better prognosis than in patients with the same risk factors who have a positive result. Also important are the number and extent of reversible thallium defects, whether or not there is thallium uptake by the lung after exercise and whether resting left ventricular function is normal.—R.A. O'Rourke, M.D.

Effects of Dipyridamole and Aminophylline on Hemodynamics, Regional Myocardial Blood Flow and Thallium-201 Washout in the Setting of a Critical Coronary Stenosis

Granato JE, Watson DD, Belardinelli L, Cannon JM, Beller GA (Univ of Virginia Health Sciences Ctr, Charlottesville)
J Am Coll Cardiol 16:1760–1770, 1990   5–35

Introduction.—Patients unable to undergo exercise imaging to detect coronary artery disease can be assessed with dipyridamole thallium-201 (^{201}Tl) scintigraphy. Aminophylline is often used to reverse the side effects of dipyridamole that result from vasodilation. In an animal study, researchers sought to characterize the interaction of intravenous dipyridamole and aminophylline on ^{201}Tl transport kinetics, regional myocardial blood flow, and systemic hemodynamics.

Method.—The experiments were performed in 23 adult dogs. Five animals without a critical coronary stenosis served as a control group to assess the duration of the vasodilating action of intravenous dipyridamole. The remaining dogs were divided into 2 groups. The 12 in group I underwent dipyridamole infusion followed by aminophylline in the presence of coronary stenosis. The 6 animals in group II underwent aminophylline pretreatment followed by dipyridamole infusion in the presence of coronary stenosis.

Results.—Arterial pressure decreased from a mean of 107 mm Hg to 94 mm Hg in 8 dogs with a critical left anterior descending coronary artery stenosis after intravenous administration of dipyridamole. Distal left anterior descending artery pressure decreased from 70 to 55 mm Hg. The endocardial-epicardial flow ratio decreased from .70 to .36 in the left anterior descending perfusion zone, and the intrinsic thallium washout was significantly prolonged. The dipyridamole-induced systemic hypotension and transmural coronary steal were reversed with intravenous aminophylline, and the thallium washout rate returned to its baseline value (Fig 5–16).

Conclusion.—Intravenous aminophylline administration in dogs

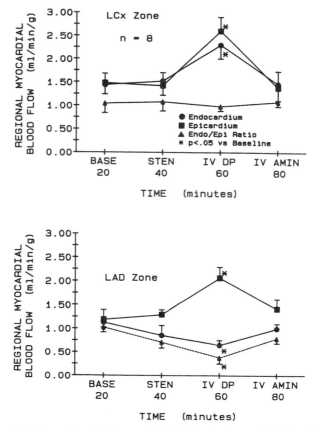

Fig 5–16.—Serial changes in regional myocardial blood flow in the normal left circumflex (LCx) coronary artery zone and in the stenotic left anterior descending coronary artery (LAD) zone at baseline (BASE), after creation of the critical LAD artery stenosis (STEN), after intravenous dipyridamole (IVDP), and after intravenous aminophylline (IV AMIN) in 8 dogs. Note that the dipyridamole-induced changes in flow are reversed by aminophylline administration. *Endo/Epi* denotes endocardial/epicardial. (Courtesy of Granato JE, Watson DD, Belardinelli L, et al: *J Am Coll Cardiol* 16:1760–1770, 1990.)

promptly reversed systemic hypotension, coronary steal, and prolonged ^{201}Tl washout after intravenous dipyridamole injection. No significant hemodynamic or coronary flow effects resulted from use of aminophylline alone. Intravenous administration of dipyridamole appears to result in a significant transmural coronary steal that is reversed by aminophylline.

▶ In this study of dogs with a severe coronary artery stenosis, intravenous dipyridamole caused a significant transmural coronary artery steal characterized by epicardial hyperemia and endocardial underperfusion. Aminophylline reversed the vasodilator effects of dipyridamole and the prolongation of myocardial thallium washout. This study shows the important interaction between aminophylline and dipyridamole on hemodynamics, regional blood flow, and ^{201}Tl washout. This is important considering the many patients being evaluated with dipyridamole ^{201}Tl imaging, many of whom are unable to perform sufficient exercise on a treadmill or bicycle ergometer.—R.A. O'Rourke, M.D.

Tolerance and Safety of Pharmacologic Coronary Vasodilation With Adenosine in Association With Thallium-201 Scintigraphy in Patients With Suspectd Coronary Artery Disease

Abreu A, Mahmarian JJ, Nishimura S, Boyce TM, Verani MS (Baylor College of Medicine)
J Am Coll Cardiol 18:730–735, 1991   5–36

Background.—Many patients suspected of having coronary artery disease cannot perform exercise in conjunction with thallium scintigraphy. Pharmacologic vasodilation with adenosine is a safer alternative than dipyridamole, but adenosine can cause myocardial ischemia by means of coronary steal, and it also reduces the velocity of atrioventricular nodal conduction.

Objective.—The safety of adenosine infusion was examined in 607 patients who either were suspected of having coronary artery disease or were being evaluated after myocardial infarction. After trials of lower doses, adenosine was infused at a rate of 140 µg/kg/minute for 6 minutes.

Observations.—The heart rate nearly always rose during adenosine infusion. Systolic blood pressure declined in 85% of the patients but increased paradoxically in 12.6% of the group. Diastolic blood pressure fell significantly. Nearly 10% of the patients had first-degree atrioventricular block during the infusion and 3.6% had second-degree atrioventricular block (2 of them with a slow ventricular rate). Significant ST depression was seen in 12.5% of the patients.

Clinical Effects.—Ten patients had severe chest pain during the infusion. Three patients had the infusion slowed or stopped because of hypotension. One patient had dyspnea and bronchospasm, and was given aminophylline.

Conclusions.—Most side effects of infused adenosine are mild and brief, and marked effects can readily be controlled by limiting the rate of infusion or discontinuing it. Adenosine can be safely used in patients with recent myocardial infarction; stepwise infusion is safest.

▶ Adenosine thallium-201 (^{201}Tl) scintigraphy is being performed as an alternative to dipyridamole ^{201}Tl imaging for the assessment of myocardial ischemia during pharmacologic stress. The shorter half-life of adenosine suggests that it may be a safer method of producing coronary artery steal in patients with severe coronary artery stenosis. Therefore, this study in 607 patients provides important data concerning the side effects of this potent coronary artery vasodilator. Although the incidence of side effects may actually be greater with the use of adenosine, most side effects ceased rapidly after stopping the adenosine infusion. Whether or not adenosine is as safe or safer than dipyridamole for detecting patients at risk from coronary artery ischemia remains to be definitely established.—R.A. O'Rourke, M.D.

Assessment of Post-Infarction Jeopardized Myocardium by Vasodilation—Thallium-201 Tomography: Impact on Risk Stratification

Nienaber CA, Spielmann RP, Salge D, Clausen A, Montz R, Bleifeld W (University Hospital Eppendorf, Hamburg, Germany)
Eur Heart J 11:1093–1100, 1990

5–37

Background.—Quantitative spatial assessment of the ischemic myocardium in patients after MI is gaining in clinical importance. Thallium-201 (^{201}Tl) tomography, and its correlation with the angiographic monitoring of heart structure and clinical outcome, were assessed in 80 patients after MI. The ^{201}Tl method was studied as a possible method for risk stratification.

Methods.—The 80 consecutive patients (mean age, 58 years) had chest pain after a documented MI. All patients underwent dipyridamole ^{201}Tl imaging in which .56 mg of dipyridamole per kg was given intravenously over a 2-minute period. Continuous monitoring was recorded, beginning 5 minutes after ^{201}Tl injection and repeated using delayed images after 180 minutes. A large field-of-view gamma camera was used to acquire the tomographic images.

Findings.—Of the 80 patients, 78 were followed. An ischemic reaction occurred in 57 patients based on the vasodilation-redistribution ^{201}Tl tomography, with 9 patients having peri-infarction ischemia and 48 demonstrating additional ischemia at a distance. Significant changes in heart rate and systolic and mean blood pressure occurred during the intravenous infusion of dipyridamole. Peak alterations were observed 4 minutes after dipyridamole administration. The ^{201}Tl tomographic perfusion imaging showed the largest total defect size in patients with ischemia at a distance. The spatial extent of the reversible perfusion defect stratified the groups so that ischemia at a distance was related significantly to a reversible defect of 19%, whereas peri-infarction redistribution covered 11.7%. The number of significantly diseased blood vessels was 2.3 in patients who had ischemia at a distance and 2.5 in those with peri-infarction ischemia. The total number of events during the study was 62, with a high incidence of 96% in subjects who had distant ischemia. This was significantly higher than the cumulative event rate in patients with peri-infarction ischemia and with no ischemia.

Conclusions.—These findings indicate that tomographic vasodilation-redistribution using ^{201}Tl imaging appears to be safe in postinfarction patients. This method can promote quantitative assessment of fixed and reversible perfusion defects and provide a useful risk stratification to predict cardiac events.

▶ In 1981 it was shown that chest pain associated with ECG evidence of ischemia outside of the area of a recent MI ("at a distance") was associated with a poorer prognosis than "peri-infarct ischemia" or postinfarction chest pain associated with ECG changes in the area of a recent MI. This study using ^{201}Tl tomography in patients after a recent acute MI indicates that the pattern of "ischemia at a distance" as detected by myocardial perfusion imaging also

indicates postinfarction patients at higher risk of further cardiac events.—
R.A. O'Rourke, M.D.

Quantitative Thallium-201 Single-Photon Emission Computed Tomography During Maximal Pharmacologic Coronary Vasodilation With Adenosine for Assessing Coronary Artery Disease
Nishimura S, Mahmarian JJ, Boyce TM, Verani MS (Baylor Coll of Medicine;
The Methodist Hosp, Houston)
J Am Coll Cardiol 18:736–745, 1991   5–38

Background.—Noninvasive tests such as dipyridamole thallium imaging have proved useful in the detection and risk assessment of patients with coronary artery disease. Recently, intravenous adenosine, with its ultrashort half-life, has been used along with thallium-201 (^{201}Tl) scintigraphy in those with suspected disease. The use of visual and quantitative ^{201}Tl tomography combined with intravenous adenosine in a large group of patients also undergoing coronary angiography was investigated.

Methods.—A consecutive group of 101 patients underwent ^{201}Tl adenosine tomography followed closely in time by coronary arteriography. Fifty-nine patients underwent angiography about 6 days before tomography, 40 underwent angiography about 6.2 days after tomography, and 2 patients underwent both procedures on the same day. Reasons for the thallium tomography included chest pain assessment, shortness of breath, postmyocardial infarction risk stratification, and coronary artery disease screening.

Findings.—Overall, patients experienced significant changes in hemodynamics, including a decrease in systolic and diastolic blood pressures and a rise in heart rate during thallium tomography. A total of 84 of the 101 patients had side effects, most commonly chest pain, which usually stopped 1 to 2 minutes after discontinuation of the adenosine infusion. Twenty-four patients experienced ischemic ECG changes, with 20 related to a reversible Tl^{201} myocardial perfusion defect. The quantitated sensitivity appeared similar for both techniques: 86% for tomography and 88% for angiography. The specificity was lower for the tomography group (83%) than for the angiography group (95%). The diagnostic sensitivity for patients without myocardial infarction with single-, double-, and triple-vessel disease was 76%, 86%, and 90%, respectively.

Conclusions.—These findings demonstrate that quantitative ^{201}Tl single-emission computed tomography has adequate sensitivity and specificity for its use in the diagnosis of coronary artery disease. It also appears beneficial in the localization of coronary stenosis and the affected vascular regions.

▶ This study indicates that adenosine ^{201}Tl myocardial imaging is an accurate noninvasive method for diagnosing the presence and localizing coronary artery disease. It also indicates that adenosine ^{201}Tl scintigraphy may be a suitable alternative test in patients who cannot exercise and in those whose medication cannot be discontinued before the test because of recent myocardial ischemic events. The diagnostic sensitivity and specificity of adenosine ^{201}Tl single-photon emission computed tomography is equal to that obtained with exercise ^{201}Tl imaging in similar patients.—R.A. O'Rourke, M.D.

Additional recent publications concerning myocardial perfusion imaging are listed as follows:

1. Coyne EP, Belvedere DA, Vande Streek PR, et al: Thallium-201 scintigraphy after intravenous infusion of adenosine compared with exercise thallium testing in the diagnosis of coronary artery disease. *J Am Coll Cardiol* 17:1289–1294, 1991.
2. Nguyen T, Heo J, Ogilby JD, et al: Single photon emission computed tomography with thallium-201 during adenosine-induced coronary hyperemia: Correlation with coronary arteriography, exercise thallium imaging and two-dimensional echocardiography. *J Am Coll Cardiol* 16:1375–1383, 1990.
3. Brown KA: Prognostic value of thallium-201 myocardial perfusion imaging in patients with unstable angina who respond to medical treatment. *J Am Coll Cardiol* 17:1053–1057, 1991.
4. Takeishi Y, Tono-oka I, Ikeda K, et al: Dilatation of the left ventricular cavity on dipyridamole thallium-201 imaging: A new marker of triple-vessel disease. *Am Heart J* 121:466, 1991.
5. Go RT, Marwick TH, MacIntyre WJ, et al: A prospective comparison of rubidium-82 PET and thallium-201 SPECT myocardial perfusion imaging utilizing a single dipyridamole stress in the diagnosis of coronary artery disease. *J Nucl Med* 31:1899–1905, 1990.
6. Burns RJ, Galligan L, Wright LM, et al: Improved specificity of myocardial thallium-201 single-photon emission computed tomography in patients with left bundle branch block by dipyridamole. *Am J Cardiol* 68:504–508, 1991.
7. Bonow RO, Dilsizian V, Cuocolo A, et al: Identification of viable myocardium in patients with chronic coronary artery disease and left ventricular dysfunction. *Circulation* 83:26–37, 1991.
8. Freeman MR, Langer A, Kanwar N, et al: Quantitative analysis of exercise SPECT thallium in the detection of coronary disease. *Am J Cardiac Imag* 4:231–238, 1990.
9. Doi YL, Chikamori T, Takata J, et al: Prognostic value of thallium-201 perfusion defects in idiopathic dilated cardiomyopathy. *Am J Cardiol* 67:188–193, 1991.
10. Civelek AC, Shafique I, Brinker JA, et al: Reduced left ventricular cavitary activity ("black hole sign") in thallium-201 SPECT perfusion images of anteroapical transmural myocardial infarction. *Am J Cardiol* 68:1132–1137, 1991.
11. Hecht HS, Shaw RE, Chin HL, et al: Silent ischemia after coronary angioplasty: Evaluation of restenosis and extent of ischemia in asymptomatic patients by tomographic thallium-201 exercise imag-

ing and comparison with symptomatic patients. *J Am Coll Cardiol* 17:670–677, 1991.

12. Svane B, Bone D: Thallium-201 single photon emission computed tomography in patients with symptoms of heart disease and non-significant coronary artery lesions. *Acta Radiol* 31:463–468, 1990.

13. Kiat H, Van Train KF, Maddahi J, et al: Development and prospective application of quantitative 2-day stress-rest Tc-99m methoxy isobutyl isonitrile SPECT for the diagnosis of coronary artery disease. *Am Heart J* 120:1255–1266, 1990.

14. O'Connor MK, Hammell T, Gibbons RJ: In vitro validation of a simple tomographic technique for estimation of percentage myocardium at risk using methoxyisobutyl isonitrile technetium 99m (sestamibi). *Eur J Nucl Med* 17:69–76, 1990.

15. Stewart RE, Heyl B, O'Rourke R, et al: Demonstration of differential post-stenotic myocardial technetium-99-m-teboroxime clearance kinetics after experimental ischemia and hyperemic stress. *J Nucl Med* 32:2000–2008, 1991.

Positron Emission Tomography

Noninvasive Quantification of Regional Myocardial Blood Flow in Coronary Artery Disease With Oxygen-15-Labeled Carbon Dioxide Inhalation and Positron Emission Tomography

Araujo LI, Lammertsma AA, Rhodes CG, McFalls EO, Iida H, Rechavia E, Galassi A, De Silva R, Jones T, Maseri A (Hammersmith Hosp, London, England)
Circulation 83:875–885, 1991   5–39

Background.—For noninvasive and quantifiable assessment of regional myocardial blood flow, the tracer $H^{15}O$ water shows great promise. It diffuses freely and is almost totally extracted from blood over a considerable range of flow rates. It is metabolically inert, and its extraction is unaffected by profound perturbations of cell metabolism. A study was done to validate the use of ^{15}O carbon dioxide, which is transformed to $H^{15}O$ water in the lungs, for positron emission tomography (PET) studies of myocardial blood flow (MBF).

Methods.—In the initial phase, MBF estimated by PET and inhaled ^{15}O carbon dioxide was compared with values obtained in invasive studies with γ-labeled microspheres. In 9 closed-chest dog preparations, flow rates were manipulated from .6 to 6.1 mL/g/min by intravenous dipyridamole administration. Arterial input and myocardial time-activity curves were fitted to a 1-tissue-compartment tracer movement model. Four men and 4 women with effort angina and significant coronary stenoses but no evidence of past myocardial infarction and 11 normal men inhaled ^{15}O carbon dioxide and underwent the same PET protocols used in the dog studies.

Results.—The correlation between PET and microsphere measures of MBF was .91 in the dog studies (Fig 5–17). In control humans, MBF assessed by ^{15}O carbon dioxide inhalation and rapid multiple-slice dynamic

PET MBF and Microspheres MBF in Dogs

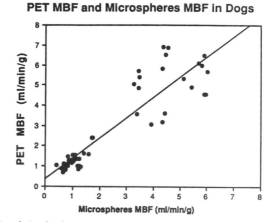

Fig 5–17.—The relationship between MBF measured by PET and that measured by γ-labeled microspheres in the validation studies. (Courtesy of Araujo LI, Lammertsma AA, Rhodes CG, et al: *Circulation* 83:875–885, 1991.)

PET scanning was .88 mL/g/min initially and 3.52 mL/g/min after dipyridamole administration. Values were uniform throughout the left ventricle. In cardiac patients, normal and stenotic arteries had comparable resting average flow rates of 1.01 and .93 mL/g/min, respectively, but stenotic arteries hardly responded to dipyridamole challenge. Flows in stenotic arteries rose to 1.32 mL/g/min compared with 2.86 mL/g/min in regions with unconstricted arteries.

Discussion.—Inhalation of ^{15}O carbon dioxide combined with PET scanning is a desirably noninvasive method of determining regional MBF. It yields results comparable to those obtained with γ-labeled microspheres over a range of flow rates. Disadvantages include "noise" from the high level of activity in the cardiac chambers and a generally noisier image than that attained with other flow tracers.

▶ This combined animal and human study indicates that myocardial blood flow measurements as determined by PET using ^{15}O carbon dioxide correlates well with measurements of myocardial blood flow as determined by radiolabeled microspheres and that this technique is a valid and clinically applicable method for quantitating and noninvasively measuring regional myocardial blood flow in patients.—R.A. O'Rourke, M.D.

Coronary Vasodilation Is Impaired in Both Hypertrophied and Nonhypertrophied Myocardium of Patients With Hypertrophic Cardiomyopathy: A Study With Nitrogen-13 Ammonia and Positron Emission Tomography

Camici P, Chiriatti G, Lorenzoni R, Bellina RC, Gistri R, Italiani G, Parodi O, Salvadori PA, Nista N, Papi L, L'Abbate A (University of Pisa; Pescia Hospital [PT], Pistoia, Italy)

J Am Coll Cardiol 17:879–886, 1991

5–40

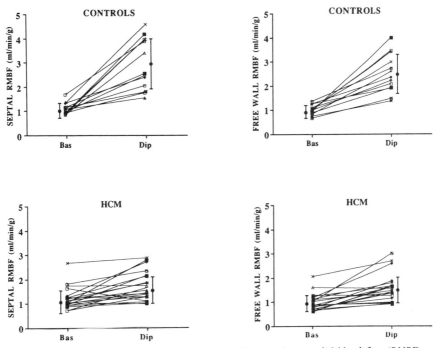

Fig 5–18.—Individual values of septal and free wall regional myocardial blood flow (*RMBF*) at baseline (*Bas*) study and after dipyridamole (*Dip*) infusion in controls (**top panels**) and patients with hypertrophic cardiomyopathy (*HCM*) (**bottom panels**). After dipyridamole, regional myocardial blood flow in patients with hypertrophic cardiomyopathy increased significantly less than in controls, both in the hypertrophied septum and the nonhypertrophied left ventricular free wall. (Courtesy of Camici P, Chiriatti G, Lorenzoni R, et al: *J Am Coll Cardiol* 17:879–886, 1991.)

Introduction.—Regional myocardial blood flow was measured by nitrogen 13 ammonia and positron emission tomography (PET) to determine whether coronary reserve was abnormal in nonhypertrophied myocardium of patients having hypertrophic cardiomyopathy. Abnormalities of the myocardium and coronary bed may not be associated with gross tissue hypertrophy.

Methods.—Myocardial blood flow measurements were made at rest (baseline) and after intravenously administered dipyridamole in 23 patients with asymmetric septal hypertrophy and in 12 controls. A series of PET images was obtained for each subject.

Results.—Baseline values for myocardial blood flow in controls and in patients with hypertrophic cardiomyopathy did not differ significantly (Fig 5–18). After infusion of dipyridamole, the increase in regional myocardial blood flow was significantly less in patients with hypertrophic cardiomyopathy than in the controls, both in the septum and the free wall. Patients with hypertrophic cardiomyopathy and history of chest pain had more significant impairment of coronary reserve than those without such history.

Discussion.—Reduction in coronary reserve may not be primarily the result of myocardial hypertrophy. These results demonstrate abnormal coronary vasodilator reserve not only in the hypertrophied interventricular septum, but also in the nonhypertrophied left ventricular free wall. Myocardial hypertrophy may be an independent marker of the disease and ischemia may be more important than previously thought.

▶ In this study, nitrogen-13 ammonia and PET were used to measure regional myocardial blood flow before and after intravenous dipyridamole in normal subjects and in patients with hypertrophic cardiomyopathy. The results suggest that coronary vasodilator reserve is abnormal not only in the hypertrophied intraventricular septum but also in nonhypertrophied segments of the left ventricle and in patients with hypertrophic cardiomyopathy, particularly in those with a history of chest pain. Baseline regional coronary artery resistance was significantly lower in patients with a history of chest pain, both in the septum and in the free wall.—R.A. O'Rourke, M.D.

Additional recent publications concerning positron emission tomography are listed below:

1. Gupta NC, Esterbrooks D, Mohiuddin S, et al: Adenosine in myocardial perfusion imaging using positron emission tomography. *Am Heart J* 122:293, 1991.
2. Marwick TH, MacIntyre WJ, Salcedo EE, et al: Identification of ischemic and hibernating myocardium: Feasibility of post-exercise F-18 deoxyglucose positron emission tomography. *Catheter Cardiovasc Diagn* 22:100–106, 1991.
3. Hicks RJ, Herman WH, Kalff V, et al: Quantitative evaluation of regional substrate metabolism in the human heart by positron emission tomography. *J Am Coll Cardiol* 18:101–111, 1991.
4. Nienaber CA, Ratib O, Gambhir SS, et al: A quantitative index of regional blood flow in canine myocardium derived noninvasively with N-13 ammonia and dynamic positron emission tomography. *J Am Coll Cardiol* 17:260–269, 1991.

Transthoracic, 2D, and Doppler Echocardiography

Value and Limitations of Doppler Pressure Half-Time in Quantifying Mitral Stenosis: A Comparison With Micromanometer Catheter Recordings
Smith MD, Wisenbaugh T, Grayburn PA, Gurley JC, Spain MG, DeMaria AN (Univ of Kentucky; VA Med Ctr, Lexington, Ky)
Am Heart J 121:480–488, 1991   5–41

Introduction.—Mitral pressure half-time measurement is used as a noninvasive test for estimation of the mitral valve area. Although this method is commonly used, no longitudinal large-scale study has been conducted for since catheterization half-time was introduced in 1968. This technique was compared with the Doppler method of estimating mitral valve area using valve areas calculated from the Gorlin equation in patients with clinically significant mitral stenosis.

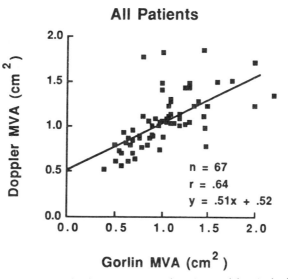

All Patients

Doppler MVA (cm^2)

Gorlin MVA (cm^2)

n = 67
r = .64
y = .51x + .52

Fig 5–19.—Linear regression plot that compares Doppler estimates of the mitral valve area (*MVA*) in square centimeters versus valve area from the Gorlin equation at catheterization. Overall, the correlation yielded *r* = .64, with standard error = .23 cm^2. (Courtesy of Smith MD, Wisenbaugh T, Grayburn PA, et al: *Am Heart J* 121:480–488, 1991.)

Methods.—Eighty consecutive patients with stenosis in native mitral valves underwent catheterization with micromanometer catheters for left ventricular (LV) pressure measurements during 4 years. Thirteen of the 80 patients were excluded; cardiac catheterization was performed in 67 patients using a percutaneous approach. Transseptal catheterization was done from the femoral percutaneous approach using a standard technique. The mitral valve area was calculated using a modified Gorlin equation with thermodilution cardiac output measurements.

Results.—The study group included 44 women and 23 men. At the time of the study, 44 patients were in sinus rhythm (group I—0 to 1+ mitral regurgitation; group II—2 to 4+ mitral regurgitation); 23 had atrial fibrillation (group III—0 to 1+ mitral regurgitation; group IV—2 to 4+ mitral regurgitation); 39 had no mitral regurgitation. Continuous-wave Doppler pressure half-times ranged from 120 to 422 ms; catheterization pressure half-times ranged from 120 to 637 ms. Predicted mitral valve area by the Doppler pressure half-time method showed a mean of 1.05 cm^2, whereas the catheterization-derived areas had a mean of 1.03 cm^2 (Fig 5–19), for a fair correlation (*r* = .64). Correlations of the Doppler-derived mitral valve area compared with the catheterization-derived valve area were good in group I and poor in group II. The best correlation was in patients in sinus rhythm without significant mitral regurgitation (group I). The results correlated poorly in groups II and IV. The opening pressure in the initial pressure gradient was not an independent predictor of the half-time or of the mitral valve area. No significant difference was observed between the 2 heart rate measurements.

Conclusions.—These findings indicate that both catheterization and

Doppler pressure half-times fairly predict the Gorlin-derived mitral valve area in patients with clinical mitral stenosis. The relationship between pressure half-time and valve area is best represented by an exponential equation. The catheterization-derived Gorlin valve areas are adversely affected by the occurrence of atrial fibrillation and significant mitral regurgitation.

▶ In this particular study there was only a fair correlation between the catheter-derived mitral valve area and the mitral valve area as determined from the Doppler pressure half-time. The pressure half-time by continuous-wave Doppler echocardiography provides a reliable assessment of mitral valve area in patients with sinus rhythm who have no significant mitral regurgitation. The lack of a closer relationship between the 2 methods of measuring mitral valve area in patients with mitral stenosis is likely multifactorial. It must be pointed out that in this particular study, the 2 methods of measuring mitral stenosis valve area were not performed simultaneously.—R.A. O'Rourke, M.D.

Importance of Two-Dimensional Echocardiographic Assessment of Left Ventricular Systolic Function in Patients Presenting to the Emergency Room With Cardiac-Related Symptoms
Sabia P, Abbott RD, Afrookteh A, Keller MW, Touchstone DA, Kaul S (Univ of Virginia, Charlottesville)
Circulation 84:1615–1624, 1991   5–42

Background.—Although many clinical and ECG variables are diagnostically and prognostically valuable in evaluating patients in the emergency department who have cardiac symptoms, the usefulness of evaluating left ventricular (LV) systolic function in this setting is unknown. Two-dimensional echocardiography (2DE) was used to study the relationship between LV systolic function and cardiac events occurring during or soon after emergency department presentation, as opposed to those occurring later.

Methods.—The subjects were 171 consecutive patients seen in the emergency department with cardiac-related symptoms. Eighty-eight were men, mean age 59 years, and 83 were women, mean age 62 years. For each patient, 1 of the physicians obtained a complete history and physical examination, 12-lead ECG and serum enzyme measurements, and 2DE study. Emergency department physicians treated the patient without knowledge of the results of 2DE. All patients were contacted at 2 years for follow-up. Cardiac events occurring within 48 hours of presentation were considered early and those occurring thereafter were considered late.

Results.—Some major cardiac event occurred during follow-up in 32% of the patients—of these 55 events, 32 were early and 23 were late. Age-adjusted rate of early events was 26.9% for patients with LV systolic dysfunction (LVSD) compared with 3.3% for patients without LVSD. Rate of late cardiac events was 23.9% for those with LVSD and 6.4%

for those without. An ECG, which was diagnostic of myocardial infarction, was the most important confounder in predicting early events, other than advanced age. For late events, advanced age and history of hypertension were important confounders. However, after controlling for other risk factors, the only parameter associated with both types of events was LVSD. The presence or absence of LVSD greatly improved the prediction of cardiac events based on combination of historical, clinical, ECG, and 2DE findings.

Conclusions.—In the emergency department, LVSD as shown by 2DE is a valuable diagnostic and prognostic finding in patients with cardiac-related symptoms. The physician may wish to admit patients with LVSD in whom an acute event is suspected. The absence of LVSD can ease the decision to discharge, especially in those with a normal ECG. Those with the finding of LVSD should be followed aggressively.

▶ In many studies, the presence of moderate-to-marked impairment in LV systolic function has been associated with a poorer prognosis, particularly in patients with coronary artery disease. In this study of 171 consecutive patients seen in an emergency department with cardiac-related symptoms, the 2-year prognosis was much worse in those with evidence of left ventricular systolic dysfunction as determined by 2DE. The prediction of early or late cardiac events as derived from a combination of history, clinical, electrocardiographic and 2DE findings was significantly improved when the presence or absence of LV systolic dysfunction was included as a parameter for determining a favorable or unfavorable 2-year prognosis.—R.A. O'Rourke, M.D.

Stress Echocardiography and the Human Factor: The Importance of Being Expert

Picano E, Lattanzi F, Orlandini A, Marini C, L'Abbate A (University of Pisa, Italy)
J Am Coll Cardiol 17:666–669, 1991   5–43

Background.—Stress echocardiography is now used to diagnose coronary artery disease. It is a low cost, easily available, and noninvasive tool to combine with exercise or drug stimuli for cardiac imaging. A study was conducted to determine the diagnostic accuracy of the stress echocardiographic technique, as used in the dipyridamole echocardiographic test, in relation to the experience of the physician interpreting the results of this method.

Methods.—Twenty physician observers viewed and gave their interpretations of the videotapes of dipyridamole echocardiographic studies. All 20 observers were cardiologists who had completed their training in echocardiography. The 20 physicians were classified as beginners if they had obtained and interpreted fewer than 20 stress echocardiograms and as experts if they had obtained and interpreted at least 100 such procedures. Ten observers (5 beginners and 5 experts) continued in a longitudinal study in which they were trained; they then assessed another 50 dipyridamole-enhanced echocardiographic studies. The initial groups of recordings came from 19 women and 31 men (mean age, 55 years) who experienced chest pain with effort. The second group of patient recordings came from 16 women and 34 men (mean age, 54 years) who also had chest pain with effort. All 100 patients undergoing dipyridamole echocardiography had coronary angiography 1 week before the study. Two-dimensional echocardiographic and 12-lead ECG monitoring was combined with dipyridamole infusion over a 2-minute period.

Findings.—Of the 50 patients first assessed, 33 had angiographically verified coronary artery disease; in the second 50 patients, 34 had documented coronary artery disease. The diagnostic accuracy of the 10 beginning observers was significantly lower than that of the 10 expert observers, affecting both the sensitivity and specificity of the method. False positive results occurred more often in subjects without disease. In the pretraining videotapes in the longitudinal study, the 5 beginners had significantly reduced diagnostic accuracy compared with the 5 more expert physicians. In the posttraining videotape assessments, the accuracy gap was not significantly different between the 2 groups. After training, the beginner group improved significantly, but the expert group did not.

Implications.—Although stress echocardiography appears easy to learn, a significant training period should be conducted. If the physician has had no specific training or previous exposure to interpretation of echocardiography, stress echocardiography should not be attempted.

▶ Not surprisingly, this study indicates that interpretations of stress echocardiographic studies by echocardiographers without specific training severely underestimates the diagnostic potential of the method. It also suggests that the learning curve for stress echocardiography (dipyridamole echocardiographic testing) requires no more than 100 stress tests interpreted with an experienced supervisor. This is similar to the training period required to obtain Doppler ultrasound skills by an operator experienced in M-mode and 2-D echocardiography.—R.A. O'Rourke, M.D.

Echocardiographic Demonstration of Decreased Left Ventricular Dimensions and Vigorous Myocardial Contraction During Syncope Induced by Head-Up Tilt
Shalev Y, Gal R, Tchou PJ, Anderson AJ, Avitall B, Akhtar M, Jazayeri MR (Univ of Wisconsin Med School, Milwaukee)
J Am Coll Cardiol 18:746–751, 1991   5–44

Introduction.—The head-up tilt test has served as a diagnostic examination for unexplained syncope or presyncope. The way in which hypotension and bradycardia caused by the head-up tilt actually occurs is not totally understood. Echocardiography was used to assess the left ventricular dimension and its function during the head-up tilt test.

Methods.—Eleven control subjects and 18 patients with recurrent unexplained syncope had 2-dimensional echocardiography (2DE) during a head-up tilt test. If the patients had a normal baseline head-up tilt test, the patient returned to the supine position and received an infusion of intravenous isoproterenol to achieve a 20% increase in heart rate. Nine patients with a positive test received a 10-mg bolus injection of metoprolol intravenously.

Results.—The 11 control subjects completed the 15-minute head-up tilt test without any symptoms or problems. Four patients had a negative head-up tilt test result, 9 had a positive test at baseline, and 5 developed syncope after isoproterenol infusion. Controls and patients having a negative test response demonstrated an end-systolic decrease within 1 minute of moving upright. Those with a positive test at baseline had a decrease in left ventricular end-systolic and end-diastolic areas, both of which continued to fall during the upright position. Those with a positive test after isoproterenol had a similar decrease in these 2 parameters, but the end-systolic area continued to gradually and significantly fall during the upright position. In those receiving metoprolol, the fractional shortening at the end of the head-up tilt was significantly lower than during the initial studies of syncope in both groups experiencing positive head-up tilt test results.

Implications.—These findings indicate that vigorous myocardial contraction and a significant fall in left ventricular end-systolic dimensions can induce syncope. This left ventricular hypercontractility may be active in causing syncope produced by the head-up tilt test.

▶ In this study, 2DE was used as a technique for assessing left ventricular volumes and function in control subjects compared with patients who had recurrent unexplained syncope. Syncope induced by head-up tilt was associated with a greater decrease in LV end-systolic dimension and a much greater increase in LV fractional shortening than in patients not experiencing syncope during baseline head-up tilt or after isoproterenol challenge. This study indicates the usefulness of 2DE for assessing cardiac function during maneuvers that reproduce the patient's symptoms.—R.A. O'Rourke, M.D.

Additional recent publications concerning transthoracic 2D and Doppler echocardiography are listed below:

1. Huwez FU, Pringle SD, Macfarlane PW: A comparison of left ventricular mass and volume using different echocardiographic conventions. *Int J Cardiol* 30:103–108, 1991.
2. Markiewicz W, Moscovitz M, Reisner S, et al: Diagnostic and prognostic value of oral dipyridamole test using echocardiography. *Isr J Med Sci* 26:601–605, 1990.
3. Kircher B, Abbott JA, Pau S, et al: Left atrial volume determination by biplane two-dimensional echocardiography: Validation by cine computed tomography. *Am Heart J* 121:864–871, 1991.
4. Agati L, Arata L, Luongo R, et al: Assessment of severity of coronary narrowings by quantitative exercise echocardiography and comparison with quantitative arteriography. *Am J Cardiol* 67:1201–1207, 1991.

5. Doud DN, Jacobs WR, Moran JF III, et al: The natural history of left ventricular spontaneous contrast. *J Am Soc Echocardiog* 3:465–470, 1990.

6. Appleton CP, Carucci MJ, Henry CP, et al: Influence of incremental changes in heart rate on mitral flow velocity: Assessment in lightly sedated, conscious dogs. *J Am Coll Cardiol* 17:227–236, 1991.

7. Gorcsan J III, Snow FR, Paulsen W, et al: Noninvasive estimation of left atrial pressure in patients with congestive heart failure and mitral regurgitation by Doppler echocardiography. *Am Heart J* 121:858–863, 1991.

8. Jaffe WM, Dewhurst TA, Otto CM, et al: Influence of Doppler sample volume location on ventricular filling velocities. *Am J Cardiol* 68:550–552, 1991.

9. Picard MH, SanFilippo AJ, Newell JB, et al: Quantitative relation between increased intrapericardial pressure and Doppler flow velocities during experimental cardiac tamponade. *J Am Coll Cardiol* 18:234–242, 1991.

10. Tramarin R, Torbicki A, Marchandise B, et al: Doppler echocardiographic evaluation of pulmonary artery pressure in chronic obstructive pulmonary disease. A European multicentre study. *Eur Heart J* 12:103–111, 1991.

11. Mehta RH, Helmcke F, Nanda NC, et al: Uses and limitations of transthoracic echocardiography in the assessment of atrial septal defect in the adult. *Am J Cardiol* 67:288–294, 1991.

12. Chafizadeh ER, Zoghbi WA: Doppler echocardiographic assessment of the St. Jude medical prosthetic valve in the aortic position using the continuity equation. *Circulation* 83:213–223, 1991.

13. Utsunomiya T, Ogawa T, Doshi R, et al: Doppler color flow "proximal isovelocity surface area" method for estimating volume flow rate: Effects of orifice shape and machine factors. *J Am Coll Cardiol* 17:1103–1111, 1991.

14. Bengur AR, Snider AR, Vermilion RP, et al: Left ventricular ejection fraction measured with Doppler color flow mapping techniques. *Am J Cardiol* 68:669–673, 1991.

15. Baumgartner H, Schima H, Kühn P: Importance of technical variables for quantitative measurements by color Doppler imaging. *Am J Cardiol* 67:314–315, 1991.

Transesophageal Echocardiography

Safety of Transesophageal Echocardiography: A Multicenter Survey of 10,419 Examinations

Daniel WG, Erbel R, Kasper W, Visser CA, Engberding R, Sutherland GR, Grube E, Hanrath P, Maisch B, Dennig K, Schartl M, Kremer P, Angermann C, Iliceto S, Curtius JM, Mügge A (Hannover Medical School, Germany; University Clinic, Mainz, Germany; University Clinic, Freiburg, Germany; Academic Medical Center, Amsterdam; University Clinic, Münster, Germany; et al)

Circulation 83:817–821, 1991

5–45

Background.—An unimpeded, high-quality view of the heart and great vessels has made transesophageal echocardiography (TEE) a popular technique when conventional transthoracic echocardiography is inconclusive. Because TEE is semi-invasive and may involve some discomfort and risk for the patient, a multicenter survey was executed to assess the risk and practicality of this technique.

Methods.—Questionnaires were completed by the cardiology divisions at 15 European institutions that had used adult TEE for at least 1 year and had retained records on patients and sequelae of TEE. Among these centers, 10,419 TEE studies were done, an average of 694 per center (range 106 to 2,977), compared with 160,431 transthoracic echocardiograms done during the same period.

Results.—Eighty-eight percent of patients were awake during the 10- to 20-minute procedure. All but 1 center used local pharyngeal anesthesia. Only 54 physicians performed TEE. Of these, only 54% had formal experience with endoscopy. In the 1.9% of cases in which the probe could not be inserted, physician inexperience and/or lack of patient cooperation was the most frequent cause. Centers that had performed 200 or fewer TEE examinations had almost triple the failure rate of other centers. In only 18 of 10,218 examinations did significant complications (pulmonary or cardiac complications or pharyngeal bleeding) occur. They resolved spontaneously when the probe was removed in 17 patients. In an additional 65 examinations, patient intolerance of the probe mandated interruption of the procedure.

Conclusion.—The TEE procedure has a reasonably low level of risk when performed by physicians trained in endoscopic procedures in a setting with appropriate facilities. It can be a valuable source of information when traditional transthoracic echocardiography proves inadequate.

▶ This large, retrospective multicenter study indicates that TEE is associated with an acceptable low risk when performed by experienced operators under appropriate safety conditions. Pulmonary, cardiac, or bleeding complications necessitating interruption of the transesophageal echocardiographic examinations were observed in only .18% of cases. Death occurred in only 1 patient out of 10,218 studies performed. The complication rate is in the range comparable to complication rates reported in large series of patients undergoing gastroduodenoscopy examinations, who have a mortality rate of approximately .0004%.—R.A. O'Rourke, M.D.

Diagnosis of Noninfective Cardiac Mass Lesions by Two-Dimensional Echocardiography: Comparison of the Transthoracic and Transesophageal Approaches
Mügge A, Daniel WG, Haverich A, Lichtlen PR (Hannover Medical School, Hannover, Germany)
Circulation 83:70–78, 1991   5–46

Background.—The diagnostic accuracy of transthoracic echocardiog-

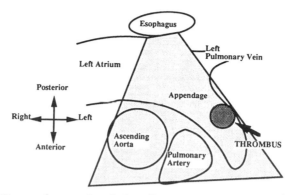

Fig 5–20.—Diagram of transesophageal echocardiogram demonstrating thrombotic material (*arrow*) within the left atrial appendage (LAA). Thrombus was subsequently proven by surgery. (Courtesy of Mügge A, Daniel WG, Haverich A, et al: *Circulation* 83:70–78, 1991.)

raphy was compared with that of transesophageal echocardiography in detecting cardiac and paracardiac masses. The study included 46 patients with cardiac thrombi, 15 with atrial myxomas, and 32 with other cardiac or paracardiac tumors. Diagnoses were later proven by surgery, autopsy, CT, MRI, or angiography.

Methods.—All patients underwent conventional transthoracic echocardiography and, within 24 hours after the precordial examination, transesophageal echocardiographic investigation.

Results.—Transthoracic and transesophageal approaches both provided accurate diagnoses in all 15 myxomas. The transesophageal echocardiogram clearly identified the point of attachment at the septum in all 15; the transthoracic echocardiogram identified it in 12. All left atrial appendage thrombi were visible on the transesophageal echocardiogram (Fig 5–20) but did not appear on the precordial echocardiogram. However, left ventricular apical thrombi were predicted more frequently by precordial echocardiography. All 6 left-sided pericardiac or paracardiac tumors were correctly identified by both techniques. Only 9 of 14 right-sided tumors were identified by transthoracic echocardiography, whereas the transesophageal view correctly identified all 14.

Conclusions.—Cardiac tumors, particularly lesions around the right heart, were more accessible when imaged from the esophagus. These data indicate the clinical superiority of transesophageal cardiography in diagnosing patients in whom cardiac masses are suspected or need to be excluded to ensure the safety of clinical procedures.

▶ In this study comparing transthoracic and transesophageal echocardiography in the detection of noninfective cardiac and paracardiac masses, atrial myxomas were identified equally by both techniques, but transesophageal echocardiography was much better in identifying atrial thrombi and other cardiac or paracardiac tumors. As might be anticipated, transthoracic echocardiography was a better technique for detecting left ventricular apical thrombi.—R.A. O'Rourke, M.D.

Assessment of Left Atrial Appendage Function by Transesophageal Echocardiography: Implications for the Development of Thrombus

Pollick C, Taylor D (Vancouver General Hospital; University of British Columbia, Vancouver)

Circulation 84:223–231, 1991   5–47

Background.—The trabecular left atrial appendage (LAA) is a remnant of the original embryonic left atrium that develops during the third week of gestation. Its function is unknown. The predilection of the LAA for thrombus formation has been known since 1909. An LAA thrombus is a known potent risk factor for stroke, but the pathogenesis of LAA thrombus has not been defined. The cause of LAA thrombus formation was investigated by examining the appearance and function of the LAA in health and in various cardiac diseases.

Patients.—During a 6-month study period, 118 patients underwent 2-dimensional transesophageal echocardiography, and in 82 of them adequate visualization of the LAA allowed detailed measurements. There were 40 men and 42 women, aged 22–78 years. Primary indications for transesophageal echocardiography included prosthetic valve evaluation, stroke, congenital heart disease, and endocarditis.

Findings.—Sixty-three patients were in sinus rhythm, and 5 of them had LAA thrombus. Nineteen patients had atrial fibrillation or atrial flutter, of whom 4 had LAA thrombus, 3 had LAA spontaneous contrast, and 1 had both. There were 2 characteristic locations of LAA thrombus: at the LAA apex, either alone or with extension into the body of the LAA, or attached to the lateral LAA wall (Fig 5–21). In sinus rhythm, the LAA behaved as a highly contractile muscular pump that displayed a characteristic pattern of emptying quite distinct from that of the main body of the left atrium. In sinus rhythm with thrombus, LAA contraction was decreased and the LAA was usually also dilated. In atrial fibrillation or flutter without LAA contrast or thrombus, the LAA displayed passive filling and emptying as a result of compression from the adjacent left ventricle onto the medial LAA wall. In atrial fibrillation or flutter with LAA contrast or thrombus, or both, the LAA invariably behaved as a static pouch.

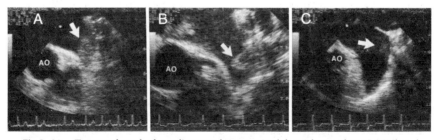

Fig 5–21.—Transesophageal echocardiograms demonstrating left atrial appendage (*LAA*) thrombus in 3 patients with atrial fibrillation. **A,** thrombus (*arrow*) extends from apex into body of LAA; **B,** thrombus (*arrow*) is attached to lateral wall; **C,** thrombus (*arrow*) is attached to lateral wall. *Abbreviation: AO,* aorta. (Courtesy of Pollick C, Taylor D: *Circulation* 84:223–231, 1991.)

Conclusion.—A severaly hypokinetic and enlarged LAA appears to predispose to thrombus formation in the same way a left ventricular aneurysm predisposes to thrombus formation.

▶ This imaging study indicates that the left atrial appendage is a highly contractual pump with a pattern of contraction quite distinct from that of the main body of the left atrium. It shows that left atrial appendage thrombus formation is associated with decreased left atrial appendage contraction as well as with dilatation of the appendage.—R.A. O'Rourke, M.D.

Transesophageal Doppler Echocardiography Evaluation of Coronary Blood Flow Velocity in Baseline Conditions and During Dipyridamole-Induced Coronary Vasodilation
Iliceto S, Marangelli V, Memmola C, Rizzon P (University of Bari, Italy)
Circulation 83:61–69, 1991   5–48

Background.—The proximal coronary artery anatomy and coronary blood flow velocity (CBFV) may be assessed by transesophageal echocardiography. To assess the potential of this technique for evaluating CBFV and variations in CBFV induced by coronary-active drugs, high-quality pulsed-wave Doppler recordings were made in 15 patients.

Methods.—The patients were 11 men and 4 women, mean age 56.6 years, undergoing diagnostic coronary angiography. The CBFV was evaluated by transesophageal Doppler before and 2 minutes after cessation of dipyridamole infusion, .56 mg/kg in 4 minutes. Aminophylline, 240 mg, was injected, and CBFV was measured again after 2 minutes. Maximal and mean diastolic and systolic velocities were measured at each step, along with ratio between maximal diastolic velocity recorded before and after dipyridamole administration.

Results.—The left anterior descending coronary artery was normal in 9 patients (designated group A), and stenotic (75% or greater) in 6 patients (designated group B). Group A patients had significant increases in all CBFV parameters during dipyridamole infusion, with return to near baseline after aminophylline infusion. None of the CBFV parameters increased after dipyridamole infusion in group B patients. Ratio of dipyridamole to baseline maximal diastolic velocity was 3.22 in group A and 1.46 in group B. Ratio of mean diastolic velocity was 3.04 in group A and 1.48 in group B.

Conclusions.—Transesophageal Doppler echocardiography can be used to evaluate CBFV as well as changes induced by coronary-active drugs. This technique may be useful in assessing coronary blood flow reserve.

▶ This study shows that transesophageal Doppler echocardiography can be used in certain patients to assess the effects of vasoactive drugs and to evaluate coronary blood flow reserve in the left anterior descending coronary artery. Peak and mean systolic velocities increased after dipyridamole infusion in patients without stenosis of the left anterior descending coronary artery and reverted to baseline levels with subsequent administration of aminophylline. No increase in mean or peak systolic velocity occurred with dipyridamole in patients with critical coronary artery stenosis involving the left anterior descending artery. The frequency with which this technique will be applied clinically to patients undergoing assessment for coronary artery disease remains to be established. However, currently available invasive approaches including Doppler catheters, thermodilation, and digital angiography have both technical difficulties and limitations.—R.A. O'Rourke, M.D.

Additional recent publications concerning transesophageal echocardiography are listed below:

1. Black IW, Hopkins A, Lee CL, et al: The clinical role of transoesophageal echocardiography. *Aust NZ J Med* 20:759–764, 1990.
2. Porembka DT, Hoit BD: Transesophageal echocardiography in the intensive care patient. *Crit Care Med* 19:826–835, 1991.
3. Muhiudeen IA, Kuecherer HF, Lee E, et al: Intraoperative estimation of cardiac output by transesophageal pulsed Doppler echocardiography. *Anesthesiology* 74:9–14, 1991.
4. O'Shea JP, Southern JF, D'Ambra MN, et al: Effects of prolonged transesophageal echocardiographic imaging and probe manipulation of the esophagus—an echocardiographic-pathologic study. *J Am Coll Cardiol* 17:1426–1429, 1991.
5. Glance LG, Keefe DL, Carlon GC: Transesophageal echocardiography for assessing the cause of hypotension. *Crit Care Med* 19:1213–1214, 1991.
6. Castello R, Pearson AC, Lenzen P, et al: Evaluation of pulmonary venous flow by transesophageal echocardiography in subjects with a normal heart: Comparison with transthoracic echocardiography. *J Am Coll Cardiol* 18:65–71, 1991.
7. Klein AL, Obarski TP, Stewart WJ, et al: Transesophageal Doppler echocardiography of pulmonary venous flow: A new marker of mitral regurgitation severity. *J Am Coll Cardiol* 18:518–526, 1991.
8. Yamagishi M, Yasu T, Ohara K, et al: Detection of coronary blood flow associated with left main coronary artery stenosis by transesophageal Doppler color flow echocardiography. *J Am Coll Cardiol* 17:87–93, 1991.
9. Lanzieri M, Michaelson S, Cohen IS: Transesophageal echocardiography in the diagnosis of mitral bioprosthetic obstruction. *Crit Care Med* 19:979–981, 1991.

Intravascular Ultrasound Imaging

Intravascular Ultrasound Imaging of Human Coronary Arteries In Vivo: Analysis of Tissue Characterizations With Comparison to In Vitro Histological Specimens

Tobis JM, Mallery J, Mahon D, Lehmann K, Zalesky P, Griffith J, Gessert J, Moriuchi M, McRae M, Dwyer M-L, Greep N, Henry WL (Univ of California, Irvine; VA Hosp, Long Beach, Calif; InterTherapy Inc, Costa Mesa, Calif)
Circulation 83:913–926, 1991

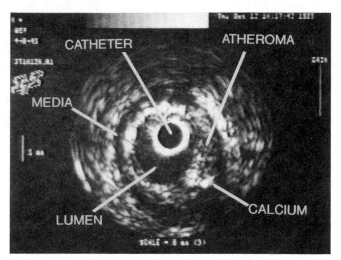

Fig 5–22.—Representative intravascular ultrasound image from the midportion of the LAD coronary artery from a patient after ballon angioplasty, taken from a section that appeared normal on angiography. (Courtesy of Tobis JM , Mallery J, Mahon D, et al: *Circulation* 83:913–926, 1991.)

Background.—Currently available in vivo imaging techniques, including contrast coronary angiography and chest fluoroscopy, are inadequate to thoroughly characterize the histologic traits of atherosclerosis. The usefulness of intravascular ultrasound imaging in identifying the composition of human arterial atherosclerotic plaques was assessed.

Methods.—Under fluoroscopic control, an intra-arterial ultrasound device (30 real-time cross-sectional images per second) with a 20-MHz transducer on the distal end of a 1.2-mm diameter cable was inserted into a 1.6-mm introducer sheath. Studies were done on 27 patients immediately after standard coronary balloon angioplasty for symptomatic angina. The ultrasound apparatus was successfully introduced in 22 patients in whom 9 right coronary arteries, 5 circumflex branches, 7 left anterior descending (LAD) coronary arteries, and 1 saphenous vein were studied. In addition, 20 segments from human coronary, iliac, carotid, and femoral arteries were imaged for comparison with their histologic sections and the in vivo imaging results.

Results.—The most striking finding was the amount of residual atheroma in the dilatation site detected by ultrasound. The mean cross-sectional area of the lumen was 5 mm^2, and 63% of the area within the media, a mean of 8.7 mm^2, was filled with atheroma. In angiographically normal segments (Fig 5–22), atheroma filled a mean 4.7 mm^2 of the available arterial space. Calcium was found in 73% of the arteries by ultrasound and in only 5% by angiography. The in vitro ultrasound studies accurately characterized the composition of arterial samples as defined in histologic sections.

Discussion.—Compared with ultrasound, contrast angiography may underestimate the presence of atheroma by overestimating the residual lumen after angioplasty. The good correlation of histologic and ultrasound measurements suggests that ultrasound provides a more accurate representation than angiography.

▶ Recently, there has been great interest and several clinical reports of the use of intravascular ultrasound imaging of normal and abnormal coronary arteries, particularly in patients undergoing use of balloon coronary angioplasty. This preliminary study demonstrates the capability of intravascular ultrasound for providing real-time, cross-sectional images of the coronary artery lumen and wall in vivo.

In cases where the arteriogram and the ultrasound image correlate poorly, 2 sources of in vitro data suggest that the ultrasound image provides a more accurate representation. In several studies, excellent correlations were obtained between the lumen cross-sectional area measured from ultrasound images and direct measurements from histologic cross-sections. Also, an in vitro study using an acrylamide cast of a phantom model demonstrated that contrast angiography overestimates the true lumen cross-sectional area compared with intravascular ultrasound when the lumen is not elliptical but is irregular.—R.A. O'Rourke, M.D.

Intravascular Ultrasound Imaging of Human Coronary Arteries After Percutaneous Transluminal Angioplasty: Morphologic and Quantitative Assessment
Werner GS, Sold G, Buchwald A, Kreuzer H, Wiegand V (Georg-August-University, Goettingen, Germany)
Am Heart J 122:212–220, 1991   5–50

Background.—Although angiography is the diagnostic method of choice to assess coronary arteries, intravascular ultrasound has recently been used to detect and quantify the mechanical effects of certain intravascular therapies. The present study investigated the use of a new 4.8 F intravascular ultrasound probe in measuring the morphological changes induced by percutaneous transluminal angioplasty in the human coronary artery.

Methods.—Sixteen patients were examined with the intravascular ultrasound probe after undergoing percutaneous transluminal coronary angioplasty. An LZT (lead/zirconium/titanium) crystal attached to the tip of a motor-driven shaft was used with the probe. The optimum focus of this crystal had a range of 1.5 mm and gave a lateral resolution of 300 to 450 μm and an axial resolution of 150 to 300 μm, with a maximum depth penetration of 1 cm. The outer diameter of the ultrasound catheter and an accompanying artifact restricted its use to a minimum vessel diameter of 3 mm.

Findings.—The ultrasound morphology of a normal and a diseased coronary artery in the patient with a single-vessel disorder showed that a ring of intimal layer encircled the normal vessel lumen. The thickening of this layer compared with the media indicated early atherosclerosis. In the 16 patients undergoing ultrasound imaging, the procedure failed in 2. Of the 14 successful procedures, the vessel lumen appeared irregular in 8. In 11 of the 14, an intimal-layer separation and plaque was found by the ultrasound technique. The results of the ultrasound examination closely correlated with the results of the angiogram, but the ultrasound technique seemed to measure larger dimensions and luminal area. No severe complications occurred during the intravascular procedure.

Conclusions.—The authors conclude that the morphology of the vessel lumen is better measured by the ultrasound technique. The intravascular imaging can also aid in plaque detection, morphology, and composition.

▶ This quantitative comparison between coronary arteriography and the ultrasound measurement showed a close correlation for coronary vessel sites distal to the point of coronary angioplasty for both vessel diameter and for luminal area. In 11 cases, the correlation of angiographic and sonographic measurements of the dilated coronary artery segments was good for the assessment of the vessel diameter but poor for the determination of the luminal area. The difference reflected the complex morphology of the vessel lumen after angioplasty, which could be better assessed by the cross-sectional ultrasound technique than by contrast arteriography.—R.A. O'Rourke, M.D.

Comparison of Intravascular Ultrasound, External Ultrasound and Digital Angiography for Evaluation of Peripheral Artery Dimensions and Morphology

Sheikh KH, Davidson CJ, Kisslo KB, Harrison JK, Himmelstein SI, Kisslo J, Bashore TM (Duke Univ Med Ctr, Durham, NC)
Am J Cardiol 67:817–822, 1991   5–51

Background.—Because external ultrasound (US) can accurately determine vessel dimensions and forms, and it provides cross-sectional arterial images, it was compared with intravascular US to better determine the accuracy of this newer technique. Shortcomings of other methods were disclosed.

Methods.—Fifteen patients underwent intravascular US, external 2-dimensional US, Doppler color-flow imaging, and digital angiography at 29 femoral artery sites. Peripheral artery dimensions and presence and composition of arterial plaque were determined.

Results.—Intravascular US determinations of lumen diameter correlated well with those of external US and angiography, but Doppler color flow underestimated true lumen size. The disclosure of plaque and its composition was similar with intravascular and external US. Angiography did not adequately identify sites of plaque, nor did it accurately determine plaque composition as did intravascular and external US techniques.

Conclusions.—Comparisons of intravascular US findings with those of external US disclose a good correlation between the 2, surpassing Doppler color flow in estimating lumen size and angiography in identifying plaque sites and evaluating plaque composition. Catheter-based intravascular US appears to be a safe and reliable method for determining peripheral artery dimensions and forms.

▶ This study shows a good correlation between intravascular ultrasound and external ultrasound in estimating the lumen size of peripheral arteries; intravascular ultrasound surpassed Doppler color flow in estimating the lumen size and was better than arteriography at identifying plaque sites and evaluating plaque composition.—R.A. O'Rourke, M.D.

An additional recent publication concerning intravascular ultrasound imaging is listed below:

1. Nissen SE, Gurley JC, Grines CL, et al: Intravascular ultrasound assessment of lumen size and wall morphology in normal subjects and patients with coronary artery disease. *Circulation* 84:1087–1099, 1991.

Exercise and Exercise Testing

Comparison of Silent and Symptomatic Ischemia During Exercise Testing in Men

Miranda CP, Lehmann KG, Lachterman B, Coodley EM, Froelicher VF (Long Beach Veterans Affairs Med Center, Long Beach; Univ of California at Irvine, Calif)
Ann Intern Med 114:649–656, 1991   5–52

Background.—Research has shown that patients with known coronary artery disease and exercise-induced angina and/or ST-segment depression had the same 7-year survival as those with symptomatic and asymptomatic episodes of ischemia. It has also shown that the risk for developing an acute myocardial infarction or sudden death in patients with symptomatic or asymptomatic exercise-induced ST-segment depression is related to the severity of the underlying coronary artery disease and presence of left ventricular dysfunction rather than symptoms. Angina and ST-segment depression were compared during exercise testing as markers for coronary artery disease.

Methods.—Four hundred sixteen men referred for assessment of symptoms and/or postmyocardial infarction testing were studied. Two hundred had no clinical or electrocardiographic evidence of previous myocardial infarction, and 216 had a previous myocardial infarction. All did a standard exercise test and had diagnostic coronary angiography with ventriculography within a mean 32 days of the test.

Results.—Among the men without a previous myocardial infarction, 80 had no ischemia, 23 had angina pectoris only, 40 had silent ischemia, and 57 had ST-segment depression and angina pectoris. Exercise-induced ST-segment depression was a better marker than exercise-induced angina for the presence of any coronary artery disease among patients without previous myocardial infarction. Men with symptomatic exercise-induced ischemia had a higher prevalence of severe coronary artery disease than those with only silent ischemia. Among the survivors of previous myocardial infarction, ST-segment depression was again a better marker for the presence of severe coronary artery disease than was angina alone. The prevalence of severe coronary artery disease in men with no ischemia plus myocardial infarction was 10%; in men with angina pectoris only plus myocardial infarction, 9%; in men with silent ischemia plus myocardial infarction, 23%; and in men with ST-segment depression and angina pectoris plus myocardial infarction, 32%.

Conclusions.—Exercise-induced ST-segment depression is better than exercise-induced angina as a marker for coronary artery disease. In addition, symptomatic ischemia during exercise testing is superior to silent ischemia as a marker for severe coronary artery disease.

▶ Angina pectoris, electrocardiographic ST-segment depression or the combination may occur during ECG exercise stress testing. Several previous studies have indicated that both typical exercise-induced angina and exercise ST segment depression indicate a poorer long-term prognosis in patients with similar degrees of coronary artery disease than the absence of either or both of these findings during stress. The current study in a large number of patients indicates that exercise-induced ST segment depression is a better marker for coronary artery disease than is exercise-induced angina. Postinfarction patients with both ST-segment depression and angina pectoris during exercise testing had the highest prevalence rates of severe coronary artery disease.—R.A. O'Rourke, M.D.

The Threshold for Myocardial Ischemia Varies in Patients With Coronary Artery Disease Depending on the Exercise Protocol

Garber CE, Carleton RA, Camaione DN, Heller GV (Mem Hosp of Rhode Island, Pawtucket; Brown Univ, Providence; Univ of Connecticut, Storrs)
J Am Coll Cardiol 17:1256–1262, 1991   5–53

Background.—Angina pectoris and myocardial ischemia are presumed to occur at a fixed heart rate–systolic blood pressure product in a given patient. Recently, the notion of a fixed threshold has been challenged. The effects of varying exercise intensity on the ischemic threshold were studied.

Methods.—Thirty-three patients with coronary artery disease and provokable myocardial ischemia underwent 2 exercise tests 2 to 7 days apart. After a symptom-limited incremental treadmill exercise, the patients underwent a 20-minute submaximal treadmill test at an intensity of about 70% of the peak heart rate achieved during the incremental test.

Results.—Angina pectoris developed in 16 patients during the incremental exercise test. Seventeen were asymptomatic. At least .1 mV of ST-segment depression developed in all patients during incremental testing at a mean exercise duration of 5.3 minutes, a rate-pressure product of 19,130, and oxygen uptake of 19.6 mL/kg/min. During submaximal exercise testing, 85% of the patients had significant ST-segment depression. Eighty-six percent of these were asymptomatic, including 10 patients with previous anginal symptoms during incremental testing. During the submaximal test, the average time to onset of .1 mV ST-segment depression was 8.1 minutes. These changes occurred at a rate-pressure product of 15,250 and an oxygen uptake of 14.3 mL/kg/min. They were significantly lower than values noted during the graded exercise. Six patients had angina pectoris during both tests, although 2 had no accompanying ST-segment depression during submaximal testing.

Conclusions.—Myocardial ischemia, with or without accompanying angina pectoris, can occur at a lower rate-pressure product and oxygen uptake during submaximal, steady-state exercise compared with symptom-limited incremental exercise. The ischemic threshold appears to vary under different exercise conditions.

▶ This study provides further evidence that angina pectoris and myocardial ischemia occur at variable thresholds in the same patient on different occasions and that the heart rate-systolic blood pressure product, an indirect index of the myocardial oxygen demand at which myocardial ischemia occurs, differs at the onset of myocardial ischemia during different types of exercise testing. This is not surprising considering the changes in coronary vascular tone that often contribute to an inadequate myocardial oxygen supply and that the heart rate and systolic blood pressure attained during exercise testing are only 2 of several determinates of the increase in myocardial oxygen requirement.—R.A. O'Rourke, M.D.

Symptom-Limited Exercise Testing Causes Sustained Diastolic Dysfunction in Patients With Coronary Disease and Low Effort Tolerance
Fragasso G, Benti R, Sciammarella M, Rossetti E, Savi A, Gerundini P, Chierchia SL (Istituto Scientifico H San Raffaele, Milan, Italy)
J Am Coll Cardiol 17:1251–1255, 1991   5–54

Background.—Exercise stress testing is considered to be safe and is used routinely for noninvasively assessing coronary artery disease. However, provoking severe ischemia may cause delayed recovery in myocardial function. A study was done to explore the possibility that maximal exercise testing may induce prolonged impairment of left ventricular (LV) function.

Methods.—The subjects were 15 patients with angiographically proved coronary disease and 9 age-matched control subjects with atypical chest pain and normal coronary arteries. They underwent radionuclide ventriculography at rest, at peak exercise, during recovery, and 2 and 7 days after exercise. Ejection fraction, peak filling and peak emptying rates, and LV wall motion were analyzed.

Results.—The control subjects had a normal exercise test at maximal work loads. In addition, they all had improved LV function on exercise. Patients with coronary disease developed 1-mm ST depression at a mean

217 seconds at a work load of 70 W and a rate-pressure product of a mean 18,530 mm Hg × beats/min. Exercise was stopped when angina or equivalent symptoms began, but diagnostic ST depression developed much earlier than symptoms in all patients. At peak exercise, patients had a reduction in ejection fraction and peak emptying and filling rates. Ejection fraction and peak emptying rate normalized during the recovery period. However, peak filling rate continued to be depressed throughout that period and was still diminished 2 days later.

Conclusions.—Maximal exercise may produce sustained impairment of diastolic function in patients with severe impairment of coronary flow reserve. Exercise testing in such patients should be done with caution. A more conservative diagnostic approach based on development of ST changes instead of symptom occurrence is recommended.

▶ The data in this study "suggest" that myocardial stunning can occur when ischemia is caused by a transient increase in myocardial oxygen requirements. However, LV systolic function is more reliably measured by noninvasive techniques than is diastolic function. However, LV diastolic function is often abnormal when measurements of systolic function are normal; studies in dog models of global myocardial ischemia indicate a slower return of accurate, invasively measured parameters of diastolic LV function after cessation of myocardial ischemia (coronary artery stenoses plus atrial pacing) despite an almost immediate return to normal of significant LV systolic-depressed function.— R.A. O'Rourke, M.D.

Additional recent publications concerning exercise and exercise testing are listed below:

1. Mark DB, Shaw L, Harrell FE Jr, et al: Prognostic value of a treadmill exercise score in outpatients with suspected coronary artery disease. *N Engl J Med* 325:849–853, 1991.
2. Aursnes I, Benestad AM, Sivertssen E, et al: Degree of coronary artery disease predicted by exercise testing. *J Intern Med* 229:325–330, 1991.
3. Ballegaard S, Meyer CN, Trojaborg W: Acupuncture in angina pectoris: Does acupuncture have a specific effect? *J Intern Med* 229:357–362, 1991.
4. Siscovick DS, Ekelund LG, Johnson JL, et al: Sensitivity of exercise electrocardiography for acute cardiac events during moderate and strenuous physical activity. *Arch Intern Med* 151:325–330, 1991.
5. Panza JA, Quyyumi AA, Diodata JG, et al: Prediction of the frequency and duration of ambulatory myocardial ischemia in patients with stable coronary artery disease by determination of the ischemic threshold from exercise testing: Importance of the exercise protocol. *J Am Coll Cardiol* 17:657–663, 1991.
6. Pedersen F, Sandoe E, Lærkeborg A: Prevalence and significance of an abnormal exercise ECG in asymptomatic males. Outcome of thallium myocardial scintigraphy. *Eur Heart J* 12:766–769, 1991.
7. Douglas PS, O'Toole ML, Woolard J: Regional wall motion abnor-

malities after prolonged exercise in the normal left ventricle. *Circulation* 82:2108–2114, 1990.

8. Hsu T-S, Lee Y-S: Endpoints of treadmill exercise testing for functional evaluation of patients with mitral stenosis. *Int J Cardiol* 31:81–87, 1991.

9. Gardner AW, Skinner JS, Smith LK: Effects of handrail support on claudication and hemodynamic responses to single-stage and progressive treadmill protocols in peripheral vascular occlusive disease. *Am J Cardiol* 68:99–105, 1991.

10. Morrison DA, Stovall JR, Barbiere C: Left and right ventricular systolic function and exercise capacity with coronary artery disease. *Am J Cardiol* 67:1079–1083, 1991.

11. Myers J, Buchanan N, Walsh D, et al: Comparison of the ramp versus standard exercise protocols. *J Am Coll Cardiol* 17:1334–1342, 1991.

12. Rudas L, Pflugfelder PW, Kostuck WJ: Comparison of hemodynamic responses during dynamic exercise in the upright and supine postures after orthotopic cardiac transplantation. *J Am Coll Cardiol* 16:1367–1373, 1990.

13. Wangsnes KM, Gibbons RJ: Optimal interpretation of the supine exercise electrocardiogram in patients with right bundle branch block. *Chest* 98:1379–1382, 1990.

14. Ray CA, Cureton KJ, Ouzts IIG: Postural specificity of cardiovascular adaptations to exercise training. *J Appl Physiol* 69:2202–2208, 1990.

15. Simari RD, Miller TD, Zinsmeister AR, et al: Capabilities of supine exercise electrocardiography versus exercise radionuclide angiography in predicting coronary events. *Am J Cardiol* 67:573–577, 1991.

Signal-Averaged ECG

Spectral Turbulence Analysis of the Signal-Averaged Electrocardiogram and Its Predictive Accuracy for Inducible Sustained Monomorphic Ventricular Tachycardia

Kelen GJ, Henkin R, Starr A-M, Caref EB, Bloomfield D, El-Sherif N (St Vincent's Med Ctr, Staten Island, NY; State Univ of New York Health Science Ctr, Brooklyn, NY; Veterans Administration Med Ctr, Brooklyn, NY)
Am J Cardiol 67:967–975, 1991 5–55

Background.—A retrospective study was designed to assess the accuracy of a noninvasive frequency analysis method for predicting patients with inducible sustained monomorphic ventricular tachycardia (VT). Measurements, calculations, and observations in this method were performed on the QRS complex as a whole, without assumptions as to abnormally high or low frequency overall.

Methods.—Electrocardiograms were studied of 142 subjects who were divided into 4 groups based on the presence or absence of time-domain late potentials and inducibility of sustained monomorphic VT at electrophysiologic study. Subjects also underwent time-domain and frequency-domain analysis. Spectrocardiograms, or 3-dimensional frequency plots, were derived for each patient. Data were analyzed for normal groups and for inducible sustained monomorphic VT groups and the criterion for abnormality was established that gave the best total predictive accuracy.

Results.—The frequency analysis technique correctly classified all 74 totally normal control subjects and 97% of the patients with late potentials by time-domain analysis and inducible sustained monomorphic VT. Classification of patients with late potentials but no evidence of sustained monomorphic VT was accurate in 86% of cases, and in 60% of those with inducible sustained monomorphic VT but absence of time-domain late potentials. Frequency analysis proved accurate in 94% of the cases as compared with 73% of time-domain late potential analysis.

Discussion.—A high degree of spectral turbulence of the overall QRS signal during sinus rhythm may be a more accurate sign than time-domain or frequency-domain analysis for the anatomical-electrophysiologic substrate of re-entrant tachyarrhythmias. Spectral turbulence analysis can be used on patients irrespective of the QRS duration and the presence or absence of bundle branch block.

▶ There has been considerable interest in the usefulness of the signal-averaged ECG for determining which patients are likely to develop potentially lethal ventricular tachyarrhythmia during their clinical course. Whereas most studies have used the time-domain analysis of the signal-averaged ECG, more recent studies have used a frequency-domain analysis, which is applicable to patients with bundle branch block as well as those with normal conduction. In the risk stratification of postmyocardial infarction patients, the presence of late potentials (a positive result) on the signal-averaged ECG indicates an increased risk of spontaneous ventricular tachyarrhythmias during follow-up, particularly in patients with other indicators such as recurrent myocardial ischemia or impaired left ventricular function. In the postinfarction dog model (as indicated in the 1990 YEAR BOOK OF CARDIOLOGY) a signal-averaged electrocardiogram that is positive for late potentials tends to correlate with inducible ventricular monomorphic ventricular tachycardia during electrophysiologic testing. In the above article, the frequency analysis technique was accurate in 94% of the cases with inducible sustained monomorphic ventricular tachycardia as compared with 73% with time-domain late potential analysis.

Although these results are impressive, additional clinical studies of the usefulness of the signal-averaged ECG comparing the 2 methods of analysis are indicated.—R.A. O'Rourke, M.D.

Standards for Analysis of Ventricular Late Potentials Using High Resolution or Signal-Averaged Electrocardiography: A Statement by a Task Force Committee Between the European Society of Cardiology, American Heart Association, and the American College of Cardiology
Breithardt G, Cain ME, El-Sherif N, Flowers N, Hombach V, Janse M, Simson MB, Steinbeck G (European Soc of Cardiology, Rotterdam, The Netherlands; American Heart Assoc, Dallas; American College of Cardiology, Bethesda, Md)
Eur Heart J 12:473–480, 1991   5–56

Introduction.—Abnormal microvolt-level waveforms, or "late potentials," are recorded in the terminal QRS complex in 60% to 90% of subjects prone to sustained ventricular tachycardia and in up to 7% of normal subjects. Several systems of high-resolution ECG are available. Reentrant mechanisms are implicated in the formation of late potentials. Myocardial activation may be delayed by a lengthened excitation pathways and/or slowed conduction velocity.

Technical.—The signal-averaging technique involves aligning a new beat against previous beats before averaging. Adequate noise reduction is critical in properly analyzing high-resolution ECGs. Controversy continues over which cutoff is best. It consequently is recommended that the high-pass corner frequency be programmable by the user.

Data Analysis.—Most studies are based on analyzing a vector magnitude of the filtered leads, the "filtered QRS complex." In frequency analysis, a sequence generated by sampling a time-domain signal is represented in the frequency domain by taking the fast Fourier transform. Ensemble signal-averaging assumes that signals of interest are reproducible throughout the averaging process. Pilot studies suggest that ventricular late potentials may be detected using beat-to-beat analysis of ECG signals.

Clinical Uses.—Features of the high-resolution ECG may distinguish postinfarction patients with and without sustained ventricular tachycardia. Attempts to categorize patients with remote infarction for the risk of nonstained ventricular tachycardia appear promising. High-resolution ECG also may help to assess patients with unexplained syncope and detect acute rejection of a cardiac transplant. Myocardial reperfusion may be recognized after thrombolytic treatment of acute infarction.

▶ The Task Force report by the committee representing 3 organizations important to cardiology provides a current assessment of the usefulness of the high-resolution or signal-averaged ECG for determining the risk of developing sustained ventricular tachyarrhythmias in patients recovering from myocardial infarction without bundle branch block.—R.A. O'Rourke, M.D.

Additional recent publications concerning signal-averaged ECG are listed below:

1. Freedman RA, Fuller MS, Greenberg GM, et al: Detection and localization of prolonged epicardial electrograms with 64-lead body surface signal-averaged electrocardiography. *Circulation* 84:871–883, 1991.
2. Vaitkus PT, Kindwall E, Marchlinski FE, et al: Differences in electrophysiological substrate in patients with coronary artery disease and cardiac arrest or ventricular tachycardia. Insights from endocardial mapping and signal-averaged electrocardiography. *Circulation* 84:672–678, 1991.
3. Lombardi F, Finocchiaro ML, Vecchia LD, et al: Signal averaging of pre- and post-extrasystolic beats in patients with ventricular arrhythmias. *Eur Heart J* 12:481–487, 1991.

4. Emmot W, Vacek JL: Lack of reproducibility of frequency versus time domain signal-averaged electrocardiographic analyses and effects of lead polarity in coronary artery disease. *Am J Cardiol* 68:913–917, 1991.

Miscellaneous Topics

Patterns of Global and Regional Systolic and Diastolic Function in the Normal Right Ventricle Assessed by Ultrafast Computed Tomography

Marzullo P, L'Abbate A, Marcus ML (Univ of Iowa, Iowa City; University of Pisa, Italy)

J Am Coll Cardiol 17:1318–1325, 1991   5–57

Background.—To date, no author has published a detailed assessment of global and regional systolic function and diastolic filling of the human right ventricle. Ultrafast CT was used to provide a noninvasive physiologic evaluation of global and regional systolic and diastolic function in the normal right ventricle.

Methods.—Ten normal men, with a mean age of 26 years, participated. Early diastolic filling data were fit to a third order polynomial curve. The peak rate of diastolic filling and time to peak filling were determined globally and regionally at 3 ventricular levels in each ventricle.

Results.—The right and left ventricular stroke volumes did not differ statistically, nor did the peak filling rates as referenced to the stroke volume. Time to peak filling rate did not differ between the 2 ventricles. However, reference of stroke volumes and absolute peak filling rates to end-diastolic volumes showed lower dynamic values for the right ventricle. Basal and apical right ventricular ejection fractions and peak filling rates were similar regionally. They were statistically different from midventricular levels. Right ventricular apical and midventricular levels had lower values for systolic and diastolic function compared with the same regional values for the left ventricle.

Conclusions.—There is a close volumetric and temporal match between systolic and diastolic function of the 2 ventricles when global measures are referred to stroke volume. When referenced to end-diastolic volume, the right ventricle can be viewed as a lower dynamic chamber. Regionally, segmental ventricular ejection fraction and peak filling rate are typically nonuniform across the right ventricle. When compared with segmental left ventricular function, right ventricular mid and apical segments have lower regional dynamics.

▶ In this study, the noninvasive technique of ultrafast (fast cine) CT was used to evaluate global and regional right ventricular systolic function as well as right ventricular diastolic filling in 10 normal men. Because precise estimates of right ventricular volume and function have been difficult to obtain because of the configuration of the right ventricle, which is not well approximated by simple geometric formulas, the information presented in this study relating right to left ventricular function globally and regionally is of particular interest. Ultrafast CT may provide a reliable means of assessing global and regional right ventricular dynamics in patients with cardiac and pulmonary diseases, and further clinical research applications of this technique for assessing right ventricular anatomy and function are likely.— R.A. O'Rourke, M.D.

A Randomized Comparison of the Nephrotoxicity of Iopamidol and Diatrizoate in High Risk Patients Undergoing Cardiac Angiography

Taliercio CP, Vlietstra RE, Ilstrup DM, Burnett JC, Menke KK, Stensrud SL, Holmes DR Jr (Mayo Clin and Found, Rochester, Minn)
J Am Coll Cardiol 17:384–390, 1991   5–58

Background.—Hospital-acquired acute renal insufficiency is often caused by renal dysfunction after exposure to radiocontrast media, which can be composed of the salts of negatively charged, iodinated, organic compounds. New radiocontrast agents have lower osmolality, but their relative nephrotoxicity is not known. A randomized, double-blind trial was undertaken to compare the relative nephrotoxicity of iopamidol and diatrizoate in patients at high risk because of preexisting renal insufficiency; all were undergoing cardiac angiography.

Methods.—Patients seen consecutively at the Mayo Clinic from February 1987 through March 1989 were considered if their serum creatinine level was more than 1.5 mg/dL and they were not on dialysis, did not have heart failure or severe aortic stenosis, were not receiving nephrotoxic medication, and gave signed consent. Before coronary angiography, the patients were optimally hydrated. They then received the contrast material after a blood sample was taken to determine the serum creatinine level. The patients were randomized, double-blind, into the 2 contrast media groups: iopamidol or diatrizoate. Cardiac catheterization was performed according to the Sones or Judkins technique. A follow-up blood sample was obtained the morning after angiography.

Findings.—Of the 307 patients recruited, serum creatinine levels were determined immediately before angiography in 305; 294 provided serum samples 24 hours after the procedure, and 191 did so 24 hours to 1 week after angiography. The mean age of participating patients was 68 years, and the mean recruitment serum creatinine concentration was 2.02 mg/dL. The mean serum creatinine level increased significantly 24 hours after angiography, with an increase of more than .5 mg/dL in 5% of those given iopamidol and 11% given diatrizoate. Patients given diatrizoate had a highly more significant increase in the serum creatinine level than patients given iopamidol. Acute renal failure occurred in 5 patients. Patients receiving the lower doses of contrast agent had significantly less severe baseline dysfunction. Insulin-dependent diabetic patients had significantly greater maximal increases in the serum creatinine level after angiography than did other study patients. Overall, a significantly greater change in the serum creatinine level was observed after diatrizoate administration in insulin-requiring diabetics and in those with preexisting severe renal insufficiency.

Conclusions.—Iopamidol appears less nephrotoxic than diatrizoate in high-risk patients undergoing cardiac angiography. Thus iopamidol may be preferred for use in some individuals with advanced renal impairment.

▶ In this study of a relatively large number of patients, the use of a nonionic, low osmolar radiocontrast agent was compared with use of a conventional radiocontrast agent with subsequent follow-up evaluation of renal function. Although the change in renal function after angiography was less pronounced with the nonionic agent, there was no significant difference between agents in the likelihood of patients developing clinically severe acute renal dysfunction. Although the nonionic agent is less nephrotoxic, the difference is small and of no major importance in the majority of high-risk patients.—R.A. O'Rourke, M.D.

Altered β Adrenergic Receptor Function in Subjects With Symptomatic Mitral Valve Prolapse

Anwar A, Kohn SR, Dunn JF, Hymer TK, Kennedy GT, Crawford MH, O'Rourke RA, Katz MS (Audie L Murphy Mem Veterans Hosp, San Antonio, Texas)
Am J Med Sci 302:89–97, 1991   5–59

Introduction.—Approximately 6% of females in the United States have mitral valve prolapse (MVP). The incidence of MVP in males is much lower. Although several physicians have attributed the symptoms of MVP to a hyperadrenergic state or some other autonomic nervous system dysfunction, the mechanisms underlying autonomic dysfunction in MVP are not completely understood. The molecular mechanisms underlying the β-adrenergic hyperresponsiveness seen in symptomatic MVP were investigated.

Patients.—The study group consisted of 12 women, aged 23–39 years, and 14 asymptomatic age- and sex-matched controls without MVP. All symptomatic women had auscultatory and echocardiographic evidence of MVP. Study participants exercised on an upright exercise bicycle until 85% of age-predicted maximum heart rate was reached. Blood samples for the study of adrenergic parameters were obtained at baseline and immediately after the termination of exercise. Eight women with MVP and 8 normal controls underwent isoproterenol infusion studies at a later date.

Results.—The β-adrenergic receptor function during rest and exercise in women with symptomatic MVP differed from that in controls. At rest, the proportion of high-affinity receptors in women with MVP was greater than that in normal controls, even though both groups had equivalent receptor densities. In women with MVP, the increase in high-affinity receptors was associated with increased β-adrenergic responsiveness as reflected by greater isoproterenol stimulation of cyclic adenosine monophosphate compared with controls (Fig 5–23). During exercise, the proportion of high-affinity receptors in women with MVP decreased to that observed in controls, while equivalent receptor densities were main-

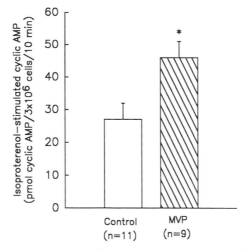

Fig 5–23.—Isoproterenol-stimulated cyclic adenosine monophosphate (AMP) accumulation by intact lymphocytes from control and mitral valve prolapse (MVP) subjects during rest. Cyclic AMP responses are expressed as the difference between isoproterenol (10^{-5}M) stimulated and basal (unstimulated) cyclic AMP. *Mitral valve prolapse value is significantly different from control value, $P < .02$. (Courtesy of Anwar A, Kohn SR, Dunn JF, et al: *Am J Med Sci* 302:89–97, 1991.)

tained in the 2 groups. The similar high-affinity receptor values were associated with similar cyclic adenosine monophosphate responses to isoproterenol. Women with MVP and normal controls had similar baseline plasma catecholamine concentrations at rest and similar increases during exercise.

Conclusion.—In the absence of abnormal plasma catecholamine concentrations, the hyperadrenergic state seen in women with MVP at rest may be attributable to an alteration in β-adrenergic receptor function. Exercise appears to desensitize high-affinity β-receptors and thus preserve normal adrenergic responsiveness.

▶ This study in patients with symptomatic mitral valve prolapse demonstrated altered β-adrenergic receptor function during rest and exercise without abnormalities in plasma catecholamine levels. Under resting conditions, the portion of high affinity β-receptors and the cyclic AMP responses to isoproterenol were increased in patients with mitral valve prolapse. Isoproterenol infusion also elicited abnormal heart rate response and transient arrhythmias in mitral valve prolapse subjects, although the role of β-receptor dysfunction in the heightened response to isoproterenol remains to be determined.—R.A. O'Rourke, M.D.

Identification and Characterization of a Ouabain-Like Compound From Human Plasma
Hamlyn JM, Blaustein MP, Bova S, DuCharme DW, Harris DW, Mandel F, Mathews WR, Ludens JH (Univ of Maryland School of Medicine, Baltimore; University of Padua, Italy; Upjohn Labs, Kalamazoo, Mich)
Proc Natl Acad Sci USA 88:6259–6263, 1991   5–60

Background.—Amphibians possess bufodieneolides, and a receptor for cardiotonic steroids is conserved on the surface of most mammalian cells. A large number of Na,K-ATPase inhibitors are detectable in mammalian preparations. Recently, an endogenous ouabain-like compound (OLC) was found in human plasma. This compound interacts with the cardenolide receptor on the Na^+ pump, and its pattern of inhibition closely resembles that of digitalis glycosides.

Quantification.—The endogenous OLC has been purified and structurally identified by mass spectroscopy as indistinguishable from ouabain. Immunoreactive OLC was found in the plasma of many mammals, and was found to occur in high concentrations in both human and bovine adrenal glands. The section of immunoreactive OLC by cultured bovine adrenocortical cells was reduced in the presence of an increased external K^+ concentration, and this effect did not merely reflect hypertonicity.

Implications.—Circulating OLC may modulate intracellular Na^+ and influence Na^+ gradient-dependent processes such as pH homeostasis and the intracellular Ca^{++} concentration. Altered levels of circulating OLC might have a role in some forms of hypertension.

▶ The authors have purified and identified by mass spectroscopy an endogenous substance from human plasma that is indistinguishable from the cardenolide ouabain. The circulating compound may modulate intracellular Na^+ and affect numerous Na^+ gradient-dependent processes including intracellular calcium and pH homeostasis in many tissues. The clinical significance of this circulating substance remains to be evaluated in normal subjects and in patients with heart failure.— R.A. O'Rourke, M.D.

The following references include additional important articles concerning cardiovascular function and noninvasive methods not previously cited:

1. Pietras RJ, Wolfkiel CJ, Veselik K, et al: Validation of ultrafast computed tomographic left ventricular volume measurement. *Invest Radiol* 26:28–34, 1991.
2. Gaudio C, Tanzilli G, Mazzarotto P, et al: Comparison of left ventricular ejection fraction by magnetic resonance imaging and radionuclide ventriculography in idiopathic dilated cardiomyopathy. *Am J Cardiol* 67:411–415, 1991.
3. Wikström M, Martinussen HJ, Wikström G, et al: Magnetic resonance imaging of acute myocardial infarction in pigs using Gd-DTPA. *Acta Radiol* 31:619–624, 1990.
4. Scholz TD, Grover-McKay M, Fleagle SR, et al: Quantitation of the extent of acute myocardial infarction by phosphorus-31 nuclear magnetic resonance spectroscopy. *J Am Coll Cardiol* 17:1380–1387, 1991.

6 Cardiac Surgery

Introduction

Although the news from cardiac surgery cannot compete with the dissolution of the Soviet Empire, there has been substantial progress in some areas.

Most patients now take aspirin after coronary bypass surgery. Several studies show no particular advantage in starting medication before operation, and there is an apparent disadvantage of increased perioperative bleeding. It is apparent that progressive atherosclerotic involvement of saphenous vein grafts is a continuing problem and that it is not significantly ameliorated simply with risk factor alteration after surgery. Whether or not the inflammatory response involving infiltration of macrophages is specifically related to progressive arteriosclerosis is at present uncertain. There continues to be a great interest in alternative arterial conduits for coronary bypass, and several centers report early favorable results using the inferior epigastric artery as a free graft. With the increasing number of patients undergoing reoperations for progressive coronary occlusive disease after coronary bypass surgery, there is a great interest in alternative techniques for myocardial protection during reoperative surgery. Use of the conduits for administration of cardioplegic agents as well as for retrograde perfusion are having apparently favorable results.

The use of composite valve and graft repair techniques for diseases of the aortic valve and ascending aorta continues to increase. Variations on the technique originally described by Bentall continue to be developed. Attempts also continue in the area of the aortic valve reconstructive operations for both aortic stenosis and insufficiency. Although some favorable results have been reported, there has not been a general acceptance of reconstructive procedures, particularly for aortic insufficiency. The use of intraoperative echocardiographic analysis has been a great advantage in both valvular and congenital heart surgery.

Further variations of the Fontan operation continue to emerge with certain specific advantages and various conditions. A number of interesting papers have appeared.

"Cerebroplegia" is gradually emerging as an alternative to profound systemic hypothermia for CNS protection during circulatory arrest. This appears to be a very promising technique. A very interesting paper has been written by the group at UCLA, who suggest that often there is a decreased benefit from cardiac transplantation in patients who have survived a prolonged interval on the waiting list for a new heart. Total lymphoid irradiation has produced some favorable benefit in otherwise intractable allograft projection for some patients.

Papers on these and other areas of continuing interest constitute this year's section on Cardiac Surgery. I hope the reader will find these articles as instructional as I have.

John J. Collins, Jr., M.D.

Coronary Surgery

Immediate Postoperative Aspirin Improves Vein Graft Patency Early and Late After Coronary Artery Bypass Graft Surgery: A Placebo-Controlled, Randomized Study
Gavaghan TP, Gebski V, Baron DW (St Vincent's Hospital, Sydney; Sydney University, New South Wales, Australia)
Circulation 83:1526–1533, 1991   6–1

Background.—Perioperative antiplatelet therapy improves the patency of autologous saphenous vein grafts implanted during coronary artery bypass grafting (CABG). Aspirin can be used, although its efficiency depends on dosage and time of administration. In a prospective, double-blind, randomized, placebo-controlled trial, 324 mg/day of aspirin, initiated within 1 hour of CABG, was given to 237 patients. Early and late graft patency were investigated.

Results.—The early (1 week) vein graft occlusion rate was 1.6% in patients receiving aspirin and 6.2% in those receiving placebo. The late (1 year) vein graft occlusion rate was 5.8% with aspirin treatment and 11.6% with placebo (Fig 6–1). New graft occlusion was also less common in patients receiving aspirin therapy. Mean chest tube blood loss during the first day and red blood cell transfusion requirements were not significantly different for the placebo and aspirin groups. The reoperation rate was 4.8% for the aspirin group and 1% for the placebo group.

Conclusion.—Administration of aspirin immediately after CABG improves early graft patency. Continued administration of aspirin protects

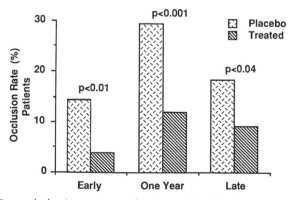

Fig 6–1.—Bar graph showing percentage of patients with graft occlusion in placebo-treated and aspirin-treated groups. Angiographic results at 1 week and 1 year are presented. Late patient group with both angiograms and new occlusion evident only after early angiography. (Courtesy of Gavaghan TP, Gebski V, Baron DW: *Circulation* 83:1526–1533, 1991.)

against re-occlusion for at least 1 year. Aspirin use was associated with a slightly higher reoperation rate.

▶ The efficacy of postoperative aspirin therapy begun very early after coronary bypass surgery observed in this study is remarkable, with nearly twice as many patients having early occlusion in the placebo group. It certainly deserves careful consideration. It is interesting that the rate of reoperation was considerably higher for the aspirin group despite the fact that the observed blood loss and transfusion requirements were not significantly different. I don't know how to explain that. In the VA cooperative study reported by Goldman et al. (1), there was no advantage of aspirin therapy started preoperatively compared with starting treatment 6 hours after surgery, although the reoperation rate for bleeding was greater when aspirin was given before surgery.—J.J. Collins, Jr., M.D.

Reference

1. Goldman S, Copeland J, Moritz T, et al: Starting aspirin therapy after operation: Effects on early graft patency. *Circulation* 84(2):520–526, 1991.

Cytokinetic Study of Aortocoronary Bypass Vein Grafts in Place for Less Than Six Months
Amano J, Suzuki A, Sunamori M, Tsukada I, Numano F (Hokushin General Hospital, Nagano Prefecture, Japan; Tokyo Medical and Dental University)
Am J Cardiol 67:1234–1236, 1991   6–2

Introduction.—Autogenous saphenous vein grafts used for arterial bypass have a higher early and late attrition than arterial grafts, but they are still used because of the limited number of available arterial grafts. The late histologic features of these venous grafts have been well described, but the cell components and kinetics of the early stage have not.

Methods.—Atherosclerotic changes in these grafts within 6 months of implantation were studied in 7 patients who underwent saphenous vein grafting for coronary artery revascularization but died at 4 days to 6 months after the operation. Specimens of vein graft and aorta were subjected to histologic examination and immunocytochemical analysis. Cell components were analyzed with the use of monoclonal antibodies specific for smooth muscle cells (HHF35) and macrophages.

Results.—In the patient who died on day 4, migration of macrophages into the intima and media was already seen. A patient who died at 1 week showed focal endothelial deprivation and increased extracellular matrix in the intima. At 1 month, grafts showed mild-to-moderate focal intimal thickening beneath the endothelium, which became prominent at 2 months, at which time foam cells were seen in the subendothelium and media. Some grafts were nearly occluded at 5–6 months by severe intimal thickening resulting from smooth muscle cell proliferation. At 1 month, grafts showed sporadic macrophages in each layer and no

HHF35-positive foam cells. The numbers of these cells increased at 2 months in a similar distribution. At 5–6 months, there were abundant and circumferential macrophages in the media, and fibrous intimal thickening was ubiquitous in smooth muscle cells.

Conclusion.—Macrophage recruitment and intimal thickening occur early after implantation of saphenous vein grafts into the coronary circulation. The rapid progression and severity of these changes contribute to the development of early failure of these grafts.

▶ That a diffuse inflammatory change with macrophage infiltration is observed in transplanted autologous vascular grafts should not be terribly surprising. On the other hand, the question of the precise contribution of these cells to the development of vein graft atherosclerosis is intriguing, particularly when macrophage infiltration appears to be an early stage of atherosclerosis in experimental animals fed an atherogenic diet or even rodents undergoing cardiac transplantation. The relationship between the physiology and the immunology of vascular endothelium probably holds the mystery of atherosclerosis, but unlocking the secret is not so simple.—J.J. Collins, Jr., M.D.

Coronary Bypass Graft Fate: Long-Term Angiographic Study
Fitzgibbon GM, Leach AJ, Kafka HP, Keon WJ (Univ of Ottawa)
J Am Coll Cardiol 17:1075–1080, 1991   6–3

Introduction.—Graft atherosclerosis is the most important factor in the outcome of coronary bypass vein grafts. The appearance and progression of atherosclerosis in coronary bypass vein grafts up to 5 years postoperatively was previously reported. The same considerations in 741 grafts 6.5 to more than 11.5 years postoperatively were studied.

Methods.—The study included 22 patients who had 741 grafts that were studied by angiography early, after 1 year, and at least 6.5 years after operation. The mean interval to the latest examination was 9.6 years. A 5-year examination was performed in 565 grafts. The perioperative mortality rate was 1.7% for the 1,202 first operations and 5.4% for the 149 reoperations. Of the group of 889 patients from which the study sample was drawn, the 6.5-year survival rate was 92.7%. A hemodynamic grading system was used in which A represented good patency and O occlusion, with the intermediate grade of B representing stenosis of the lumen to less than 50%. Another morphological system was used to define irregularities and classify lesions into high- or low-profile types.

Results.—Graft occlusion rates were 8% at the early examination, 20% at 5 years, 41% at 10 years, and 45% at the final examination. There was a striking increase in B grade patency at 7.5 years, followed by a decrease at 10 years. No atherosclerosis was considered to be present at the early examination; however, 8% were involved at 1 year, 38% at 5 years, and 75% at 10 years. There was an association between involvement of more vessel wall area and greater protrusion of lesions into the lumen. As time went on, graft disease involvement increased, and many grafts became occluded. Even grafts that appeared healthy at one examination could be found diseased and abruptly occluded at subsequent examinations; at 5 years, 82% of severely diseased grafts had been normal at 1 year. At 1 year, 590 patent grafts were free of disease, 30% of these were occluded at the late examination and 76% of the patent grafts were diseased. Of these diseased grafts, 50% had diffuse disease and 35% were narrowed by more than half. At the final examination, only 17% of patent grafts were healthy.

Conclusion.—The long-term outcome of coronary bypass grafts is severely limited by the occurrence of graft atherosclerosis. Modification of risk factors may be insufficient to prevent this problem. Newer drugs that normalize dyslipidemias or the calcium channel blockers may have promise.

▶ This carefully performed evaluation of vein graft patency and the development of graft atherosclerosis is another excellent contribution from the University of Ottawa. The data speak for themselves. We do not control vein graft atherosclerosis in a satisfactory fashion. The question is how to improve. Certainly, risk factor modification does not seem to have as great an effect as was originally anticipated. No difference in patency rates after 10 years was found by Meeter et al. between single and sequential vein grafts in a study from Rotterdam (1).—J.J. Collins, Jr., M.D.

Reference

1. Meeter K, Veldkamp R, Tijssen JGP, et al: Clinical outcome of single versus sequential grafts in coronary bypass operations at ten years' follow-up. *J Thorac Cardiovasc Surg* 101:1076–1081, 1991.

Long-Term Results of Coronary Bypass Surgery: Analysis of 1698 Patients Followed 15 to 20 years
Lawrie GM, Morris GC Jr, Earle N (Baylor College of Medicine; Methodist Hosp, Houston)
Ann Surg 213:377–387, 1991   6–4

Background.—Five-year, 10-year, and 10- to 15-year follow-up results of a series of coronary bypass surgery patients have been previously reported. The clinical and angiographic outcomes at 15 to 20 years were assessed.

Patients.—The subjects were 1,698 patients who underwent coronary artery bypass with autogenous saphenous vein during a 7-year period. Mean follow-up times were 15.2 years for survivors and 8.6 years for nonsurvivors. Mean age at the time of operation was 53.9 years, and 88% of patients were men. The mean number of grafts per patient was 1.9. Five percent of patients died within 30 days of operation. Ninety-six percent of patients had angina. Disease was confined to a single vessel in 18% of patients, 2 vessels in 38% and 3 vessels in 32%, and left main

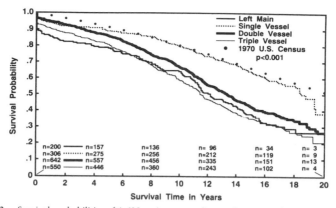

Fig 6–2.—Survival probabilities of 1,698 patients according to the extent of coronary disease before operation. (Courtesy of Lawrie GM, Morris GC Jr, Earle N: *Ann Surg* 213:377–387, 1991.)

stenosis was present in 12%. Left ventricular quality was good in 70% and poor in 30%.

Outcome.—Survival rates were 40% for single-vessel disease, 26% for double-vessel disease, 20% for triple-vessel disease, and 25% for left main stenosis (Fig 6–2). Sixty-seven percent of patients were asymptomatic and 26% were improved at 20-year follow-up. Forty-nine percent of patients were receiving nitrates, and 26% were receiving β-blockers. Graft patency rates were 81% at 0 to 5 years, 68% at 6 to 10 years, 60% at 11 to 15 years, and 46% at 16 to 20 years. Nineteen percent of patients had a repeat coronary bypass. Their survival was 62%, compared with 37% for patients who did not have reoperation. Major determinants of survival were age at operation, extent of disease, ventricular quality (Fig 6–3), history of stroke, and preoperative congestive heart failure. Of the surviving patients, 76% had at least 1 patent graft, and the probability of freedom from reoperation was .62.

Conclusions.—Long-term results of an early experience with coronary

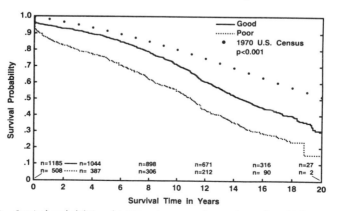

Fig 6–3.—Survival probabilities of 1,698 patients according to the quality of left ventricular function before operation. (Courtesy of Lawrie GM, Morris GC Jr, Earle N: *Ann Surg* 213:377–387, 1991.)

bypass surgery show that most patients have done well at up to 20 years of follow-up. With current techniques, long-term results will probably become even more favorable.

▶ This very large series of patients reported by Drs. Lawrie, Morris, and Earle provides a useful overall view of the effect of coronary bypass surgery. It is interesting that the incidence of symptomatic recurrence in these patients parallels the observations of others concerning the progression of graft atherosclerosis.—J.J. Collins, Jr., M.D.

Technique for Use of the Inferior Epigastric Artery as a Coronary Bypass Graft
Mills NL, Everson CT (The Cardiology Ctr, New Orleans)
Ann Thorac Surg 51:208–214, 1991   6–5

Background.—Late patency of the saphenous vein graft is less than that of arterial grafts, prompting use of the inferior epigastric artery (IEA) as a coronary arterial bypass graft.

Techniques.—A paramedian incision is made to harvest the IEA, stopping about 5 cm above the level of the inguinal ligament (Fig 6–4). Posterior peritoneal branches are ligated adjacent to the IEA, and electrocautery serves to free interdigitations of the rectus muscle from its sheath. The IEA is harvested as a

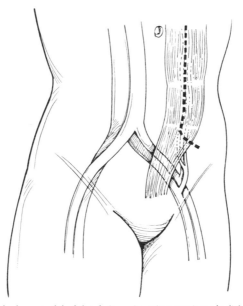

Fig 6–4.—Incision for harvest of the left inferior epigastric artery is made slightly lateral to the midline of the rectus muscle and is angled toward the femoral vessels. The incision stops well above the femoral crease. (Courtesy of Mills NL, Everson CT: *Ann Thorac Surg* 51:208–214, 1991.)

pedicle with its 2 accompanying veins. Finally, the vessel is dissected to its origin and suture-ligated. If the artery follows a lateral path, exposure is facilitated by dissecting the lateral border of the rectus muscle. Distal anastomoses are sutured using a 5 to 6-mm coronary arteriotomy and 8-0 polypropylene suture material, starting at the heel of the graft and proceeding circumferentially around the toe; both ends terminate in the midportion of the arteriotomy. The proximal anastomoses are made either to the ascending aorta, or end-to-side to an internal mammary artery or saphenous vein graft. The IEA-internal mammary proximal anastomoses may be made before cardiopulmonary bypass is instituted.

Clinical Experience.—Eighteen patients had IEA grafts made to 19 coronary arteries. Graft length ranged from 11.5 to 17 cm. No deaths occurred during follow-up for 1–18 months. There was 1 late wound infection before the routine use of Jackson-Pratt drains. No hernias have resulted from the dissection, and there is no evidence of rectus muscle necrosis. Three postoperative angiograms demonstrated widely patent IEA grafts within 10 days of surgery.

▶ Dr. Noel Mills has been an enterprising pioneer in the development of alternative techniques to vein graft bypass for coronary occlusive disease. Success in these operations is highly dependent on expert technique. The experience of the authors in harvesting the inferior epigastric artery is extremely welcome and may obviate pursuing a "learning curve" for surgeons adopting this technique. Early experience with inferior epigastric artery grafts has also been reported by Barner et al. (1) and by Milgalter and Laks (2).—J.J. Collins, Jr., M.D.

References

1. Barner HB, Naunheim KS, Fiore AC, et al: Use of the inferior epigastric artery as a free graft for myocardial revascularization. *Ann Thorac Surg* 52:429–437, 1991.
2. Milgalter E, Laks H: A technique to harvest the inferior epigastric arteries for coronary bypass procedures. *J Cardiol Surg* 6(2):306–309, 1991.

Technical Considerations for Myocardial Protection During the Course of Coronary Artery Bypass Reoperation: The Impact of Functioning Saphenous Vein and Internal Mammary Artery Grafts

Mills NL, Everson CT, Hockmuth DR (The Cardiology Ctr, New Orleans)
J Cardiac Surg 6:34–40, 1991   6–6

Introduction.—Coronary bypass grafting (CABG) for reoperation in the presence of functioning saphenous vein or internal mammary artery (IMA) grafts at risk for distal embolization presents a challenge to the surgeon. Particularly problematic are patients who have previously experienced postoperative pericardiotomy syndrome, mediastinitis, or other problems associated with adhesions. Standard cardioplegia to areas supplied by functional grafts may be difficult to deliver and require alteration. Alternate techniques have been developed for myocardial protection during CABG reoperation in patients with functioning saphenous vein or IMA grafts.

Methods.—Coronary bypass grafting reoperation in the presence of a functioning IMA graft carries definite hazards. Not only is there a danger of dividing or damaging the IMA graft, especially after 2 or more operations, but myocardial injury as a result of effecting a large temperature gradient between the myocardial bed supplied by the IMA and the remaining myocardium may be incurred. Often, such hazards may be avoided by performing a left thoracotomy in conjunction with moderate-to-deep hypothermia and periods of low flow or circulatory arrest. Myocardial temperature measurements in multiple areas are mandatory to avoid zones of rewarming, especially with completely occluded aortic-to-coronary grafts and functioning pedicle grafts. The previous commonly used technique of "cold fibrillating heart" may be safely used in the absence of left ventricular hypertrophy when relatively brief periods of cross-clamping or distal anastomotic time are anticipated. In some cases, standard cardioplegia with a clamped mammary graft may be possible without incurring any increased risk, depending on the status of the native circulation and coronary collateral.

Conclusion.—The new technical challenges involving myocardial protection during reoperation for CABG can be attributed to the use of new conduits, extensive endarterectomies, and the presence of functioning grafts that are at high risk for distal embolization.

▶ The operative risk of reoperation coronary bypass is not entirely related to adequate myocardial protection. However, it seems likely that well over half of the early mortality in these difficult operations is related to inadequate myocardial protection, producing either severe intraoperative ischemia or significant reperfusion damage. The considerations described by Dr. Mills and associates should be studied in detail by all surgeons involved in these procedures.—J.J. Collins, Jr., M.D.

Multiple Reoperative Coronary Artery Bypass Grafting

Accola KD, Craver JM, Weintraub WS, Guyton RA, Jones EL (Emory Univ Atlanta, Ga)
Ann Thorac Surg 52:738–744, 1991   6–7

Introduction.—An increasing number of patients are undergoing reoperative coronary bypass surgery; the number is expected to approach 14,000 annually in the early 1990s. Data were reviewed on 53 patients who had a third or (in 4 patients) a fourth coronary bypass procedure in 1980–1990. The patients represented .3% of all those who had coronary bypass surgery in this period.

Methods.—The mean interval between the first and second operations was 5.3 years, between the second and third, 4.9 years, and from the third to the fourth, 4.65 years. The average number of grafts placed was 2.6. Internal mammary artery grafts were used in most patients.

Results.—Postoperatively, 10 patients required balloon pump support. Although there were no intraoperative deaths, 4 patients died postoperatively, 1 of heart failure. In 6 patients, there was ECG evidence of perioperative myocardial infarction, 13 patients had perioperative dysrhythmias, and 2 had a stroke. In 3 patients, reoperation was necessary because of bleeding. The postoperative 3-year myocardial infarction-free survival rate was 70%.

Conclusion.—Multiple reoperations for coronary artery disease carry an increased risk of morbidity and early death, but nevertheless should be considered for patients who have revascularizable distal vessels and adequate ventricular function.

▶ The Cardiac Surgical Unit at Emory has a vast experience in both primary and reoperation coronary bypass operations. Their experience with multiple reoperations confirms the substantially increased hazard observed in most cardiac surgical units. Considerations of the modifications suggested by Mills et al. (see Abstract 6–6) may help to eventually reduce the risk of this type of technically demanding operation.—J.J. Collins, Jr., M.D.

The Vascular Resistance of Arterial Stenoses in Series

Kilpatrick D, Webber SD, Colle J-P (University of Tasmania, Hobart, Australia; Centre Hospitalier Universitaire Bordeaux, France)
Angiology 41:278–284, 1990   6–8

Introduction.—The significance of paired stenoses in the clinical setting is often controversial. To further clarify this issue, fiberoptic laser Doppler anemometry (FOLDA) was used to measure intravascular velocities within stenoses.

Experimental Design.—An in vitro system for measuring pressure and flow across narrowings in vessels was constructed. All experiments were performed using citrated human blood. A reservoir of adjustable height was used to simulate flow at a constant perfusion pressure, and a mechanical stirring device was used to keep the blood continuously agitated within this reservoir. Soft polyethylene tubing was used to simulate freshly dissected arteries. However, some experiments were also done with freshly dissected sheep carotid arteries. Paired stenoses were created by external constriction of the tubing or arteries. The severity of the first stenosis was calculated before the second stenosis was created. Pressure gradients across each of the paired stenoses were measured while both the severity and the distance between the stenoses were altered. The individual resistances were then compared with the combined resistance.

Results.—Resistance at a stenosis is a nonlinear function of the severity of the stenosis. The resistance at a stenosis is a complex function of perfusion pressure and cross-sectional area (Fig 6–5). The resistance at a stenosis cannot be accurately predicted from a single plane angiographic image. In the case of multiple stenoses, an approximate assessment of their combined effect can be obtained by adding up the resistance values

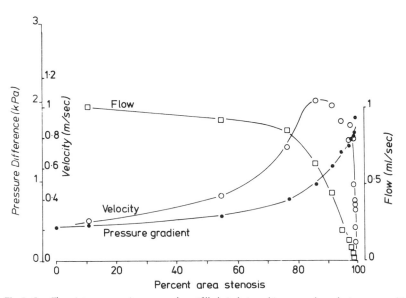

Fig 6–5.—Flow (*open squares*), pressure drop (*filled circles*), and intravascular velocity measured by FOLDA (*open circles*) for an incremental stenosis with constant pressure perfusion. In this experiment the stenosis was increased from zero to occlusion in graded steps. (Courtesy of Kilpatrick D, Webber SD, Colle J-P: *Angiology* 41:278–284, 1990.)

of the 2 stenoses, but not the degree of the stenoses. The nonlinear relationship between stenosis resistance and stenosis severity means that if 1 stenosis is more severe than the other, the combined effect of the 2 stenoses can be considered the same as the effect of the more severe stenosis acting by itself. The distance between 2 paired stenoses does not alter their combined effect.

Conclusions.—The clinical significance of the findings is that, in most cases, the effect of a combined stenosis is effectively the same as that of the more severe stenosis. The resistance to flow at each stenosis can be added up to produce a combined resistance, but the nonlinear nature of the resistance at a stenosis means that for all practical purposes the anatomical data are insufficient for predicting the stenotic resistance.

▶ From time to time it is useful to consider the physics of vascular obstructions upon which we frequently operate. It is remarkably difficult to characterize in accurate terms the significance of the complex series of obstructions that represent most native atherosclerotic disease. The efforts of Kilpatrick and his associates are certainly helpful. Reading this interesting paper requires considerable thought, but there are certain useful conclusions. In particular, the usual practice of placing grafts distal to the most severe stenosis but not necessarily to all of the stenotic areas is well defended by this basic research.—J.J. Collins, Jr., M.D.

Valve and Ascending Aorta

Preservation of Aortic Valve in Type A Aortic Dissection Complicated by Aortic Regurgitation

Fann JI, Glower DD, Miller DC, Yun KL, Rankin JS, White WD, Smith LR, Wolfe WG, Shumway NE (Stanford Univ, Stanford, Calif; Duke Univ, Durham, NC)
J Thorac Cardiovasc Surg 102:62–75, 1991   6–9

Introduction.—Operative treatment is best for patients with type A aortic dissection, but the guidelines for aortic valve resuspension as opposed to aortic valve replacement (AVR) are not well described. The AVR may expose these patients unnecessarily to the risks of prosthetic valves. The clinical experience at 2 university medical centers were reviewed to compare valve resuspension with AVR in patients with type A dissection complicated by aortic regurgitation.

Methods.—Surgery was performed in 252 patients for spontaneous type A aortic dissection. The dissection was acute in 67% of patients and chronic in 33%. An aortic valve procedure was necessary in addition to the ascending aorta repair or replacement in 121 patients. Valve resuspension was performed in 46 patients, of whom 39 had acute and 7 had chronic dissection. In 75 patients, 36 with acute and 39 with chronic dissection, AVR was performed. The mean follow-up was 4 years, and longest follow-up 20 years.

Results.—Operative mortalities were 13% with valve resuspension and 20% for AVR; the difference was not significant. For patients who had the aortic procedure only, operative mortality was 32%. Aortic valve replacement was performed in patients with coexistent aortic valve disease, Marfan's syndrome, annuloaortic ectasia, and failed resuspension. The overall actuarial survival rate was 59% at 5 years, 40% at 10 years, and 25% at 15 years. Survival for valve resuspension patients was 67%, 52%, and 26%; for AVR patients, 70%, 39%, and 21%; and for patients who had an ascending aortic procedure only, 51%, 37%, and 23%. Significant, independent predictors of early or late death were old age, previous cardiac or aortic surgery, more preoperative complications of dissection, and earlier operative date. Neither the type of valve procedure nor the treating institution were significant predictors. Late AVR was needed in 2 valve resuspension patients, 4 patients with initial AVR, and 5 of the isolated aortic repair patients; freedom from AVR at 10 years was 80%, 73%, and 91%, respectively.

Conclusions.—In patients with type A aortic dissection and aortic regurgitation, aortic valve resuspension appears to be a satisfactorily durable repair. For this reason, along with avoidance of the complications of prosthetic valves and the need for indefinite anticoagulation, most patients should have the native valve preserved whenever possible. Patients with Marfan's syndrome and gross annuloaortic ectasia are exceptions.

Sixteen-Year Experience With Aortic Root Replacement: Results of 172 Operations
Kouchoukos NT, Wareing TH, Murphy SF, Perrillo JB (Washington Univ, St Louis)
Ann Surg 214:308–320, 1991   6–10

Objective.—One hundred seventy-two aortic root replacements were performed in 168 patients during a 16-year interval that concluded in 1990.

Technique.—In 1981 an open technique replaced the inclusion/wrap technique used in the first 105 procedures. In the open procedure, after excision of the aortic valve and completion of the sutures between the annulus and the prosthetic valve, buttons of graft opposite the coronary ostia are excised. The aortic wall next to the coronary ostia is sutured to those openings.

Results.—The hospital mortality rate was 5%. The only significant independent predictor of early death was the duration of cardiopulmonary bypass. The mean duration of follow-up was 81 months. Actuarial survival rate was 61% at 7 years and 48% at 12 years. There was no significant difference in survival rate between the inclusion/wrap and open technique; however, the frequency of reoperation was significantly less with the open procedure (Fig 6–6). Actuarial freedom from thromboembolism for 152 patients with prosthetic valves was 82% at 12 years.

Conclusion.—The results reported support the continued use of composite graft replacement of the aortic root for annuloaortic ectasia, persistent aneurysm of the sinuses of Valsalva, and for patients with ascending aortic dissection. The open technique is associated with fewer reoperations and has become the method of choice. The use of aortic

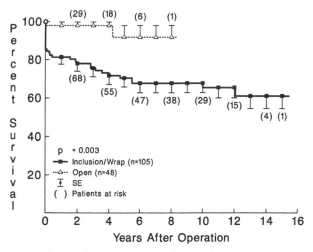

Fig 6–6.—Actuarial freedom from reoperation on the ascending aorta or aortic arch for any cause according to operative technique for the patients receiving prosthetic grafts. (Courtesy of Kouchoukos NT, Wareing TH, Murphy SF, et al: *Ann Surg* 214:308–320, 1991.)

allografts and pulmonary autografts has broadened the indications for aortic root replacement.

Composite Graft Repair of Marfan Aneurysm of the Ascending Aorta: Results in 100 Patients
Gott VL, Pyeritz RE, Cameron DE, Greene PS, McKusick VA (Johns Hopkins Med Insts, Baltimore)
Ann Thorac Surg 52:38–45, 1991   6–11

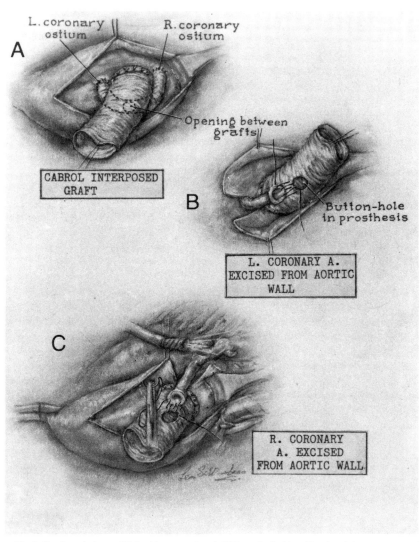

Fig 6–7.—**A,** technique of Cabrol interposed graft. This method of handling low-lying coronary ostia has been replaced by mobilization of coronary ostia as depicted in **B** and **C.** (Courtesy of Gott VL, Pyeritz RE, Cameron DE, et al: *Ann Thorac Surg* 52:38–45, 1991.)

Introduction.—Data were reviewed on 100 consecutive patients with Marfan's syndrome who underwent composite graft repair of an ascending aortic aneurysm in 1976–1989. Aortic dissection was present at the time of surgery in 22 patients. Eighteen patients had a mitral valve procedure as well.

Technique.—At surgery both hypothermic cardiopulmonary bypass and crystalloid potassium cardioplegic arrest were used. Initially the aneurysmal wall was wrapped about the graft to promote hemostasis. Subsequently the aneurysmal wall was simply tacked loosely over the graft. A Cabrol shunt between the aneurysm wrap and right atrium was used in 13 cases (Fig 6–7).

Results.—None of the 92 patients operated on electively died at surgery, but 1 of 8 who had emergency repair died during surgery. Five of the 10 late deaths occurred in the first 11 cases. Three late deaths resulted from endocarditis of the composite graft. Three other patients who had endocarditis survived after replacement of the aortic root with a cryopreserved homograft. Actuarial survival was 93% at 5 years and 76% at 10 years. One patient had successful repair of coronary dehiscence.

Discussion.—It is possible to repair Marfan aneurysms with a composite graft with low early and late mortality. Anastomosing the coronary ostia directly to the composite graft, thereby avoiding the need for an interposed graft, is the preferred procedure. Avoiding an inclusive aortic wrap has lowered the risk of late suture-line dehiscence. Late endocarditis, however, remains a serious problem.

▶ The above publications by Fann, Kouchoukos, and Gott (Abstracts 6–9— 6–11) summarize the clinical experience at 4 excellent cardiac surgical centers in the treatment of patients with aortic insufficiency and abnormalities of the ascending aorta requiring combined reconstruction. It will become evident from these abstracts that there are 3 major variations in management. For some patients, it is possible to maintain the native aortic valve by resuspension or simple isolation from the distal aneurysm. A second group of patients require composite aortic valve and ascending aorta replacement. There are 2 major variations in this procedure. The classic Bentall operation involves direct anastomosis of the coronary ostia to the prosthetic conduit, leaving the aortic wall intact. The variation strongly recommended by Kouchoukos and associates involves coronary flow by attaching an isolated button of aorta surrounding the coronary ostium to the prosthetic conduit. Whereas the opinions of the authors may be strongly expressed and well defended for espousement of their favorite variations, it is evident from careful perusal of these publications that excellent results may be obtained by the skillful use of any of these techniques. Our own experience suggests that retention of the native aortic valve should be reserved for those patients who have neither annulo-aortic ectasia nor a connective tissue disorder such as Marfan syndrome or Ehlers-Danlos syndrome.— J.J. Collins, Jr., M.D.

Aortic Valve Replacement for Aortic Stenosis in Persons Aged 80 Years and Over

Culliford AT, Galloway AC, Colvin SB, Grossi EA, Baumann FG, Esposito R, Ribakove GH, Spencer FC (New York Univ, New York)
Am J Cardiol 67:1256–1260, 1991   6–12

Background.—As the United States population ages, the risks and benefits of aortic valve replacement in patients over 80 have increasing significance. Results of aortic valve replacement in aortic stenosis with and without aortic regurgitation in patients over 80 were analyzed.

Methods.—The 12-year experience included 71 patients with a mean age of 82 who had aortic stenosis or mixed stenosis and regurgitation. Of these, 35 had aortic valve replacement alone and 36 had a concomitant coronary bypass procedure with no other valve procedure. The patients had severe cardiac limitations; 91% were in New York Heart Association class III or IV. Standard cardiopulmonary bypass (mean duration, 117 minutes) was used in all patients. Patients were followed up at office visits or by telephone for a mean of 26.5 months.

Results.—Overall hospital mortality was 12.7%, but it varied from 5.7% for the patients with valve replacement alone to 19.4% for those with combined procedures. There was 1 perioperative stroke. One-year survival from late cardiac death was 98.2%, and at 3 years the figure was 95.5%. For patients who had combined procedures, 1-year and 3-year survivals were 96.3% and 91.2%, respectively, and for those who had valve replacement alone, both survivals were 100%. Symptoms improved markedly in 83% of patients. At 1 year, 93.3% of patients were free from valve-related complications; at 3 years, the figure was 80.4%.

Conclusions.—Aortic valve replacement for aortic stenosis in patients aged 80 and older seems to have low morbidity and mortality. Mortality appears to be higher in patients who also undergo coronary artery bypass grafting. There is a low incidence of perioperative stroke and neurologic fatality. For most patients in this age group with symptoms of aortic valve dysfunction, this may be the therapy of choice.

▶ There can be no doubt that extremely advanced age influences the expected results of cardiac surgical operations. However, in patients whose general health is otherwise fine, the operative risk of valve replacement for aortic stenosis is remarkably low. Furthermore, and of equal importance, rehabilitation in patients who survive operation is excellent, with a satisfactory return to lifestyle for the great majority of patients.—J.J. Collins, Jr., M.D.

Patient Age and Results of Balloon Aortic Valvuloplasty: The Mansfield Scientific Registry Experience

Reeder GS, Nishimura RA, Holmes DR Jr, the Mansfield Scientific Aortic Valvuloplasty Registry Investigators (Mayo Clin and Found, Rochester, Minn)
J Am Coll Cardiol 17:909–913, 1991   6–13

Background.—Some studies have suggested that the results of balloon aortic valvuloplasty are better in younger than in older patients. Patients of both age groups from the Mansfield Scientific Aortic Valvuloplasty Registry were studied to compare the results of this procedure in older vs. younger patients.

Methods.—Four hundred ninety-two patients were divided into 3 age groups. There were 59 patients less than 70 years of age, 168 aged 70 to 79 years, and 265 aged 80 or more. The criteria for success were an increase in valve area of 25% or less, a decrease in pressure gradient of 50% or more, or both in a patient who did not require valve replacement. Older patients had more severe stenosis, and patients aged 80 years or more had a higher incidence of congestive heart failure. There were more female patients in the older age groups.

Results.—Success rates were 83% to 89%, with no significant differences among age groups. Neither was there any significant difference in final valve area after normalization for body surface area. Average increase in valve area was about .32 cm^2. Rate of in-hospital death ranged from 4.2% to 9.4%, with no significant differences between groups. At 7 months, the overall mortality rate was 23%.

Conclusions.—Results of balloon aortic valvuloplasty are similar in older and younger patients, regardless of the initially more severe disease found in older patients. The procedure remains palliative and mortality remains substantial. Rates of in-hospital and other complications do not differ significantly between age groups.

▶ This interesting report by Reeder and associates indicates that age alone does not seem to adversely influence the results of balloon angioplasty. This is similar to what has been observed with valve replacement surgery. However, it is worthwhile, to note that the expected duration of rehabilitation is much more favorable in patients undergoing valve replacement.—J.J. Collins, Jr., M.D.

Indications and Limitations of Aortic Valve Reconstruction

Duran C, Kumar N, Gometza B, Halees ZA (King Faisal Specialist Hosp and Research Ctr, Riyadh, Saudi Arabia)
Ann Thorac Surg 52:447–454, 1991   6–14

Objective.—The value of conservative surgery for aortic regurgitation was examined in a series of 251 consecutive patients operated on between 1988 and 1990, 144 of whom had valve replacement and 107, a conservative procedure. The mean age was 23 years; most of the patients had rheumatic valve disease.

Surgery.—Nearly 40% of the patients undergoing conservative surgery had isolated lesions, but one fifth required triple-valve surgery. Sixty-nine patients underwent annular and leaflet plasties (Fig 6–8). Twenty-five patients had cusp extension with glutaraldehyde-treated bovine pericardium, and 13 others had cusp extension with autologous pericardium.

Results.—The hospital mortality rate was 2%, with both deaths occur-

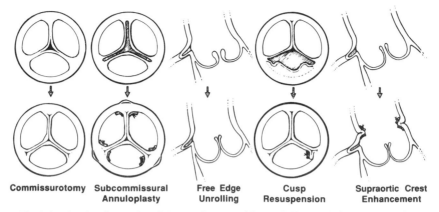

| Commissurotomy | Subcommissural Annuloplasty | Free Edge Unrolling | Cusp Resuspension | Supraortic Crest Enhancement |

Fig 6–8.—Aortic valve repair techniques. (Courtesy of Duran C, Kumar N, Gometza B, et al: *Ann Thorac Surg* 52:447–454, 1991.)

ring in the repair group. There were no late deaths and no embolic events. Only 5% of the patients underwent anticoagulation. Twelve patients undergoing repair procedures required reoperation, usually because of mitral dysfunction. Two patients having cusp extension surgery were reoperated on because of mitral dysfunction. The echocardiographic results were superior in patients having cusp extension during a maximum follow-up of 30 months.

Discussion.—Conservative surgery is feasible in a high proportion of younger rheumatic patients with aortic regurgitation. Anticoagulation is not necessary. Cusp extension appears to be the most reliable procedure, but whether glutaraldehyde-treated pericardium will prove durable remains to be seen. More frequent intraoperative echocardiography may reduce the need for reoperation.

▶ Carlos Duran and associates continue their excellent work in the development of surgical repair for patients with aortic insufficiency. Although the long-term results are not yet definable, there certainly is evidence that some patients may be very well served by aortic valve reconstruction. As the results of valve replacement continue to improve, the place of conservative operations on the aortic valve is not well established. Long-term results will have to be superb to justify the increased technical complexity of this procedure, with its attendant risk of early failure. Favorable results with aortic valvuloplasty have also been reported by Cosgrove and associates (1). For interested surgeons, the study of Anderson and associates (2) is useful reading.—J.J. Collins, Jr., M.D.

References

1. Cosgrove DM, Rosenkranz ER, Hendren WG, et al: Valvuloplasty for aortic insufficiency. *J Thorac Cardiovasc Surg* 102:571–577, 1991.
2. Anderson RH, Devine WA, Yen Ho S, et al: The myth of the aortic annulus: The anatomy of the subaortic outflow tract. *Ann Thorac Surg* 52:640–646, 1991.

Closing Click of St. Jude Medical and Duromedics Edwards Bileaflet Valves: Complaints Created by Valve Noise and Their Relation to Sound Pressure and Hearing Level

Moritz A, Steinseifer U, Kobina G, Neuwirth-Riedl K, Wolters H, Reul H, Wolner E (University of Vienna; Helmholtz Institute for Biomedical Engineering, Aachen, Germany; General Hospital Klagenfurt, Austria)
Eur Heart J 12:673–679, 1991   6–15

Introduction.—The metallic click produced by mechanical heart valve prostheses often annoys patients. The present study was designed to determine whether the sounds produced by different bileaflet prostheses correlate with patients' complaints.

Patients and Methods.—Seventy-three patients with a mean age of 56 years had received a Duromedics Edwards (DE) or a St. Jude Medical (SJM) bileaflet valve prosthesis. The groups were matched for valve position, tissue annulus diameter, and body surface area. Sound pressure levels were measured by using a precision sound-level meter.

Observations.—Analysis of closing sounds revealed a noise peak at 0-4 kHz, representing vibrations of the decelerated column of blood, and another peak at 16 kHz caused by deceleration of the occluder itself. The DE prostheses were louder at 10 cm than were the SJM valves. The DE prostheses produced significantly higher sound pressure levels in all frequency ranges. Patients with symptoms were younger than those without. For both valve types developed sound energy increased with valve size in the aortic position (Fig 6–9), but not in the mitral valve. The cardiac rhythm did not influence the developed sound pressure.

Conclusions.—The use of pyrolytic carbon for occluders has changed the frequency peak of the closing click to 16 kHz. The intensity of the closing click correlates with patients' complaints of sound emission, and this is a valid consideration when selecting a prosthesis.

▶ The great majority of prosthetic cardiac valves implanted currently throughout the world are bileaflet carbon valves. Every surgeon has recognized the increasing number of patients who complain of the noise generated by the closure of the valve. This interesting study documents the difference in closing

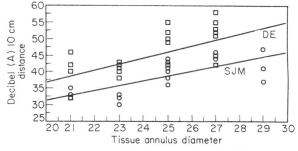

Fig 6–9.—In aortic valves, sound pressure increased with valve size. This was more apparent for DE (*squares*) than for SJM (*circles*) valves. (Courtesy of Moritz A, Steinseifer U, Kobina G, et al: *Eur Heart J* 12:673–679, 1991.)

sound of the carbon valve and its greater intensity justifying the observation that these valves are more likely to produce audible closing signals than were prostheses using silicon rubber poppets. For most patients, the noise of the prosthesis is a minor irritation, but for a few it can be a very vexing annoyance.—J.J. Collins, Jr., M.D.

Comparative Study of the Hydrodynamic Function of the CarboMedics Valve

Butterfield M, Fisher J, Davies GA, Spyt TJ (University of Leeds, Leeds, England)
Ann Thorac Surg 52:815–820, 1991   6–16

Introduction.—The CarboMedics valve prosthesis was designed to limit turbulence by eliminating pivot guards, struts, and orifice projections. The valve can be precisely positioned through its ability to rotate relative to the sewing ring. The pivot recess was designed to facilitate washout. The Dacron sewing ring is coated in carbon to limit pannus formation. The opening leaflet angle of 78 degrees allows for rapid synchronous closure.

Methods.—Hydrodynamic studies were conducted to compare the function of the mitral and aortic CarboMedic valve prostheses with those of similar-sized St. Jude and Björk-Shiley Monostrut valves. The valves were tested under 5 conditions of pulsatile flow.

Results.—Each of the CarboMedics valves demonstrated good hydrodynamic function, despite relatively high energy loss across the 19-mm aortic valve. Function was comparable to that of the St. Jude Medical valve. Leakage volumes were significantly larger for both of these designs than for the Björk-Shiley Monostrut valve. Total energy loss for the Björk-Shiley prosthesis was less than for the bileaflet valves in the aortic position.

Conclusion.—The CarboMedics valve should function as well as previous carbon prosthetic bileaflet heart valves, although closed valve regurgitation remains a problem.

▶ Both the St. Jude and CarboMedics prostheses have a greater diastolic regurgitant volume than many surgeons appreciate. It is enough to produce a definable pattern by echocardiographic examination as well as a faint whisp of regurgitation in contrast aortography or ventriculography. The pattern of transvalvar regurgitation is quite characteristic, and differentiation from perivalvular leak should not be difficult in most instances. Auscultation of a diastolic murmur for an aortic valve or a systolic murmur for a mitral prosthesis in the absence of perivalvular leak is extremely unusual, if it ever occurs.—J.J. Collins, Jr., M.D.

Obstruction of Mechanical Heart Valve Prostheses: Clinical Aspects and Surgical Management

Deviri E, Sareli P, Wisenbaugh T, Cronje SL (Johannesburg Hospital; University of Witwatersvand, Johannesburg)
J Am Coll Cardiol 17:646–650, 1991   6–17

Introduction.—In 1980–1989, 100 patients with a median age of 32 years underwent a total of 106 operations for obstructed mechanical valve prosthesis. Obstruction was caused by thrombus alone in 61 valves, pannus in 7, and both causes in 44.

Patients.—Similar numbers of patients had an obstructed aortic and mitral prosthesis. A Björk-Shiley valve was implicated in 51 valves, a St. Jude valve was implicated in 41, and a Medtronic-Hall prosthesis was implicated in 20. The median time from valve replacement to diagnosis of obstruction was 4 years. Most patients were receiving inadequate anticoagulant therapy; 63% were in New York Heart Association functional class IV.

Treatment and Results.—A total of 81 affected valves were replaced. In the other patients, declotting was performed and pannus was excised as required. In all patients, surgery was performed on an urgent basis, even if the patient was clinically stable. The operative mortality was 13.7% in patients with aortic obstruction and 12.2% in those with an obstructed mitral prosthesis.

Conclusion.—Prosthetic valve obstruction is most often caused by thrombus. The clinical presentation varies widely. Prompt operative treatment carries a relatively low mortality rate. In the short term, declotting and excision of pannus have given results comparable to those of replacing the valve prosthesis. Attempted thrombolysis will fail in a significant number of patients with pannus formation.

▶ The remarkably high incidence of obstruction observed in the patients reported by Deviri and associates has not been appreciated in our practice. However, there is no question that encroachment of pannus may produce obstruction, particularly in prosthetic devices of small diameter in either the aortic or mitral position, more commonly the aortic.—J.J. Collins, Jr., M.D.

Failure of Hancock Pericardial Xenografts: Is Prophylactic Bioprosthetic Replacement Justified?
Bortolotti U, Milano A, Guerra F, Mazzucco A, Mossuto E, Thiene G, Gallucci V (University of Padova, Italy)
Ann Thorac Surg 51:430–437, 1991   6–18

Introduction.—Bioprosthetic pericardial valves made of bovine pericardium, introduced in 1970 as an alternative to porcine valves because of their superior hemodynamic performance, have shown an extremely high early mechanical failure rate. These findings, together with the observation that dysfunction of pericardial xenografts can occur suddenly, underline the importance of close monitoring of bovine graft recipients and suggest the need for prophylactic graft replacement in asymptomatic patients with clinical evidence of structural valve deterioration. The outcome of 97 Hancock pericardial xenografts (HPX) was assessed after a 7-year follow-up.

Patients.—Between 1981 and 1984, 48 men and 36 women with a mean age of 55.7 years received a total of 97 HPX bioprosthesis. Fifty-four patients had aortic valve replacement (AVR), 17 had mitral valve replacement (MVR), and 13 had combined mitral and aortic valve replacement (MAVR). Surviving patients were monitored by biannual 2-dimensional transthoracic echocardiography.

Results.—There were 8 hospital deaths, including 4 after AVR, 1 after MVR, and 3 after MAVR. Of 76 patients discharged, 21 died in the late postoperative period. Actuarial survival at 7 years was 66% after AVR, 64% after MVR, and 41% after MAVR. During follow-up, 32 patients required reoperation, 21 of them after AVR, 4 after MVR, and 7 after MAVR. Indications for reoperation after AVR included a paraprosthetic leak in 1, endocarditis in 3, and structural deterioration in 17. Two patients with deterioration of the AVR died before reoperation. One of the 8 patients with MAVR also died before operation. Of the current survivors, 78% have clinical evidence of valve failure. At 7 years, the actuarial freedom from structural deterioration of the HPX is 25% after AVR, 29% after MVR, and 0% after MAVR.

Conclusion.—The extremely poor durability of the HPX justifies prophylactic replacement of this device in asymptomatic patients with clinical evidence of HPX dysfunction and confirms the need for closer noninvasive monitoring of patients with an implanted HPX.

▶ While use of the Hancock pericardial xenograft has not been common in the United States, these data from Bortolotti and associates indicate that serious consideration needs be given to prophylactic replacement of these devices. The Ionescu-Shiley xenograft has also been found to be less satisfactory than predicted, and most surgeons no longer use it (1).—J.J. Collins, Jr., M.D.

Reference

1. Masters RG, Pipe AL, Bedard JP, et al: Long-term clinical results with the Ionescu-Shiley pericardial xenograft. *J Thorac Cardovasc Surg* 101:81–89, 1991.

Replacement of the Aortic Valve or Root With a Pulmonary Autograft in Children
Gerosa G, McKay R, Ross DN (National Heart Hospital, London)
Ann Thorac Surg 51:424–429, 1991   6–19

Background.—In addition to its other advantages, the pulmonary autograft is living autogenous tissue that may function indefinitely and grow as the patient grows. Pulmonary autografts were used for replacement of the aortic valve or aortic root in 34 children.

Methods.—The patients were 27 boys and 7 girls with a mean age of 14 years. The operations were done over a 21-year period. The procedure was done using cardiopulmonary bypass and moderate hypothermia. The valve was taken with a supporting cuff of myocardium, and the right

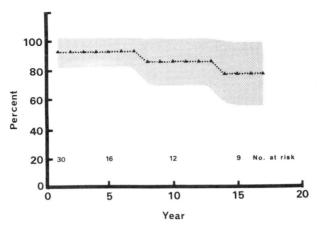

Fig 6–10.—Linearized actuarial survival after aortic valve or root replacement with pulmonary autograft. *Shaded area* represents the 95% confidence interval. (Courtesy of Gerosa G, McKay R, Ross DN: *Ann Thorac Surg* 51:424–429, 1991.)

ventricular outflow tract was reconstituted with an aortic homograft, usually fresh, or a pulmonary homograft, most often cryopreserved. Average bypass time was 133 minutes. Frozen valves were stored in liquid nitrogen vapor, and ABO cross-matching was not done routinely.

Results.—Hospital mortality was 11.8%, and late mortality was 13.3%. One patient died of unknown causes 4 months after operation. At 10 years, actuarial late survival was 85.7%, and at 15 years it was 77.1% (Fig 6–10). Sixteen percent of patients required reoperation, usually because of bacterial endocarditis. After 214 patient-years of follow-up, all survivors were in New York Heart Association functional class I and none were taking cardiac medication.

Conclusions.—Pulmonary autograft appears to give good results in children. The graft has undoubted viability and compatibility and thus appears less prone to calcification and degeneration. No serious or progressive incompetence was noted in the present series. In young patients, the graft may continue to grow postoperatively.

▶ The use of pulmonary autografts, particularly in children, for aortic valve replacement is strongly defended by these data from the National Heart Hospital and Mr. Donald Ross. Unfortunately, the substantial increase in the complexity of operation does result in a higher operative mortality than is common with other types of aortic valve replacement procedures. This aspect has put a damper on the enthusiasm of other surgeons throughout the world.—J.J. Collins, Jr., M.D.

Extreme Obstruction to Left Ventricular Outflow by a Bioprosthesis in the Mitral Valve Position
Roberts WC, Dollar AL (Natl Heart, Lung, and Blood Inst, Natl Insts of Health, Bethesda, Md)
Am Heart J 121:607–608, 1991

Background.—Mitral valve replacement may be complicated by obstruction to left ventricular outflow, usually because a large prosthesis was used in a patient with a relatively small left ventricle. This preventable complication may be fatal.

Case Report.—Woman, 72, had a precordial murmur for several years. Atrial fibrillation and congestive heart failure developed at age 70 and the patient was treated medically. When her exertional dyspnea worsened and nocturnal dyspnea appeared at age 72, mitral valve replacement was done. The patient was 65 inches tall and weighed 110 pounds at this time. A 29-mm Carpentier-Edwards bioprosthesis was used to replace the patient's floppy valve. In the recovery room, severe hypotension developed, which worsened despite vasopressor treatment. The patient died of cardiac arrest 3 hours postoperatively. During resuscitative efforts, the chest was opened and the posterior wall of the left ventricle was seen to be ruptured. The heart weighed 425 g and the ventricular cavities were of normal size, but left ventricular outflow had been nearly occluded by the bioprosthesis.

Conclusions.—A case of death caused by use of a too-large substitute cardiac valve is reported. To prevent this complication, the surgeon should use small prostheses in small-sized patients, regardless of the type of hemodynamic lesion. A smaller prosthesis should be used if the left ventricular cavity is normal or near-normal in size. Left ventricular outflow obstruction may be caused by any type of prosthesis or bioprosthesis.

▶ Not only is there a major hazard from the selection of too large a valve for the mitral position, but the incidence of perivalvular leak will be significantly increased if 2 large valves are placed in the aortic position with the resultant stress on the suture line.—J.J. Collins, Jr., M.D.

Intraoperative Transesophageal Doppler Color Flow Imaging Used to Guide Patient Selection and Operative Treatment of Ischemic Mitral Regurgitation

Sheikh KH, Bengston JR, Rankin JS, de Bruijn NP, Kisslo J (Duke Univ, Durham, NC)
Circulation 84:594–604, 1991   6–21

Introduction.—In patients with mitral regurgitation, it is essential to have information on the severity of the condition at the time of cardiopulmonary bypass (CPB) operation. Particularly if coronary reperfusion has been performed, the characteristics of regurgitation may be quite different from what they were at catheterization. Mitral regurgitation is accurately assessed by transesophogeal Doppler color flow (TDCF) imaging.

Methods.—This technique was used intraoperatively to assess its usefulness in the selection and operative treatment of ischemic mitral regurgitation in 246 patients undergoing surgery for ischemic heart disease. Preoperative cardiac catheterization was performed in all patients. The 5-MHz esophageal probe transducer was placed after induction of anesthesia and endotracheal intubation, with the first images obtained before skin incision. Intraoperatively, images were preliminarily interpreted by experienced anesthesiologists or senior cardiology staff as needed. Mitral regurgitation was estimated according to the greatest length and width of the abnormal jet, relative to the left atrium.

Results.—Interobserver agreement was high, with complete concordance in 91% of patients. Estimations of the severity of mitral regurgitation by catheterization and pre-CPB TDCF were discordant in 46% of patients. Patients in whom estimations were discordant and concordant both had lower mean arterial and pulmonary capillary wedge pressures at the time of TDCF. Patients in the discordant group were more likely to have an unstable clinical syndrome at catheterization, to have thrombolytic therapy, and to have higher left ventricular end-diastolic pressures at catheterization. Based on the findings of TDCF, the operative plan was altered in 11% of patients. In most of these, coronary artery bypass alone was performed without a mitral valve procedure because of the finding of less regurgitation. Corrective surgery was performed immediately in 5 patients in whom unsatisfactory findings were noted postoperatively. The most important predictor of survival was residual regurgitation postoperatively, even more than age or left ventricular ejection fraction.

Conclusion.—In patients with ischemic mitral regurgitation, TDCF appears to be useful in guiding patient selection and operative treatment. Intraoperative TDCF should be a routine part of treatment for these patients. It may find unsuspected defects and help prevent patients leaving the operating room with high-grade mitral regurgitation.

▶ The introduction of intraoperative transesophageal imaging has been a major advance in the treatment of valvular heart disease. Not only are occasional unsuspected intracardiac clots or other abnormalities discovered, but the evaluation of the adequacy of the repair of valvular lesions is also very greatly assisted by this technique. Interestingly, the technique threatens to spawn a new area of specialization, that of the anesthetist-echocardiographer. Perhaps we will soon see a society formed, a new journal, and eventually the development of an examination for certification for these specialists. Intraoperative echocardiography also has important application in congenital heart disease, and smaller probes promise benefit even for small children and infants (1).—J.J. Collins, Jr., M.D.

Reference

1. Cyran SE, Myers JL, Gleason MM, et al: Application of intraoperative transesophageal echocardiography in infants and small children. *J Cardiovasc Surg* 32:318–321, 1991.

Outcome Probabilities and Life History After Surgical Mitral Commissurotomy: Implications for Balloon Commissurotomy

Hickey MSJ, Blackstone EH, Kirklin JW, Dean LS (Univ of Alabama at Birmingham)
J Am Coll Cardiol 17:29–42, 1991

6–22

Background.—Although a good outcome appears more likely after open than after closed surgical mitral commissurotomy, this has never been tested in a randomized trial. Early and late outcomes after both the closed and open procedures were therefore studied in a series of patients treated in the era of safe mitral valve replacement. A multivariable analysis was also done to compare outcome probability after surgical commissurotomy with that after mitral valve replacement after percutaneous balloon commissurotomy.

Methods.—The series comprised 339 patients with mitral stenosis who underwent surgical commissurotomy over a 21-year period, 236 of whom had the open and 103 the closed procedure. The 2 groups had similar characteristics. The closed procedure was always performed through a left anterolateral thoracotomy and the open procedure through a median sternotomy under cardiopulmonary bypass.

Results.—Overall 1-month survival rate was 99.7%; 1-year survival was 99%; 5-year survival, 95%; 10-year survival, 87%; and 20-year survival, 59%. Choice of surgical technique was not a risk factor, and the modes of death were similar with both techniques. There was no difference between the 2 groups in risk of a second operation, mitral valve replacement, thromboembolism, or poor function. Older age at operation, being black, high pulmonary vascular resistance, calcification of the mitral leaflet, enlargement of the left ventricle, and postoperative mitral incompetence were risk factors. Although important mitral incompetence developed in only 2 patients undergoing the closed procedure, the closed technique was a risk factor for immediate postoperative mitral incompetence. At 10 years, 78% of the patients did not require mitral valve replacement; at 20 years the figure was 47%.

Conclusions.—Surgical closed, or percutaneous balloon, mitral commissurotomy should probably be the first therapeutic choice for most patients with mitral stenosis. The equations presented can help compare outcome probability after percutaneous balloon commissurotomy with that after surgical commissurotomy, and then compare those outcomes with outcome probability after mitral valve replacement.

▶ Observations reported in this relatively large series of patients undergoing mitral commissurotomy agrees remarkably with those obtained by Harken (1) in the now distant past. As the authors point out, these results must serve as a bench mark for balloon valvuloplasty and, for open mitral commissurotomy.— J.J. Collins, Jr., M.D.

Reference

1. Ellis LB, et al: Fifteen-to-twenty-year study of one thousand patients undergoing closed mitral valvuloplasty. *Circulation* 48:357, 1973.

Mitral Valve Repair in the Extensively Calcified Mitral Valve Annulus

El Asmar B, Acker M, Couetil JP, Perier P, Dervanian P, Chauvaud S, Carpentier A (Hôpital Broussais, Paris)
Ann Thorac Surg 52:66–69, 1991

6–23

Background.—Mitral valve repair is not performed on patients with a heavily calcified mitral annulus because of the increased risk of ventricular rupture. However, mitral valve replacement is also a risky procedure. Extensive decalcification of the annulus was performed before mitral valve repair in 12 patients.

Technique.—The type of mitral disease and the degree and location of the calcification were analyzed. All patients had a calcified bloc in the posterior part of the mitral annulus, which extended further in some patients. Decalcification of the annulus was initiated by incision of the ventricular endothelium around the borders of the calcified bar. Scissors were used to excise the calcium (Fig 6–11). After removal of the calcium, interrupted mattress sutures were used to close the trench created by the decalcification. The posterior leaflet was then reattached (Fig 6–12). After annular reconstruction, other lesions were repaired.

Results.—In a series of 12 patients, there were no thromboembolic events, reoperations, or deaths. All patients are currently in New York Heart Association class I or II.

Conclusion.—Mitral valve repair can be performed successfully on patients with an extensively calcified mitral annulus, avoiding the risks associated with mitral valve replacement.

▶ This small series of patients represents a remarkable achievement in my opinion. Certainly, our results in valvuloplasty on patients with extensive calcifi-

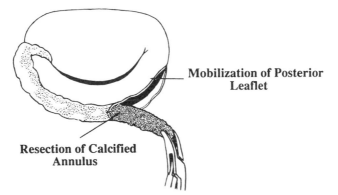

Mobilization of Posterior Leaflet

Resection of Calcified Annulus

Fig 6–11.—Mobilization of posterior leaflet and decalcification of annulus. (Courtesy of El Asmar B, Acker M, Couetil JP, et al: *Ann Thorac Surg* 52:66–69, 1991.)

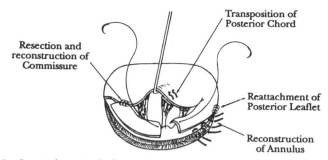

Fig 6–12.—Repair of posterior leaflet, annulus, commissure, and anterior leaflet. (Courtesy of El Asmar B, Acker M, Couetil JP, et al: *Ann Thorac Surg* 52:66–69, 1991.)

cation of the mitral annulus have not been encouraging. Whether the extensive decalcification recommended by Asmar and associates will improve results overall is difficult to say. It certainly appears to be a complex operation, and it may not be uniformly effective.—J.J. Collins, Jr., M.D.

Repair of the Flail Anterior Leaflets of Tricuspid and Mitral Valves by Cusp Remodeling

Sutlic Z, Schmid C, Borst HG (Hannover Medical School, Hannover Germany)
Ann Thorac Surg 50:927–930, 1990   6–24

Background.—Many pathologic conditions may result in chordae tendineae rupture. An alternative approach to this problem was developed.

Case Report.—Man, 30, had several attacks of leg edema and dyspnea over 3 years. Exercise tolerance had progressively declined, and he could only walk up 10 stairs. As a child, he had sustained minor thoracic trauma falling out a window. He had a grade 3/6 systolic murmur over the left sternal border in the fifth intercostal space and massive enlargement of the right atrium and ventricle on chest radiograph. Severe tricuspid insufficiency was noted on 2-dimensional echocardiography. At total cardiopulmonary bypass, a greatly enlarged tricuspid annulus was seen with tearing of the caudad ⅔ of the chordae of the anterior leaflet. The chordae tendineae of the posterior leaflet was ruptured. Flail portions of both leaflets were resected, the cut edges were united by a running 6–0 suture, and the annulus segment without leaflets was plicated (Fig 6–13). A tricuspid valve orifice measuring 3 cm² was achieved. The patient regained full exercise tolerance.

Conclusions.—A alternative treatment method to extensive chordae tendineae rupture with flail anterior leaflets is described. The case of a patient with bacterial endocarditis is also discussed and treatment illustrated (Figs. 6–14, and 6–15). Maximal use of the remaining leaflets and their chordal support provides an adequate valve orifice.

▶ This ingenious approach to anterior mitral leaflet reconstruction has yielded fine results in the patients reported. There are, however, not very many pa-

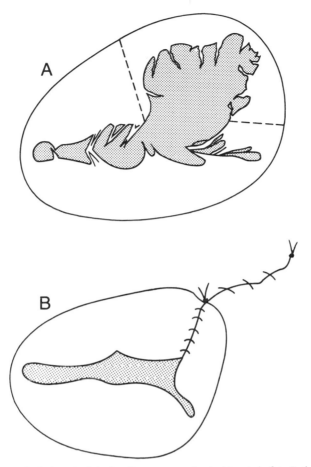

Fig 6–13.—Method of repair. **A,** broken lines correspond to incisions in leaflets. **B,** the cut edges of the remaining cusps are sutured. The portion of the annulus devoid of leaflets after resection is extensively plicated, with the plication carried out onto the atrial wall. (Courtesy of Sutlic Z, Schmid C, Borst HG: *Ann Thorac Surg* 50:927–930, 1990.)

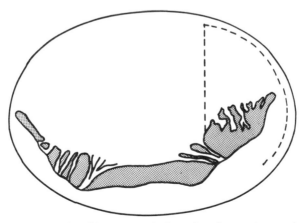

Fig 6–14.—Ruptured chordae of the anterior mitral cusp from the posterior strut chorda to the posterior commissure. Broken lines correspond to incisions in leaflets. (Courtesy of Sutlic Z, Schmid C, Borst HG: *Ann Thorac Surg* 50:927–930, 1990.)

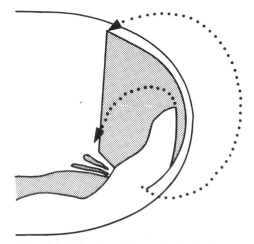

Fig 6-15.—After excision of the flail portion of the anterior leaflet, the tip of the corresponding part of the detached posterior cusp is rotated toward the torn edge of the former. (Courtesy of Sutlic Z, Schmid C, Borst HG: *Ann Thorac Surg* 50:927–930, 1990.)

tients in whom the nature of the problem is so readily defined and the condition of the leaflets so favorable for such a procedure.—J.J. Collins, Jr., M.D.

Congenital

Surgical Techniques for Hypertrophic Left Ventricular Obstructive Myopathy Including Mitral Valve Plication
Cooley DA (Texas Heart Inst, Houston)
J Cardiac Surg 6:29–33, 1991   6–25

Introduction.—The cause, pathogenesis, physiology, and anatomical features of idiopathic hypertrophic subaortic valvular stenosis (IHSS) have not been defined, and debate over its optimal treatment continues. Although the location of the obstructive element in IHSS may vary, most patients have a broad ridge of tissue, known as the hypertroph, in the outflow tract. Surgical treatment is indicated in symptomatic patients who do not respond to conservative medical treatment.

Technique.—Milder forms of IHSS are repaired by septectomy, according to Morrow, involving excision of a wedge of tissue about 15 mm in depth and extending from the aortic valve annulus above to a point below and near the attachment of the papillary muscles. To enhance the postoperative diameter of the outflow tract and prevent systolic anterior movement with possible valvular encroachment on the hypertroph, plication of the anterior leaflet of the mitral valve using interrupted sutures (Fig 6–16) has recently been used. In patients with advanced IHSS, especially those with mitral valve incompetence or midcavitary obstruction, the mitral valve is replaced with a prosthesis. To prevent posterior annular hemorrhage and enhance left ventricular contraction, the posterior leaflet and some chordal attachments of the mitral valve are preserved. A low profile,

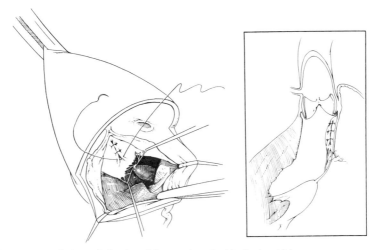

Fig 6–16.—Technique of plication of the anterior mitral leaflet in addition to septectomy to relieve outflow tract obstruction. Inset reveals the result of combined procedures. (Courtesy of Cooley DA: *J Cardiac Surg* 6:29–33, 1991.)

disk-type bileaflet prosthesis is the preferred device for mitral valve replacement in IHSS.

Patients.—Between 1970 and 1990, 192 patients with IHSS were operated on, of whom 106 had septal myomectomy alone without other procedures, 21 had repair or replacement of the mitral valve only, and 65 had combined valve replacement and myomectomy. The mitral valve was replaced in 70 patients. Of the 18 patients who had mitral valve repair, 12 had plication of the anterior leaflet.

Discussion.—The surgical techniques used earlier to treat IHSS and midcavitary hypertrophic obstruction have now been abandoned. For instance, neither the left cavitary approach nor the right ventricular approach gave optimal results. At present, most patients with IHSS are treated by a combination of left ventricular septectomy through an aortotomy with precise excision of a portion of the hypertroph. When possible, the mitral valve is repaired by plication of the anterior leaflet because it avoids the problems associated with a prosthesis, especially the need for permanent anticoagulation.

▶ This review of various operations used in the treatment of patients with hypertrophic left ventricular obstruction describes various operations that have been successful in the relief of aortic outflow obstruction. Our experience with these operations indicates that transaortic resection is probably the easiest and most successful technique. It is, however, not without some risk of aortic valve damage from retraction (1). Mitral valve replacement in these patients is both technically difficult and fraught with a higher than usual hazard of perivalvular leak. It is only rarely indicated. This very large series should be carefully studied by all surgeons operating on septal hypertrophy.—J.J. Collins, Jr., M.D.

Reference

1. Brown PS, Jr, Roberts CS, McIntosh CL, et al: Aortic regurgitation after left ventricular myotomy and myectomy. *Ann Thorac Surg* 51:585–592, 1991.

Analysis of Left Ventricular Wall Movement Before and After Reimplantation of Anomalous Left Coronary Artery in Infancy
Carvalho JS, Redington AN, Oldershaw PJ, Shinebourne EA, Lincoln CR, Gibson DG (Royal Brompton National Heart and Lung Hospital, London)
Br Heart J 65:218–222, 1991   6–26

Introduction.—An anomalous left coronary artery arising from the pulmonary artery is a rare congenital anomaly requiring reimplantation or redirection from the pulmonary artery to the aorta. Although postoperative improvement of global indices of left ventricular function has been documented, few studies have assessed the effects of persistent wall movement. Early operation may reduce the number of persistent wall motion abnormalities and reduce the risk of late sudden arrhythmic deaths.

Patients.—During a 5-year period, 5 infants were treated for an anomalous left coronary artery arising from the pulmonary artery at ages 2.8–5.7 months. Two infants underwent cardiopulmonary bypass and 3 had deep hypothermia with circulatory arrest. Direct reimplantation was possible in 4 infants. An intrapulmonary pericardial baffle was constructed in the remaining infant. There were no perioperative deaths. Four patients had cardiac catheterization and angiography at a mean of 33 months after operation. Preoperative and postoperative left ventricular angiograms were digitized frame by frame to study changes in wall motion.

Results.—The ejection fraction was severely impaired before operation but returned to normal after operation in 4 of the 5 patients. Analysis of wall motion plots showed considerable generalized hypokinesia, with no change in cavity shape before operation. The left ventricular cavity was more circular at end diastole, and there was little change in cavity shape during systole. After reimplantation, the degree of systolic shape change had increased, suggesting improvement in global systolic function. When restudied, 3 of the 4 children showed normal isometric and contour wall motion plots. One child still showed asynchronous onset of contraction and isovolumic relaxation. This child was the oldest one to be operated on.

Conclusion.—Surgical treatment of an anomalous coronary artery in infancy used to have a high mortality, and delay was therefore advocated. With direct reimplantation or redirection of the coronary artery, the chances of early survival have improved. Early surgical intervention with establishment of a dual coronary artery system now seems to be the best option for symptomatic infants with this congenital anomaly.

▶ This study documents the favorable influence of early revascularization surgery for infants with anomalous origin of the left coronary artery from the pulmonary artery. Correction is technically demanding but far preferable to prolonged delay. This anomaly is also hazardous in adults and should be corrected when discovered.—J.J. Collins, Jr., M.D.

References

1. Salloum DTJ, Montalescot G, Drobinski G, et al: Anomalous coronary arteries coursing between the aorta and pulmonary trunk: Clinical indications for coronary artery bypass. *Eur Heart J* 12:832–834, 1991.
2. Purut CM, Sabiston DC, Jr: Origin of the left coronary artery from the pulmonary artery in older adults. *J Thorac Cardiovasc Surg* 102:566–570, 1991.

Operative Survival and 40 Year Follow Up of Surgical Repair of Aortic Coarctation
Bobby JJ, Emami JM, Farmer RDT, Newman CGH (Charing Cross and Westminster Medical School, London)
Br Heart J 65:271–276, 1991   6–27

Background.—Coarctation of the aorta has been surgically corrected for more than 45 years. An experience dating back to the initial use of this procedure was analyzed to study early and late mortality.

Methods.—Over a 35-year period, 223 patients underwent surgical correction of coarctation of the aorta. One hundred fifty-six were male, and 38% were aged 5 to 15 years. About half the patients had hypertension, and many had had heart failure. Coarctation was postductal in most patients. Resection with end-to-end anastomosis was the most common technique, the subclavian flap technique being used increasingly after 1974. Eight infants with complex lesions had pulmonary artery banding, and only 2 survived. Total follow-up time was 3,288 patient-years, and it exceeded 30 years in 27 patients.

Results.—Mortality within 1 month of the operation was 12% overall, 2.6% for patients undergoing elective surgery, and 0% for patients operated on since 1968. Many of these deaths were emergency surgeries in very young infants. Fifteen patients were lost to follow-up. Twenty-two patients died during follow-up, and 17 of these deaths were attributed to the coarctation or to its repair or to associated anomalies. Preoperative hypertension appeared to be associated with increased risk of later mortality. Many of the aneurysm-related deaths occurred in patients exposed to hypertension and coarctation for 18 years or more. No patient died of cerebrovascular accident. Eighty percent of patients claimed to have no symptoms, yet many were hypertensive. The highest mortality was noted more than 20 years postoperatively.

Conclusions.—Life expectancy is evidently increased by surgical repair of coarctation of the aorta. Long-term survivors may have problems resulting from hypertension or recoarctation, but the association with duration of hypertension was not significant in this series. Doppler techniques, angiography, and MRI should allow more sensitive analyses in the future.

▶ Patients with coarctation of the aorta, although favorably affected by early repair, are still candidates for careful follow-up because of the high incidence of hypertension. Recurrence of coarctation must always be kept in mind as possibly aggravating the tendency toward hypertension.—J.J. Collins, Jr., M.D.

Coarctation: Do We Need to Resect Ductal Tissue?
Jonas RA (Children's Hosp, Boston)
Ann Thorac Surg 52:604–607, 1991   6–28

Introduction.—With the initial use of neonatal arterial switch for coarctation, there was concern about the potential for stenosis at the great vessel and circumferential artery anastomoses. However, of more than 400 such procedures, there have been no reoperations for aortic stenosis and only 9, all early in the experience, for pulmonary artery stenosis. Data on circumferential anastomoses in 100 neonates treated for aortic coarctation over a 12-year period were reviewed.

Methods.—There were 39 patients with associated complex anomalies, 32 with ventricular septal defect, and 29 with coarctation. Subclavian flap aortoplasty was performed in 70 infants, mostly after 1977, and resection and end-to-end anastomosis was done in 24, mostly before 1977. At 5 years, 93% of infants who had resection and end-to-end anastomosis were free of recoarctation, compared with 75% of those who had subclavian flap arthroplasty. These findings did not establish the superiority of resection and end-to-end anastomosis, however. Morphological factors, including length and diameter of the artery, diameter of the distal aortic arch, length of the isthmic segment, and isthmic diameter, could not predict recurrence after subclavian flap angioplasty.

Results.—Sacrifice of the left subclavian artery is a distinct disadvantage that limits the surgical options for dealing with a hypoplastic distal aortic arch. Histologic evidence suggests that the juxtaductal coarctation shelf is composed of smooth muscle of ductal origin. This tissue later fibroses and may be at risk of late aneurysm, especially with balloon dilation angioplasty. If there is a secondary coarctation membrane in the distal aortic arch, it can easily be missed with the subclavian flap procedure, but it is readily detected during resection. Cystic medial necrosis may also explain the risk of aneurysms after balloon angioplasty.

Conclusion.—No data clearly demonstrate a lower risk of recurrent coarctation with either subclavian flap procedure or resection and end-to-end anastomosis. Resection and end-to-end anastomosis are the preferred methods.

▶ Although recurrence of coarctation is possible with either resection or subclavian flap operations, the lower incidence with resection and end-to-end anastomosis seems to favor this procedure.—J.J. Collins, Jr., M.D.

Special Problems in Fontan-Type Operations for Complex Cardiac Lesions
Gildein HP, Ahmadi A, Fontan F, Mocellin R (University of Freiburg, Freiburg, Germany; Universitaire de Bordeaux, Bordeaux, France)
Int J Cardiol 29:21–28, 1990   6–29

Introduction.—Some complex congenital lesions of the heart are particularly difficult to treat, especially those in which the systemic and pulmonary venous drainage are separated, requiring septation of the right atrium. In these patients, other palliative procedures in addition to the Fontan procedure may be necessary. Data were reviewed on 4 patients with complex lesions in whom a Fontan-type procedure was successful. Each patient represents a particular surgical problem.

Patients.—One patient had a displaced trileaflet straddling and overriding the left atrioventricular valve, in addition to tricuspd atresia. Another patient was treated at age 22 for unilateral lung perfusion. The third patient was a child in whom a stenosis developed near the origin of the right pulmonary artery; the pulmonary vascular resistance could not be determined before the definitive palliative procedure was performed. The fourth patient had stenosis of the left atrioventricular valve, requiring operation at age 9 years. In each patient, echocardiography and cardiac catheterization were performed to detail the morphological and hemodynamic features, which allowed surgical planning.

Discussion.—In patients with low pulmonary vascular resistance, normal left ventricular contractility, and no left atrioventricular valve dysfunction, increased of pulmonary artery pressure is no longer a contraindication to the Fontan procedure. Neither are pulmonary or systemic venous connections or age younger than 4 years. Preserved right atrial function is desirable but not mandatory for hemodynamic exclusion of the right ventricle from the pulmonary circulation. In this case, atrial partitioning, which results in drainage of blood from the coronary sinus to the left atrium, has no adverse effect of arterial oxygen saturation and prevents myocardial damage by high right atrial pressure. In patients with unilateral lung perfusion, hyperperfusion of the right lung is risky; however, the patient's condition may justify such correction.

Conclusion.—The limits for modified Fontan procedure, including the selection criteria, are constantly being extended. In all of these patients, a shunt would have been an option, but the risk of Fontan procedure was justified by the positive long-term effect on ventricular function.

▶ Lessons from the various cases described in this presentation well illustrate both the remarkable usefulness of the Fontan operation and the usefulness of certain modifications to adapt the procedure to individual patient requirements.—J.J. Collins, Jr., M.D.

The Bidirectional Cavopulmonary Shunt

Lamberti JJ, Spicer RL, Waldman JD, Grehl TM, Thomson D, George L, Kirkpatrick SE, Mathewson JW (Children's Hosp and Health Ctr, San Diego)
J Thorac Cardiovasc Surg 100:22–30, 1990

6–30

Background.—Systemic arterial oxygen saturation can be improved, with no increase in ventricular work or pulmonary vascular resistance, by use of the bidirectional cavopulmonary shunt. This operation diverts the systemic venous return from the superior vena cava to both lungs. Seventeen patients treated with this operation were reviewed.

Methods.—The operation was performed primarily in 5 cases and secondarily in 12. There were 10 patients with hypoplastic right heart syndrome, 4 with single ventricle complex, and 3 with hypoplastic left ventricle. Median age was 13 months and median weight was 7.4 kg. The procedure was done without cardiopulmonary bypass in 7 cases. An additional procedure was done in all patients; 7 had takedown of a modified Blalock-Taussig shunt, 4 had revision of the right ventricular outflow tract, 4 had reconstruction of the pulmonary arteries, and 1 each had tricuspid valvuloplasty and a Damus procedure.

Results.—The patient undergoing the Damus procedure died perioperatively, and 1 of the patients with hypoplastic left heart syndrome required early revision. At a median follow-up of 23 months, 12 patients had an excellent result, including a 69% to 83% rise in arterial oxygen saturation. There were 3 late deaths of different causes at 4 to 53 months. One patient had a late failure and underwent conversion to a Glenn shunt. Right atrium–pulmonary artery connection was subsequently done in 5 patients.

Conclusions.—The cavopulmonary shunt procedure appears to be excellent for palliation when the modified Fontan procedure must be deferred. Low pulmonary artery pressure, in addition to normal pulmonary resistance, is critical to success. Preoperative evaluation must include precise definition of the systemic venous connections.

▶ Despite the widespread applicability of the Fontan and modified Fontan operations, there are some patients in whom bidirectional cavopulmonary shunts have a distinct advantage. Similar results have been found by Pearl et al. (1).— J.J. Collins, Jr., M.D.

Reference

1. Pearl JM, Laks H, Stein DG, et al: Total cavopulmonary anastomosis versus conventional modified Fontan procedure. *Ann Thorac Surg* 52:189–196, 1991.

Comparison of the Hemostatic Effects of Fresh Whole Blood, Stored Whole Blood, and Components After Open Heart Surgery in Children

Manno CS, Hedberg KW, Kim HC, Bunin GR, Nicolson S, Jobes D, Schwartz E, Norwood WI (Children's Hosp of Philadelphia)
Blood 77:930–936, 1991

6–31

Background.—In adult patients undergoing open-heart surgery, fresh blood has been reported to have advantages over platelet concentrates for postoperative transfusion. If the blood has been collected within 6 hours and has not been refrigerated, the function of the platelets is unimpaired, but maintaining a supply of such blood is difficult. Whether use of fresh whole blood improves hemostasis in infants and children who have undergone open-heart surgery with cardiopulmonary bypass was investigated in 161 children.

Methods.—Fifty-two children received very fresh whole blood (VFWB), which had been donated within 6 hours; 57 received whole blood collected 24 to 48 hours before transfusion and stored cold; and 52 received reconstituted whole blood. Patients were not strictly randomized to these groups; assignment depended partly on the families' ability to provide fresh blood donors. The groups were similar in age, coagulation profiles, difficulty of the surgical procedure, and cardiopulmonary bypass time.

Results.—For the VFWB group, mean 24-hour blood loss was 50.9 mL/kg; it was 44.8 mL/kg in the stored blood group, and 74.2 mL/kg in the reconstituted blood group. Among 93 children less than 2 years of age, the figures were 2.3 mL/kg for VFWB, 51.7 mL/kg for stored blood, and 96.2 mL/kg for reconstituted blood. Platelet aggregation responses to adenosine diphosphate, at both 30 minutes and 3 hours postoperatively, were more depressed in the reconstituted blood group than in the other 2 groups. None of the other coagulation tests performed could explain the higher blood loss of the reconstituted blood group.

Conclusions.—In children younger than 2 years who undergo complex cardiac surgery, transfusion of blood that is less than 48 hours old results in significantly less blood loss than docs transfusion of reconstituted blood. Blood that is less than 48 hours old and very fresh whole blood give comparable results, probably in part because of better platelet function. Use of day-old fresh blood may avoid the potential complication of graft-versus-host disease reported with the use of very fresh whole blood.

▶ In the early days of cardiac surgery, use of freshly harvested blood for transfusion ("warm walkers") was very common. For a variety of reasons, fresh blood transfusion has become much less commonly used recently. The specific usefulness of fresh transfusions should not, however, be entirely forgotten.—J.J. Collins, Jr., M.D.

Subcutaneous Fat Necrosis in Two Infants After Hypothermic Cardiac Surgery
Glover MT, Catterall MD, Atherton DJ (Hospital for Sick Children, London; Basildon Hospital, Essex, England)
Pediatr Dermatol 8:210–212, 1991   6–32

Introduction.—Subcutaneous fat necrosis (SCFN) is an infrequent disorder characterized by the appearance of red or violaceous nodules in early postnatal life, most often in a full-term or postmature infant. Changes resembling SCFN developed in 2 infants after the newborn period.

Patient 1.—Male infant, 4.5 months, was seen 2 weeks after repair of a ventricular septal defect under both core and surface cooling. The radial aspects of both upper forearms, where crushed ice had been applied, exhibited indurated lesions about 3 cm in diameter. A biopsy specimen from the indurated area demonstrated panniculitis. The lesions resolved totally over the next 3 weeks.

Patient 2.—Female infant, 5 weeks, was seen 4 weeks after balloon atrial septostomy, which was performed under surface and core cooling. Indurated plaques were seen on both posterior upper arms and the back. The lesions resolved without treatment in the next month.

Conclusion.—These infants appear to have had a disorder analogous to SCFN. If so, cold is an important stimulus of subcutaneous panniculitis, although trauma and anoxia may be contributory factors. Most infants with hypercalcemia lack evidence of calcium deposition in lesions of SCFN.

▶ The syndrome of subcutaneous fat necrosis after hypothermia in infants who have undergone cardiac surgery is probably more widespread than is usually appreciated.—J.J. Collins, Jr., M.D.

Aorta

Cold Cerebroplegia: A New Technique of Cerebral Protection During Operations on the Transverse Aortic Arch

Bachet J, Guilmet D, Goudot B, Termignon J-L, Teodori G, Dreyfus G, Brodaty D, Dubois C, Delentdecker P, Cabrol C (Universite Paris-Ouest, Suresnes, France)
J Thorac Cardiovasc Surg 102:85–94, 1991   6–33

Introduction.—Replacement of the transverse aortic arch still carries high morbidity and mortality. The dangers relate mainly to the vulnerability of the CNS during the period of arch exclusion. Profound hypothermia provides limited time for the repair, and requires prolonged cardiopulmonary bypass to rewarm the patient. Selective perfusion of the carotid arteries precludes an open, bloodless aortic repair.

Technique.—The cold cerebroplegia method aims to cool the brain independently of the rest of the body by selectively perfusing the brachiocephalic arteries with cold blood while the patient is kept at a core temperature of 25–28° C. A separate heat exchanger is used to perfuse the carotid arteries at a rate of 250–350 mL/min. Carotid perfusion is discontinued, and cardiopulmonary bypass resumes after completing the distal repair.

Results.—In 54 patients, the transverse aortic arch was replaced under cold cerebroplegia. There were no operative deaths, although 7 (13%)

patients died postoperatively. Only 1 death was the direct result of a neurologic complication. In 5 patients, there were neurologic complications that did not correlate with the duration of cerebral perfusion. All patients but 1 awoke normally within 8 hours after surgery. There were no bleeding complications. The mean duration of cardiopulmonary bypass was 2 hours, and that of circulatory arrest was 22 months.

Conclusion.—Cold cerebroplegia provides excellent cerebral protection without the need for prolonged cardiopulmonary bypass, and allows ample time for repairing the transverse aortic arch. Autoregulation is an important factor in maintaining cerebral blood flow during hypothermia.

▶ Cold cerebroplegia is not cerebroplegic. Nevertheless, the use of hypothermic profusion of the brain while the core temperature of the patient is retained at a somewhat higher level may well be extremely useful. This is a very interesting paper, and I am sure we will see an increased use of this innovative technique. Avoidance of profound systemic hypothermia is probably an advantage over the experimentally favorable procedure reported by Crittenden et al. (1).—J.J. Collins, Jr., M.D.

Reference

1. Crittenden MD, Roberts CS, Rosa L, et al: Brain protection during circulatory arrest. *Ann Thorac Surg* 51:942–947, 1991.

Rupture of Thoracic Aorta Caused by Blunt Trauma: A Fifteen-Year Experience

Cowley RA, Turney SZ, Hankins JR, Rodriguez A, Attar S, Shankar BS (Univ of Maryland, Baltimore)
J Thorac Cardiovasc Surg 100:652–661, 1990   6–34

Introduction.—Acute rupture of the thoracic aorta from blunt trauma is associated with a high rate of lethal exsanguination and a high incidence of postoperative paraplegia in survivors. There is still controversy over the protective effect of shunting during aortic crossclamping. The possible advantage of using a shunt during bypass repair of a ruptured thoracic aorta was examined retrospectively.

Patients.—During a 15-year period, 114 patients, aged 15–90 years, were admitted with acute rupture of the descending thoracic aorta caused by blunt trauma. During the first 5 years, aortic repair was done without shunt-bypass in 6 patients, all of whom survived, and with shunt-bypass in 25 patients, 19 of whom survived. One survivor operated on with shunting developed postoperative paraplegia. During the next 10 years, 25 of 83 admitted patients died of exsanguination during resuscitation, 7 died during surgery, and 12 died within 30 days of operation. Of the 51 patients who initially survived operation, 34 were operated on with shunt-bypass. Of these 34, paraplegia developed in 6 (17.6%). Seventeen of the 51 were operated on without shunt. Paraplegia developed in 4

(23.5%) of these patients. All 10 cases of paraplegia occurred in patients with aortic crossclamp times exceeding 30 minutes. Twenty-one of the 51 initial survivors had other major complications, including adult respiratory distress syndrome, severe renal failure, severe sepsis, and pseudoaneurysm at the graft-aorta anastomosis.

Conclusion.—Blunt traumatic rupture of the thoracic aorta continues to be associated with high mortality and morbidity rates. There was no advantage to using or not using a shunt in preventing paraplegia.

▶ The data of Dr. Crowley and associates from the very busy trauma service at the University of Maryland are always welcome. Consistent with previous studies, this report provides a very useful analysis of blunt aortic trauma. The conclusion that the use of an arterial shunt was not associated with a reduced incidence of paraplegia provides a highly useful bit of surgical (and medicolegal) information.—J.J. Collins, Jr., M.D.

Transplant

Decreasing Survival Benefit From Cardiac Transplantation for Outpatients as the Waiting List Lengthens
Stevenson LW, Hamilton MA, Tillisch IH, Moriguchi JD, Kobashigawa JA, Creaser JA, Drinkwater D, Laks H (Univ of California, Los Angeles)
J Am Coll Cardiol 18:919–925, 1991   6–35

Background.—Many patients are accepted for heart transplantation when they are clinically unstable, although most can be discharged from the hospital to await surgery. Current national policy bases outpatient priority solely on waiting time, and most patients undergo transplantation after having survived a significant period of jeopardy.

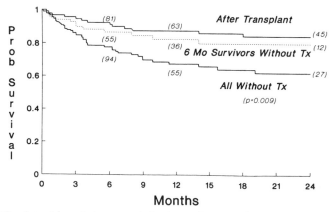

Fig 6–17.—Actuarial survival curves calculated according to Kaplan-Meier method from time of evaluation for 214 patients discharged on medical therapy after transplant evaluation, subset of 94 patients surviving first 6 months after evaluation without transplantation (Tx) and 88 patients from outpatient waiting list after transplantation. Numbers in parentheses refer to patients remaining at follow-up. *Abbreviation: Prob*, probability of. (Courtesy of Stevenson LW, Hamilton MA, Tillisch IH, et al: *J Am Coll Cardiol* 18:919–925, 1991.)

Study Plan.—The impact of waiting times was assessed by recalculating 1-year actuarial survival rates after each month without surgery for 214 potential candidates. The patients, with an average ejection fraction of .17, had individualized medical treatment after discharge. One-year survival data were also calculated for 88 outpatients who underwent transplantation.

Results.—The 1-year actuarial survival for patients discharged with individualized treatment who did not undergo transplantation was 67% (Fig 6–17). The rate for transplanted patients was 88%. Forty-three patients without transplantation died suddenly, 8 of hemodynamic decompensation. Outpatients who survived 6 months had a subsequent actuarial survival of 83% over the next year without transplantation. No criteria reliably distinguished survivors from nonsurvivors at the time of initial discharge.

Implications.—Patients who wait 6 months for a heart transplant can be expected to have a survival advantage of only 5% over the subsequent 12 months if given a transplant. Such patients should be reassessed to affirm that transplantation still is indicated. A much greater advantage accrues to transplantation in patients who remain hospitalized in critical condition until urgent transplantation is possible. Patients on a waiting list pay a substantial psychological toll. It would be helpful to be better able to select those outpatients who are at the highest risk of dying suddenly without transplantation.

▶ The innovative analysis of Stevenson and associates is instructive in several ways. First, it confirms that the impression of imminent demise in a significant number of patients selected for transplantation may be erroneous. Second, it demonstrates, as the authors suggest, that patients must have careful repeated evaluation at intervals after initial selection. This is consistent with our experience, which has shown that some patients improve and others deteriorate to the point where transplantation is inappropriate. There is a tendency to believe that the data obtained at initial evaluation remain constant. Obviously that is not true. It would be most helpful to know whether patients who survive through the first year after selection (without transplantation) have truly improved during the interval or whether they have simply maintained their previously measured functional capacity.—J.J. Collins, Jr., M.D.

Increased Rejection in Gender-Mismatched Grafts: Amelioration by Triple Therapy
Keogh AM, Valantine HA, Hunt SA, Schroeder JS, Oyer PE (Stanford Univ Hosp, Stanford, Calif)
J Heart Lung Transplant 10:106–110, 1991   6–36

Introduction.—Several studies have suggested that there is an increased incidence of graft rejection in female heart transplant recipients given cyclosporine and azathioprine immunosuppressive therapy. To determine whether gender-mismatched grafting (grafting of a male donor's heart into a female recipient) may be a factor in graft rejection, survival, rejection, and complications were studied in 313 female recipients of gender-mismatched grafts who were treated with double- or triple-agent immunosuppression.

Methods.—The 104 patients in group 1 were treated with cyclosporine and prednisone double therapy, and the 209 patients in group 2 in were treated with cyclosporine, azathioprine, and prednisone triple therapy. Of the patients, 21 in group 1 and 41 in group 2 were women. The variables of 90-day methylprednisolone sodium succinate requirements, 90-day linearized rejection rate, 90-day event-free actuarial rejection, 6-month actuarial infection-free survival, overall actuarial survival, and median time to first rejection were analyzed.

Results.—There was no difference in age between recipients of male vs. female hearts. Steroid requirements were 40% higher in female group 1 patients who received a male heart (M/F) (3,600 mg for M/F recipients vs. 2,977 mg for F/F recipients); this reflected a higher rate of rejection in the M/F recipients. The M/F recipients had a lower rejection rate and consequently a lower infection rate; this difference was not significant. There was no difference in actuarial survival. In group 2, steroid requirements, rejection rate, and infection rate were unrelated to gender mismatching.

Conclusion.—In female heart transplant recipients who receive maintenance therapy with cyclosporine and prednisone, implantation of male grafts appears to be associated with higher rejection rate and higher steroid requirements for the first 3 months. Rate of infection and actuarial survival are unaffected. Use of triple-agent immunosuppression appears to eliminate this propensity for rejection.

▶ These data seem to indicate that gender-mismatched organs do not represent a significant hazard as long as triple-agent immunosuppression is used. No difference caused by gender was found in the study of Zerbe et al. (1).—J.J. Collins, Jr., M.D.

Reference

1. Zerbe TR, Arena VC, Kormos RL, et al: Histocompatibility and other risk factors for histological rejection of human cardiac allografts during the first three months following transplantation. *Transplantation* 52:485–490, 1991.

Total Lymphoid Irradiation for Treatment of Intractable Cardiac Allograft Rejection
Hunt SA, Strober S, Hoppe RT, Stinson EB (Stanford Univ Med Ctr, Stanford, Calif)
J Heart Lung Transplant 10:211–216, 1991   6–37

Background.—Current immunosuppressive treatments maintain graft function and reverse graft rejection in most patients, but with considerable toxicity. Some patients continue to reject their grafts despite a host of different types of immunosuppressants. The results of another immunosuppressive modality—total lymphoid irradiation (TLI)—which is used to reverse recurrent cardiac allograft rejection refractive to conventional therapy, was reported.

Procedure.—Heart transplant recipients had between 1 and 6 rejection episodes before TLI was used. The TLI regimen used treatment with an upper and lower field, with the upper field, known as the "mantle," covering all major supraradiaphragmatic lymphoid regions. The heart is not specifically shielded during the procedure. The lower, or subdiaphragmatic, field appears as an inverted "Y." Peripheral blood samples were assayed for T cells using flow cytometry.

Patients.—Ten heart transplant patients received a complete TLI course. The patients included 2 women and 8 men ranging in age from 1 to 51 years. All had received maintenance immunosuppression with cyclosporine, azathioprine, prednisone, and an initial 10-day regimen of intravenous OKT3 monoclonal antibody. The TLI therapy was interrupted in 5 patients because of complications; 4 patients experienced neutropenia and 1 suffered pneumocystic and cytomegalovirus pneumonitis. Six patients received the full TLI course, and 4 received a partial TLI course. The mean duration of TLI was 47 days.

Results.—Graft rejection occurred in 6 patients after an initial resolution of the rejection episode, with recurrence appearing 40–769 days after the initiation of TLI. Three patients had no recurrence of rejection after TLI therapy. Two of the 10 patients died, 1 from cardiogenic shock during TLI and 1 from rejection recurrence after unadvised cessation of immunosuppressive therapy. The clinical course of the 3 living patients who did not complete the full TLI course appeared similar to that of the other patients.

Conclusions.—These preliminary findings suggest that TLI may aid in salvage therapy of heart transplants in cases when conventional immunosuppressive agents do not appear to work. Total lymphoid irradiation should be tested as an adjunct to immunosuppression therapy in patients susceptible to the side effects of immunosuppressive drugs.

▶ These very interesting data reported by Hunt and associates indicate that total lymphoid irradiation has a significant additional benefit to more standard immunosuppressive therapy. Whether some variation might be useful for patients without special indications remains to be seen.—J.J. Collins, Jr., M.D.

Transplant Coronary Artery Disease: Histopathologic Correlations With Angiographic Morphology
Johnson DE, Alderman EL, Schroeder JS, Gao S-Z, Hunt S, DeCampli WM, Stinson E, Billingham M (Stanford Univ Med Ctr, Stanford, Calif)
J Am Coll Cardiol 17:449–457, 1991   6–38

Introduction.—A major cause of death and of the need for retransplantation in cardiac transplant survivors is accelerated coronary artery disease. The disease is often asymptomatic and may not be apparent in annual surveillance coronary arteriograms. The arteriographic and microscopic manifestations of transplant coronary artery disease were compared to assess the accuracy of the coronary arteriogram in diagnosing graft arterial disease.

Methods.—Formalin-fixed hearts from 10 patients who had survived for more than 1 year after transplantation were available for gross and histologic examination. In all cases, graft failure or death occurred within 2 months of coronary arteriography. The coronary arteries were examined by light microscopy, and the degree of luminal-area narrowing of the histologic sections available was measured morphometrically.

Results.—Nine of the patients were men; their mean age was 39.9 years. Six had ischemic heart disease and 4 had idiopathic dilated cardiomyopathy. The mean duration of allograft viability was 52 months. The 10 grafts yielded 107 histologic sections of primary and secondary coronary artery branches for study. All 26 angiographically normal segments showed some disease by light microscopic evaluation. Mild-to-moderate fibrous intimal thickening was apparent in 73% of these segments. Discrete stenoses usually corresponded to lipid-rich intermediate of atheromatous disease. All complete occlusions were the result of fresh or organizing thrombus.

Conclusion.—Coronary arteriography is relatively insensitive for the detection of early vascular lesions in cardiac allograft coronary artery disease. Based on the histopathologic angiographic comparisons, transplant coronary artery disease has a heterogeneous appearance and is underestimated by angiography in some cases.

▶ In yet another significant report from Stanford, the impression of most cardiac transplant surgeons is confirmed. There is indeed underestimation of the extent of coronary artery disease by angiography. This is disappointing in view of the fact that the absence of symptoms in these patients makes angiography the best tool we have for determination of coronary obstructive disease in transplant recipients.—J.J. Collins, Jr., M.D.

Relationship of Immunosuppression and Serum Lipids to the Development of Coronary Arterial Disease in the Transplanted Heart

Barbir M, Banner N, Thompson GR, Khaghani A, Mitchell A, Yacoub M (Harefield Hospital, Harefield, England; Hammersmith Hospital, London)
Int J Cardiol 32:51–56, 1991   6–39

Introduction.—The development of coronary artery disease in the transplanted heart is the most serious long-term complication of heart transplantation. Its pathogenesis is unclear, but immunologic damage to the artery wall and cytomegalovirus infection may be relevant.

Methods.—The factors for coronary artery disease at 1 year after heart transplantation were investigated in 207 patients. Immunosuppression was with azathioprine and either prednisone or cyclosporine.

Results.—Coronary artery disease was present in 6.4% of patients 1 year after heart transplantation. Affected patients were older than those without coronary disease. The incidence was 23% in patients given prednisone for immunosuppression and 3% in those given cyclosporine. In a prospective series of 95 patients whose coronary vessels were angiographically normal 1 year after heart transplantation, relatively high initial total cholesterol and triglyceride levels appeared to increase the risk of coronary disease up to 4 years after transplantation.

Conclusion.—Modifying immunosuppressive therapy and serum lipid levels can potentially reduce the risk of coronary disease in the transplanted heart. The use of steroids should be avoided whenever possible.

▶ The importance of abnormal lipid profiles seems to be both magnified and accelerated in the recipients of cardiac transplants. The particular increase in the hazard of steroids is probably real, and efforts should be made to minimize steroid therapy.—J.J. Collins, Jr., M.D.

Prostacyclin in the Management of Pulmonary Hypertension After Heart Transplantation
Pascual JMS, Fiorelli AI, Bellotti GM, Stolf NAG, Jatene AD (University of São Paulo, Brazil)
J Heart Transplant 9:644 651, 1990   6–40

Introduction.—The drugs used previously to control increased pulmonary resistance do not specifically influence the pulmonary vessels, and may produce unacceptable systemic hypotension. The use of prostacyclin (PGI_2) was evaluated in 9 of 50 patients who underwent orthotopic heart transplantation, in whom severe pulmonary hypertension developed postoperatively.

Methods.—The patients had a low cardiac index, with high right atrial and pulmonary artery pressures and high pulmonary vascular resistance immediately after cardiac transplantation. Most of the patients had idiopathic or ischemic cardiomyopathy. The initial infusion rate of PGI_2 was about .5 ng/kg/min; the rate was increased as necessary to increase the

| | Derived Hemodynamic Data | | | |
Variable	Donor*	Preoperative	Before PGI2	After PGI2
PVR (dynes/sec/cm-5)	91	466 ± 191	421 ± 368	122 ± 42
SVR (dynes/sec/cm-5)	772	2089 ± 390	1318 ± 635	870 ± 263
RVSWI (gm . m/m2)	8.9	10.5 ± 2.4	9.7 ± 4.3	12.9 ± 6.1
LVSWI (gm . m/m2)	36.3	18.1 ± 4.4	23 ± 10.6	41.3 ± 16.9

Abbreviations: PVR, pulmonary vascular resistance; *SVR,* systemic vascular resistance; *RVSWI,* right ventricular systolic work index; *LVSWI,* left ventricular systolic work index.
Note: Values are mean ± SE.
*Only mean values available.
(Courtesy of Pascual JMS, Fiorelli AI, Bellotti GM, et al: *J Heart Transplant* 9:644–651, 1990.)

cardiac index to greater than 3 L/min/m^2 or to reduce the pulmonary vascular resistance to normal.

Results.—The right atrial pressure decreased from 17 to 12 mm Hg after PGI$_2$ infusion, and the pulmonary vascular resistance decreased from 421 to 122 dynes/sec/cm^{-5} (table). It was possible to withdraw other drugs within 48 hours without side effects and without hemodynamic deterioration.

Conclusion.—Prostacyclin exerts both cardiac and pulmonary vascular actions in patients in whom pulmonary hypertension develops after heart transplantation. Infusion of PGI$_2$ for 48 hours has permitted weaning of patients form inotropic drugs. Systemic vascular resistance decreases without hypotension developing.

▶ Pulmonary hypertension is one of the most serious complications for cardiac transplant recipients, because the unprepared right ventricle fails rather quickly under afterload stress. The usefulness of prostacyclin has been observed by a number of investigators. Its use is not entirely without hazard, but it appears to be the best available agent at present for management of this complication.— J.J. Collins, Jr., M.D.

Early Abdominal Complications Following Heart and Heart-Lung Transplantation

Watson CJE, Jamieson NV, Johnston PS, Wreghitt T, Large S, Wallwork J, English TAH (Addenbrooke's Hospital; Papworth Hospital, Cambridge, England)
Br J Surg 78:699–704, 1991 6–41

Introduction.—A high incidence of early abdominal complications was observed in orthotopic cardiac transplantation patients. Many of these complications resulted in significant morbidity. The complications, including their presentation and treatment, were reviewed.

Methods.—Over an 11-year period, 356 heart transplants were performed, including 73 heart-lung transplants. All patients received prednisolone, azathioprine, and cyclosporine A immunosuppression. All significant abdominal symptoms requiring consultation for 30 days posttransplantation while the patient was hospitalized were recorded.

Results.—Abdominal symptoms developed in 41(9.5%) patients, 20 of whom required surgery. Within 30 days, 41 patients died, 4 as a direct result of their abdominal symptoms. Pancreatitis occurred in 10 patients; in 2 it was diagnosed only at laparotomy and in 2 it developed in association with cytomegalovirus infection. Peptic ulcers developed in 8 patients, and pseudo-obstruction developed in 8. Of the latter, 2 patients progressed to colon perforation. Laparotomy was well tolerated. Other complications included perforated diverticulum, small bowel obstruction, and mesenteric ischemia.

Conclusion.—Immediate complications are related to cardiopulmonary bypass and the high level of initial immunosuppression. Viral infections or manifestations of rejection may later occur. Throughout the posttransplant period, complications such as gastrointestinal tract hemorrhage and diverticular perforation occur. Diagnosis and treatment must be prompt; laparotomy is appropriate if the diagnosis is doubtful.

▶ Abdominal surgical complications have long been described in patients undergoing open heart operations. The report of Watson and associates of intraabdominal illness after transplantation shows the somewhat higher incidence in these patients. However, it must be remembered that even renal transplant recipients have a significant risk of early abdominal problems. In all patients on immunosuppressive therapy, early surgical intervention has proven to be extremely important if successful management is to be attained.—J.J. Collins, Jr., M.D.

Long-Term Follow-Up of Medical Versus Surgical Therapy for Hypertrophic Cardiomyopathy: A Retrospective Study

Seiler C, Hess OM, Schoenbeck M, Turina J, Jenni R, Turina M, Krayenbuehl H-P (University Hospital, Zurich, Switzerland)
J Am Coll Cardiol 17:634–642, 1991   6–42

Background.—In patients with hypertrophic cardiomyopathy, surgical treatment of outflow tract obstruction can improve survival and symptomatic status, but more recently, medical treatment has shown beneficial effects on the long-term course. The effects of the 2 types of treatment were assessed retrospectively after follow-up ranging from 1 year to 28 years.

Methods.—Of 139 patients with hypertrophic cardiomyopathy, 60 had medical therapy (group 1) and 79 had septal myectomy (group 2). In group 1, 20 patients received propranolol, 160 mg/day; 18 patients received verapamil, 360 mg/day; and 22 patients received no therapy. In group 2, 17 patients received verapamil, 120 to 360 mg/day, after undergoing septal myectomy, and 62 patients received no postoperative medical therapy. The patients were 113 males and 26 females; mean age was 37 years. Mean follow-up was 8.9 years.

Results.—Annual mortality rates were 3.6% in group 1 and 2.4% in group 2, a nonsignificant difference. Most of the deaths occurred suddenly, and a significant proportion were attributable to congestive heart failure. Ten-year cumulative survival rates were 67% in group 1 and 84% in group 2, a significant difference. Ten-year survival rates in group 1 were 67% for those treated with propranolol, 80% for those treated with verapamil, and 65% for those who received no therapy. In group 2, 10-year survival rates were 100% for those who received verapamil and 78% for those who received no medical treatment.

Conclusions.—Combined treatment with septal myectomy and long-term verapamil administration gives the best follow-up results for patients with severe hypertrophic cardiomyopathy and large pressure gradients. In medically treated patients, verapamil appears to give better results than propranolol or no treatment. Verapamil is probably most beneficial for patients with mild symptoms and minimal or no outflow tract obstruction.

▶ This report by Seiler and associates contains several interesting considerations. First, it illustrates very well that statistical techniques influence the overall perception of the results in follow-up studies. The annual mortality rate in groups 1 and 2 was not significantly different; however, the cumulative survival (using the same data) did show a significant difference in survival at 10 years. Thus, the additive effect of a series of individually insignificant differences in mortality rate can (and do) add up to a significant difference. Great caution is necessary in interpreting mortality rates.

There seems little doubt that the surgical group fared better than the group who did not undergo surgery. Obviously, there may have been some differences in the presurgical populations, and this was not a prospective randomized study. Results in the patients operated on who subsequently received verapamil were first-rate, of course, but it is difficult to compare them with those who received no medical treatment after surgery because risk factors are not precisely known.—J.J. Collins, Jr., M.D.

Miscellaneous

Penetrating Cardiac Injuries
Attar S, Suter CM, Hankins JR, Sequeira A, McLaughlin JS (Univ of Maryland)
Ann Thorac Surg 51:711–716, 1991   6–43

Introduction.—Data were reviewed on 109 patients treated for penetrating cardiac wounds in 1967–1990. In 60 patients, there were stab wounds and in 49 there were gunshot injuries. When brought in, 38 patients were lifeless, 16 were agonal, 33 were in shock, and 22 were stable.

Methods.—Thoracotomy was performed in the emergency room in 36 of the 38 lifeless patients and 8 of the 16 who were agonal; 24 of the 33 patients in shock and 20 of the 22 who were stable had thoracotomy in the operating room. The right ventricle was injured more often than the left; 13 patients had involvement of more than 1 cardiac chamber. Most cardiac wounds were repaired with sutures over Teflon pledgets. In 3 patients, emergency coronary bypass grafting was necessary.

Results.—Of the patients who were initially in a lifeless state, 12 (31%) survived, as did 11 (69%) of those who were semiconscious but without measurable blood pressure; 26 (79%) of 33 patients with shock and 18 (82%) of 22 stable patients survived. Patients with stab wounds did much better than those with gunshot wounds. Survival was 38% after thoracotomy in the emergency room and 87% after operating room thoracotomy.

Conclusion.—Aggressive treatment, including thoracotomy in the emergency room, is warranted for patients with cardiac injury who appear to be in a lifeless or deteriorating state. Patients whose vital signs are stable and hypotensive patients who respond to attempts at resuscitation should undergo definitive repair in the operating room.

► Management of penetrating wounds of the chest is a major challenge to every emergency service. The experience of the group at the University of Maryland illustrates the remarkably good results that can be obtained by a prepared team. These data also strongly support the concept of designated trauma centers in major metropolitan areas.—J.J. Collins, Jr., M.D.

Discriminate Use of Electrocautery on the Median Sternotomy Incision: A 0.16% Wound Infection Rate
Nishida H, Grooters RK, Soltanzadeh H, Thieman KC, Schneider RF, Kim W-P (Iowa Methodist Med Ctr, Des Moines)
J Thorac Cardiovasc Surg 101:488–494, 1991   6–44

Background.—Sternotomy infection and mediastinitis have been reported in up to 5% of patients having cardiac surgery. Studies in dogs suggest that extensive electrocautery of the presternal soft tissues may be a predisposing factor to sternotomy infection.

Study Design.—The value of limiting electrocautery to pinpoint hemostasis in the sternotomy soft tissues was examined in 3,118 consecutive patients having median sternotomy for cardiac surgery in an 11-year period. All the patients lived more than a week after surgery. The presternal soft tissues were divided with a scalpel, reserving electrocautery for pinpoint hemostasis.

Results.—Mediastinal wound infection developed in 5 patients (.16%). The incidence of deep mediastinitis was .13%. No patient required major sternal débridement or muscle flap reconstruction. The only factor related to sternotomy infection was an operating time exceeding 3 hours.

Conclusion.—The selective use of electrocautery during median sternotomy appears to limit the occurrence of wound infection in patients having cardiac surgery.

► The introduction of electrocautery as a means for achieving surgical hemostasis was a major contribution by Harvey Cushing. Today, cautery is used by surgeons in every discipline taking advantage of the protein coagulation induced by heat and the specific localization and intensity control available with electric heat generation. The major problem of electrocautery in sternal incisions as well as in other areas of surgical dissection has been related to the use of currents that produce destruction far beyond the immediate area of tissue separation. Great care must be exercised to avoid charring of adjacent innocent structures in the quest for pernicious vascular leakage.—J.J. Collins, Jr., M.D.

Long-Term Results of Pectoralis Major Muscle Transposition for Infected Sternotomy Wounds
Pairolero PC, Arnold PG, Harris JB (Mayo Clin and Found, Rochester, Minn)
Ann Surg 213:583–590, 1991   6–45

Introduction.—Wound infection after sternotomy is a rare, but potentially lethal complication of thoracic surgery. The short-term results of treating infected sternotomy wounds by aggressive débridement and muscle transposition were previously reported. The long-term outcome in the same group of patients was evaluated.

Patients.—During an 11.5-year period, 79 male and 21 female patients age 5–85 years underwent surgical repair of a recalcitrant infected median sternotomy wound. Sternal drainage occurred a median of 3 weeks after sternotomy. The median time interval between onset of sternal drainage and sternal repair was 7.5 weeks. Sixty-five patients had undergone previous attempts at closure that failed. Initial treatment involved débridement of the manubrium and sternum in each patient. In addition, the manubrium and sternum were resected completely in 43 patients and partially in 33. All 76 patients had associated costochondral arches resected from the back to the ribs. The wound was closed at initial débridement in 11 patients. In the other patients, wound closure was performed a median of 14 days after initial débridement. The median number of operations in the 100 patients was 4. Hospitalization ranged from 7 to 210 days. The median follow-up was 4.2 years.

Outcome.—Forty-two patients had 59 complications, 8 of them were prolonged wound infections. There were 2 perioperative deaths, of which 1 was related to sepsis. Reconstruction was entirely with muscle transposition in 79 patients, with omental transposition in 4, and with both in 15. A total of 175 muscles were transposed. Thirty patients required mechanical ventilation beyond the second postoperative day. Twenty-six patients had a recurrent sternal infection. The median time from surgical closure to recurrence was 5.5 months. The cause of recurrence was inadequate removal of cartilage in 16 patients, bone in 6, and retained foreign body in 4. There were 30 late deaths, of which only 1 was related to recurrent infection. At the time of death or at the last follow-up visit, 92 patients had a healed chest wall.

Conclusion.—Vigorous sternal débridement and obliteration of dead space by muscle transposition remains an excellent method for managing infected sternotomy wounds.

▶ The use of muscle flaps and omentum for the management of sternal wound infections has been a major advance. Pairolero and his associates document the superb results than can be obtained.—J.J. Collins, Jr., M.D.

Left Ventricular Function Changes After Cardiomyoplasty in Patients With Dilated Cardiomyopathy
Jatene AD, Moreira LFP, Stolf NAG, Bocchi EA, Seferian P Jr, Fernandes PMP, Abensur H (Faculdade de Medicina da Universidade de São Paulo, Brazil)
J Thorac Cardiovasc Surg 102:132–139, 1991   6–46

Introduction.—Dynamic cardiomyoplasty, first applied clinically in 1985, uses electrically stimulated skeletal muscles to partially replace or

Cardiomyostimulator On and Off Data

Follow-up	CM on	CM off		CM on	CM off	
	6 month*			*12 month†*		
LVSWS (%)	16.4 ± 3.5	15.3 ± 3.3	NS	16.5 ± 2.1	14.9 ± 2.8	p = 0.04
LVEF (%)	30.5 ± 6	28.5 ± 5.6	NS	30.6 ± 3.5	28 ± 3.7	p = 0.04

Abbreviations: CM, cardiomyostimulator: *LVSWS,* left ventricular segmental wall shortening: *LVEF* left ventricular ejection fraction: *NS,* not significant.
*CM off for 4 hours.
†CM off for 24 hours.
(Courtesy of Jatene AD, Moreira LFP, Stolf NAG, et al: *J Thorac Cardiovasc Surg* 102:132–139, 1991.)

reinforce the heart muscle in patients with advanced heart failure. The long-term hemodynamic effects of this new surgical technique were examined in patients with dilated cardiomyopathy or Chagas' disease unresponsive to conventional medical therapy.

Patients and Methods.—Thirteen latissimus dorsi cardiomyoplasties were performed from May 1988 to February 1990 at the study institution. Twelve patients were men and 2 had Chagas' disease. The patients' mean age was 44.2 years. All had medical or psychosocial contraindications to cardiac transplantation. The patients were evaluated preoperatively and at the third, sixth, and twelfth postoperative months by Doppler echocardiography, radioisotopic angiography, and right-sided heart catheterization. The surgical procedure used 2 incisions, 1 for muscle flap dissection and 1 for cardiac access, and was performed without cardiopulmonary bypass.

Results.—There were no operative deaths, but 2 patients died during the late follow-up period (mean 11.5 months). At 3 months, left ventricular segmental wall shortening increased from a mean of 11.4% to 16.4%, and left ventricular stroke volume increased from 23.9 to 34.4 mL. Radioisotopic left ventricular ejection fraction improved from 20.9% to 25.4%; patients with lesser left ventricular end-diastolic dimensions showed greater increases. The left ventricular stroke work index increased from 14.6 to 23.7 gm · m/m^2, whereas pulmonary wedge pressure decreased from 24.8 to 5.8 mm Hg. These changes were essentially the same at 6 and 12 months of follow-up (table).

Conclusion.—With more than a year of follow-up, patients with dilated cardiomyopathy or Chagas' disease showed significant improvement after dynamic cardiomyoplasty. The technique helps to reverse congestive heart failure and may improve the patient's functional capacity.

▶ These interesting and excellent results reported by Jatene and associates should be encouraging to those pioneering surgeons around the world who have struggled through multiple experimental protocols and the early clinical use of cardiomyoplasty. This remains an experimental procedure, but this evidence of favorable long-term results indicates that it may all be worthwhile.— J.J. Collins, Jr., M.D.

Current Indications, Risks, and Outcome After Pericardiectomy

DeValeria PA, Baumgartner WA, Casale AS, Greene PS, Cameron DE, Gardner TJ, Gott VL, Watkins L Jr, Reitz BA (Johns Hopkins Med Insts)
Ann Thorac Surg 52:219–224, 1991   6–47

Introduction.—The optimum surgical approach to effusive and constrictive pericarditis remains controversial. The results of pericardiectomy in 60 patients performed over a 10-year period were reviewed to determine long-term survival and whether this operation improves function among long-term survivors.

Methods.—Indications for surgery were restrictive disease in 36 patients and effusive disease in 24; pain was the primary reason for intervention in 10 patients. The cause of disease was idiopathic in 45% of patients and a previous cardiac operation in 16.7%. A median sternotomy was used in 52 patients (4 required cardiopulmonary bypass) and a left anterior thoracotomy was used in 8. A limited pericardial procedure was previously performed in 9 patients, necessitating a formal pericardiectomy. The operative mortality rate was 4.2% for patients with pericardial effusion disease and 5.6% for patients with pericardial constriction.

Results.—Follow-up data were obtained for 53 patients (median follow-up, 56.9 months). The actuarial survival was 82.1% at 1 year, 71.7% at 5 years, and 59.8% at 10 years. Cox proportional hazards regression analysis demonstrated that history of malignancy, previous pericardial operation, and preoperative New York Heart Association class IV were predictors of poor survival. The most common causes of late death were complications of malignancy, myocardial infarction, and noncardiac-related sepsis. All patients who had surgery for effusion and associated pain were alive at follow-up, with improved functional capacity and no need for steroids.

Conclusion.—Complete pericardiectomy is safe and can give long-term survival and good functional results. A complete, rather than limited, procedure should be performed in patients with effusive disease that is resistant to conservative treatment. For most patients with refractory chest pain, complete pericardiectomy is safe and effective.

▶ The definition of complete pericardiectomy is a bit confusing. Actually, a considerable amount of pericardium is always left behind. Nevertheless, the authors' admonition that the free-standing pericardium be removed in the most complete fashion possible is certainly consistent with the experience of most experts in this area. It is not always easy.—J.J. Collins, Jr., M.D.

Right Atrial Versus Aortic Root Perfusion With Blood Cardioplegia

Fiore AC, Naunheim KS, Moskoff ME, Langreder SK, Barner HB (St Louis Univ Med Ctr; St Mary's Health Ctr, St Louis)
Ann Thorac Surg 52:1014–1020, 1991   6–48

Introduction.—Coronary sinus perfusion has both practical and theo-

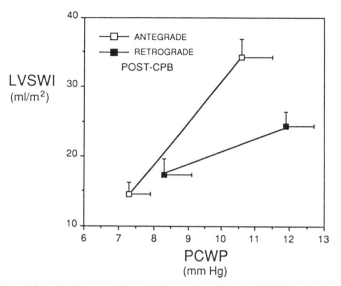

Fig 6–18.—Relationship between left ventricular stroke work index (*LVSWI*) and pulmonary capillary wedge pressure (*PCWP*) in response to volume loading. Stroke work index is improved in the antegrade group (*P* < .05). Data are shown as the mean ± SE; CPB=cardiopulmonary bypass. (Courtesy of Fiore AC, Naunheim KS, Moskoff ME, et al: *Ann Thorac Surg* 52:1014–1020, 1991.)

retical disadvantages, including delayed cardiac arrest and a risk of damaging the conduction system. One means of overcoming these disadvantages is to infuse cardioplegia directly into the right atrium.

Methods.—A total of 32 consecutive patients having elective myocardial revascularization were prospectively randomized to receive cold blood cardioplegia through the aortic root (ARC) or right atrium (RAC). The 15 patients in the ARC group and the 17 in the RAC group were comparable with respect to age, ventricular function, extent of coronary artery disease, and cross-clamp time. Revascularization was more complete in the ARC group.

Results.—The mean septal temperature and the time to electromechanical arrest were greater in the RAC group, but right ventricular temperatures were comparable. Myocardial isoenzyme release also was similar in both groups. Stroke work indices in both ventricles were equally preserved, but volume loading studies conducted just after the period of bypass suggested better left ventricular function in the ARC group (Fig 6–18).

Conclusion.—On clinical grounds alone, these methods of cardioplegia were equally effective. Right atrial cardioplegia provides no significant advantage over aortic root delivery in patients undergoing elective myocardial revascularization.

▶ Retrograde cardioplegia administered by placement of a cannula in the coronary sinus has specific hazards and disadvantages. However, in the group of patients have proximal coronary artery obstruction, some type of retrograde perfusion does seem to be useful. Infusion of cardioplegia into the right atrium in the study reported by Fiore and associates seems to have provided excellent results.—J.J. Collins, Jr., M.D.

Cardiac Surgery in the Octogenarian: Perioperative Outcome and Clinical Follow-Up
Freeman WK, Schaff HV, O'Brien PC, Orszulak TA, Naessens JM, Tajik AJ
(Mayo Clin and Found, Rochester, Minn)
J Am Coll Cardiol 18:29–35, 1991   6–49

Background.—Controversy continues about whether the large proportion of health care resources used on the very elderly is a cost-effective approach to maintaining lives of meaningful quality. It is important to carefully assess the functional outcome after cardiac surgery, as well as mere survival.

Patients.—The outcome in 191 consecutive patients aged 80 years and older who underwent cardiac surgery in 1982–1986 was reviewed. Most were in New York Heart Association functional class III or IV before operation. The mean age at operation was 82 years. Coronary artery bypass surgery was performed in 120 patients. Ninety-six had aortic valve replacement either alone or in conjunction with bypass surgery.

Outcome.—The overall 30-day cardiac mortality was 15.7%, and hospital mortality for elective surgery was 14.5%. Coronary artery bypass alone carried a mortality of only 5.6% (table). Urgent surgery in 39 patients carried a perioperative mortality of 36%. In the 155 surviving patients who were followed up for 23 months on average significant symptomatic improvement occurred in all surgical groups. Overall actuarial survival was significantly better than in age- and sex-matched control subjects.

Conclusions.—Selected octogenarians can undergo elective heart surgery without prohibitive perioperative mortality and with the expectation of significant symptomatic improvement. Many late deaths are a result of stroke in patients with atrial fibrillation.

	Hospital Mortality in 191 Patients		
Procedure	Elective Operation	Emergency Operation	Total
CAB	2/36 (5.6)	6/26 (23.1)	8/62 (12.9)
AVR	4/42 (9.5)	1/3 (33.3)	5/45 (11.1)
AVR + CAB	7/39 (17.9)	2/3 (66.7)	9/42 (21.4)
MVR ± CAB	6/21 (28.6)	4/6 (66.7)	10/27 (37.0)
Misc	3/14 (21.4)	1/1 (100)	4/15 (26.7)
Total	22/152 (14.5)	14/39 (35.9)	36/191 (18.8)

Abbreviations: AVR, aortic valve replacement; *CAB,* coronary artery bypass; *Misc,* miscellaneous; *MVR,* mitral valve repair or replacement.
Note: Deaths per patients operated on (percent mortality).
(Courtesy of Freeman WK, Schaff HV, O'Brien PC, et al: *J Am Coll Cardiol* 18:29–35, 1991.)

▶ This interesting study from the Mayo Clinic reported by Freeman and associates confirms the substantially higher 30-day mortality in elderly patients as compared to young patients undergoing operations for acquired heart disease. However, survivors did well, as has been often reported. The important message from this paper is the very substantial increase in surgical risk associated with urgent indications for surgery. This seems often unappreciated by referring cardiologists. Certainly, in our experience, the urgency of surgical indications is the strongest predictor of the probability of perioperative mortality.— J.J. Collins, Jr., M.D.

Successful Surgical Treatment of Atrial Fibrillation: Review and Clinical Update

Cox JL, Boineau JP, Schuessler RB, Ferguson TB Jr, Cain ME, Lindsay BD, Corr PB, Kater KM, Lappas DG (Washington Univ; Barnes Hosp, St Louis)

JAMA 266:1976–1980, 1991   6–50

Background.—Atrial fibrillation is the most common sustained arrhythmia other than sinus arrhythmia, but effective treatment remains unavailable. During the past decade multipoint computerized electro-

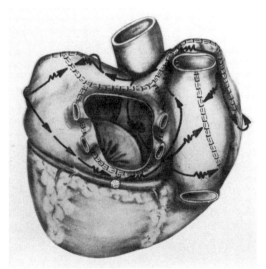

Fig 6–19.—Three-dimensional depiction of incisions used for performing maze procedure. Transmural cryolesion (white dot) of coronary sinus is seen at site of posteroinferior left atriotomy. Both atrial appendages have been excised. Only completely isolated portion of atrium is orifices of pulmonary veins. Impulse originates from region of sinoatrial node and can escape from that region only by passing inferiorly and anteriorly around base of right atrium. Impulse continues to propagate around anterior right atrium onto top of interatrial septum. There it bifurcates into 2 wave fronts, 1 passing through septum in anterior-to-posterior direction to activate posteromedial right and left atrial and other continuing around base of excised left atrial appendage to activate posterolateral left atrial wall. In this manner all atrial myocardium, except pulmonary vein orifices, is activated. Activation of this atrial myocardium is fundamental to preservation of atrial transport function after operation. (Courtesy of Cox JL, Boineau JP, Schuessler RB, et al: *JAMA* 266:1976–1980, 1991.)

physiologic mapping systems have been used for mapping experimental and human atrial fibrillation.

New Procedure.—Even if an on-line map were available, it would not be possible to ablate complex fibrillation by simply placing incisions through identified re-entrant circuits because of their transient nature. All potential macrore-entrant circuits must be interrupted. This is possible by using a "maze" procedure based on the concept of an entrance point into the atrial "box," an exit site, 1 true conduction route between these points, and several "blind alleys." The incisions used to create the electric maze are shown in Figure 6–19. The duration of the refractory period in atrial myocardium makes it unlikely that a re-entrant circuit will form between the suture lines.

Experience.—This procedure was used to treat 11 patients with paroxysmal atrial fibrillation, 9 with chronic fibrillation, and 2 with paroxysmal atrial flutter. All patients were resistant to anti-arrhythmic drugs. There were no operative deaths or permanent adverse effects. All the patients did well, but 3 had a single late episode of atrial flutter and remain controlled by a single drug. All patients are much improved clinically. Nine patients had a rate-responsive dual-chamber pacemaker implanted. The others spontaneously regained a normal cardiac rhythm.

Conclusion.—This procedure effectively relieves the irregular heart beat, hemodynamic sequelae, and risk of thromboembolism associated with atrial fibrillation.

▶ We have seen several publications from Dr. Cox and his group this year on the surgical treatment of atrial fibrillation. The series of incisions is quite remarkable, and the very careful electro-analysis of atrial conduction performed over a number of years in the laboratory by this group is wonderful indeed. Whether the use of this procedure will become widespread is difficult to predict, but further reports from the originator of the operation will be welcomed with interest. I don't think it is yet possible to predict whether this complex operation may be sufficiently simplified to allow its eventually incorporation into the armamentarium of "routine" procedures for most surgeons.—J.J. Collins, Jr., M.D.

Subject Index

A

M

Macroreentry
  in infarcted heart, 101
Magnetic resonance imaging
  white matter lesions and cognitive
    impairment in hypertensives, 155
Malformations (*see* Anomalies)
Mammary
  artery graft, functioning internal, and
    technical considerations for
    myocardial protection during
    coronary bypass reoperation, 356
Marfan aneurysm
  of ascending aorta, composite graft
    repair of, 362
Mental
  stress, effects of awareness of high
    blood pressure on adrenergic
    responses to, 132
Metformin
  for insulin resistance in hypertension, 181
Mexican-Americans
  myocardial infarction in, 26
Microalbuminuria
  in diabetes mellitus
    insulin-dependent, efficacy of
      captopril in postponing
      nephropathy in, 177
    perindopril vs. nifedipine in, 179
Micromanometer
  catheter pressure half-times in
    quantifying mitral stenosis, 322
Milrinone
  in heart failure, severe chronic, 83
Missile
  war, Iraqi, myocardial infarction and
    sudden death in Israeli civilians
    during, 36
Mitral
  commissurotomy (*see* Commissurotomy,
    mitral)
  regurgitation, ischemic, intraoperative
    Doppler color flow imaging in, 372
  stenosis (*see* Stenosis, mitral)
  valve
    annulus, extensively calcified, mitral
      valve repair in, 375
    bioprosthesis causing left ventricular
      outflow obstruction, 371
    leaflets, flail anterior, repair by cusp
      remodeling, 376
    plication for hypertrophic left
      ventricular obstructive myopathy,
      378
    prolapse, symptomatic, aerobic
      exercise in, in women, 57

prolapse, symptomatic, altered
  β-adrenergic receptor function in,
  346
repair in extensively calcified mitral
  annulus, 375
straddling, with hypoplastic right
  ventricle, crisscross atrioventricular
  relations, double outlet right
  ventricle and dextrocardia, 203
Model
  of "hibernating" myocardium, 266
Molecular
  basis for altered lipid metabolism after
    doxazosin, 172
Morbidity
  in hypertension, uncomplicated
    essential, relation to left ventricular
    mass and geometry, 153
Mortality
  (*See also* Death)
  of cardiovascular disease, long-term,
    after 5-year primary prevention
    trial, 18
  of diuretic therapy in diabetes mellitus,
    170
  in heart failure, severe chronic, effect of
    milrinone on, 83
  in hypertension
    essential, uncomplicated, relation to left
      ventricular mass and geometry, 153
    in lean patients, 152
  after thrombolytic therapy in
    myocardial infarction, effect of age
    on, 2
MRI
  white matter lesions and cognitive
    impairment in hypertensives, 155
Muscle
  disease, alcoholic heart, effects of
    abstinence on, 70
  pectoralis major, transposition for
    infected sternotomy wounds,
    long-term results, 397
  smooth (*see* Smooth muscle)
Muscular
  ventricular septal defects, congenital,
    preoperative transcatheter closure
    of, 259
Mustard procedure
  cardiac rhythm after, 195
  chronotropic impairment during
    exercise after, 229
Myocardial infarction
  angioplasty in, percutaneous
    transluminal
    death after, 9
    primary, 31
    in blacks, 38

Author Index

A SIMPLE, ONCE-A-YEAR DOSE!

Review the partial list of titles below. And then request your own FREE 30-day preview. When you subscribe to a Year Book, we'll also send you an automatic notice of future volumes about two months before they publish.

This system was designed for your convenience and to take up as little of your time as possible. If you do not want the Year Book, the advance notice makes it easy for you to let us know. And if you elect to receive the new Year Book, you need do nothing. We will send it on publication.

No worry. No wasted motion. And, of course, every Year Book is yours to examine FREE of charge for thirty days.

Year Book of **Anesthesia**® (22141)
Year Book of **Cardiology**® (22640)
Year Book of **Critical Care Medicine**® (22639)
Year Book of **Dermatology**® (22645)
Year Book of **Dermatologic Surgery**® (21171)
Year Book of **Diagnostic Radiology**® (22613)
Year Book of **Digestive Diseases**® (22625)
Year Book of **Drug Therapy**® (22630)
Year Book of **Emergency Medicine**® (22080)
Year Book of **Endocrinology**® (21174)
Year Book of **Family Practice**® (22124)
Year Book of **Geriatrics and Gerontology** (22611)
Year Book of **Hand Surgery**® (22618)
Year Book of **Hematology**® (22646)
Year Book of **Health Care Management**® (21177)
Year Book of **Infectious Diseases**® (22650)
Year Book of **Infertility** (22637)
Year Book of **Medicine**® (22638)
Year Book of **Neonatal-Perinatal Medicine** (22629)
Year Book of **Nephrology** (21175)
Year Book of **Neurology and Neurosurgery**® (22616)
Year Book of **Neuroradiology**® (21849)
Year Book of **Nuclear Medicine**® (22627)
Year Book of **Obstetrics and Gynecology**® (22636)
Year Book of **Occupational and Environmental Medicine** (22619)
Year Book of **Oncology** (22651)
Year Book of **Ophthalmology**® (22133)
Year Book of **Orthopedics**® (22644)
Year Book of **Otolaryngology – Head and Neck Surgery**® (22609)
Year Book of **Pathology and Clinical Pathology**® (21176)
Year Book of **Pediatrics**® (22130)
Year Book of **Plastic and Reconstructive Surgery**® (22635)
Year Book of **Psychiatry and Applied Mental Health**® (22649)
Year Book of **Pulmonary Disease**® (22624)
Year Book of **Sports Medicine**® (22111)
Year Book of **Surgery**® (22641)
Year Book of **Transplantation**® (21854)
Year Book of **Ultrasound** (21169)
Year Book of **Urology**® (22621)
Year Book of **Vascular Surgery**® (22612)

Mosby-Year Book, Inc. • 11830 Westline Industrial Drive • St. Louis, MO 63146